RC46 CRA (OWL)

Series editor and faculty advisor
Wilf Yeo
BMedSc, MB ChB, MD, MRCP,
Section of Clinical Pharmacology
Department of Pharmacology & Therapeutics,
Royal Hallamshire Hospital,
Sheffield

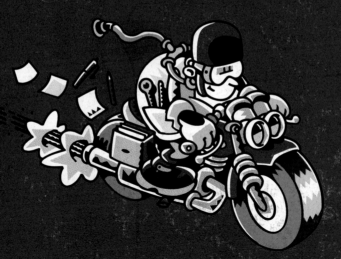

Internal Medicine

Rachael Hough
BMedSci, BMBS, MRCP
Clinical Research Fellow
Department of Clinical Oncology
Weston Park Hospital
Sheffield

Iftikhar Ul Haq
MB ChB, MBA, MRCP
Specialist Registrar in Cardiology
Northern General Hospital
Sheffield

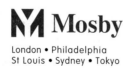
Mosby

London • Philadelphia
St Louis • Sydney • Tokyo

Managing Editor	Louise Crowe
Development Editor	Filipa Maia
Project Manager	Steven Tromans
Designer	Greg Smith
Layout	Robert Curran
Illustration Management	Danny Pyne
Illustrators	Deborah Gyan
	Sandie Hill
	Deborah Maizels
	Mick Ruddy
	Jeremy Theobald
Cover Design	Greg Smith
Production	Andrea Ford
Index	Janine Ross

ISBN 0 7234 3114 0

Copyright © Mosby International Ltd, 1999.

Published by Mosby, an imprint of Mosby International Ltd, Lynton House, 7–12 Tavistock Square, London WC1H 9LB, UK.

Printed by GraphyCems, Navarra, Spain.
Text set in Crash Course—VAG Light; captions in Crash Course—VAG Thin.

Every effort has been made to contact holders of copyright to obtain permission to reproduce copyright material. However, if any have been inadvertently overlooked, the publishers will be pleased to make the necessary arrangements at the first opportunity.

Cataloguing in Publication Data
A catalogue record for this book is available from the British Library.

Preface

Medicine is easier than you think! At the end of the day, there are only a certain number of things that can go wrong with any part of us. So, if a patient tells you about a particular symptom, or you find an abnormal sign on investigation, there are a limited number of possibilities that you need to think about. The key is to have a structured approach, remembering that common things *are* common.

In *Crash Course Internal Medicine*, we have tried to write the book we would like to have had as we faced finals and began house-jobs. The format includes a methodical approach to common symptoms, signs, and investigations. This is followed by a comprehensive, theoretical background to specific diseases and how to manage them. We have illustrated the text with diagrams, and with boxes containing hints and tips that we have found useful ourselves.

Armed with the knowledge described in this book, we hope that you will find exams and house-jobs less intimidating and more enjoyable.
Best wishes.

Ifti Ul Haq and Rachael Hough

So you have an exam in medicine and you don't know where to start? The answer is easy—start with *Crash Course*. Medicine is fun to learn if you can bring it to life with patients who need their problems solving. Conventional medical textbooks are written back-to-front, starting with the diagnosis and then describing the disease. This is because medicine evolved by careful observations and descriptions of individual diseases for which, until this century, there was no treatment. Modern medicine is about problem solving, learning methods to find the right path through the differential diagnosis, and offering treatment promptly.

This series of books has been designed to help you solve common medical problems by starting with the patient and extracting the salient points in the history, examination, and investigations. Part II gives you essential information on the physical examination and investigations as seen through the eyes of practising doctors in their specialty. Once the diagnosis is made, you can refer to Part III to confirm that the diagnosis is correct and get advice regarding treatment.

Throughout the series we have included informative diagrams and hints and tips boxes to simplify your learning. The books are meant as revision tools, but are comprehensive, accurate and well balanced and should enable you to learn each subject well. To check that you did learn something from the book (rather than just flashing it in front of your eyes!), we have added a self-assessment section in the usual format of most medical exams—multiple-choice and short-answer questions (with answers), and case studies for self-directed learning. Good luck!

Wilf Yeo
Series Editor (Clinical) and Faculty Advisor

Acknowledgements

Thanks to David for constructive comment and encouragement! *Rachael*
Thanks to Jules for help with the proofreading. *Ifti*

Figure Credits

Figure 27.14 taken from Crash Course: Cardiovascular System, by Romeshan Sunthareswaren, Mosby International, 1998.

Figure 27.36 taken from Crash Course: Nervous System and Special Senses, by David Lasserson, Carolyn Gabriel, and Basil Sharrack, Mosby International, 1998.

Figure 27.37 taken from Crash Course: History and Examination, by James Marsh, Mosby International, 1998.

Figures 33.5 and 36.3 taken from Color Atlas and Text of Clinical Medicine, by Charles Forbes and William Jackson, Mosby International, 1997.

Figures 35.1, 35.2, 35.3, 35.9, 35.14, 35.15, taken from Crash Course: Endocrine and Reproductive Systems, by Madeleine Debuse, Mosby International, 1998.

Figure 35.6 taken from Crash Course: Musculoskeletal System, by Sona Biswas and Rehana Iqbal, Mosby International, 1998.

Figures 29.16, 29.18, 29.20 adapted from Crash Course: Endocrine and Reproductive Systems, by Madeleine Debuse, Mosby International, 1998.

Figure 27.2 adapted from Clinical Examination 2e, by O Epstein, GD Perkin, D de Bono, and J Cookson, Mosby International, 1997.

Figures 29.2 and 29.3 adapted from Crash Course: Cardiovascular System, by Romeshan Sunthareswaren, Mosby International, 1998.

Figures 30.4, 30.11, 30.12, 30.13, 30.15 adapted from Color Atlas and Text of Clinical Medicine, by Charles Forbes and William Jackson, Mosby International, 1997.

Figure 36.1 adapted from Crash Course: Musculoskeletal System, by Sona Biswas and Rehana Iqbal, Mosby International, 1998.

Contents

Contents

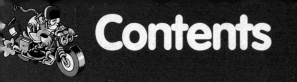

Contents

To Mum, Dad, Lubna, Farhan and Aaminah **Ifti**

To Mum, Dad, Sophy and Chris **Rachael**

x

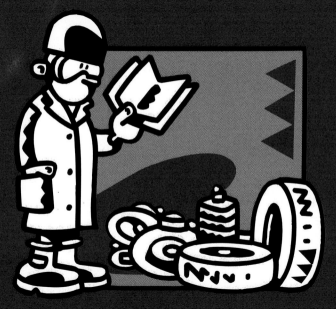

THE PATIENT PRESENTS WITH

1. Chest Pain

INTRODUCTION

Chest pain is a common cause for admission to hospital. Taking a clear history is essential in making the correct diagnosis. Different diseases present with different types of chest pain.

DIFFERENTIAL DIAGNOSIS OF CHEST PAIN

Pleuritic chest pain

This is a sharp pain that is worse on deep inspiration, coughing, or movement. The differential diagnosis includes the following:

- Pneumothorax.
- Pneumonia.
- Pulmonary embolus (PE).
- Pericarditis: retrosternal.
- Bornholm disease (Coxsackie B unilateral infection of respiratory muscles).

Dull central chest pain

The differential diagnosis of dull central pain includes the following:

- Angina: crushing.
- Myocardial infarction (MI): crushing.
- Dissecting aortic aneurysm: tearing interscapular pain.
- Oesophagitis: burning.
- Oesophageal spasm.

Chest wall tenderness

The differential diagnosis of chest wall tenderness includes the following:

- Rib fracture.
- Shingles (herpes zoster): pain precedes rash.
- Costochondritis (Tietze's syndrome).

Atypical presentations (or any of the above)

The differential diagnosis in atypical presentations (or in any of the above) includes anxiety and referred pain

from vertebral collapse causing nerve root irritation or intra-abdominal pathology (e.g. pancreatitis, peptic ulcer, or the biliary tree).

HISTORY IN THE PATIENT WITH CHEST PAIN

A careful history of the chest pain will generally be suggestive of the likely underlying problem. The focus should then turn to any associated symptoms and risk factors.

What type of chest pain does the patient have?

Onset and progression of pain

Cardiac ischaemic pain typically builds up over a few minutes and may be brought on by exercise, emotion, or cold weather. In angina the pain resolves on resting or with GTN. In unstable angina the pain may come on at rest and commonly waxes and wanes, becoming severe at times. In MI the pain is severe, often associated with systemic symptoms such as nausea, vomiting, and sweating, and lasts for at least 30 minutes. Spontaneous pneumothorax and pulmonary embolism usually causes sudden onset of pleuritic pain (the patient often remembers exactly what they were doing at the time).

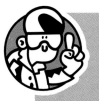

Always ask the patient what they were doing when the pain came on. This generally gives valuable information!

Site and radiation of pain

Cardiac ischaemia and pericarditis cause retrosternal pain. In ischaemia, the pain often radiates to the jaw or arms, while dissecting aortic aneurysm causes a tearing interscapular pain, and pulmonary disease causes unilateral pain which the patient can often localize specifically. Oesophageal disease can also cause retrosternal pain and may mimic cardiac pain. Referred pain from vertebral collapse or shingles will follow a dermatome pattern.

Nature of pain
The precise nature of the pain gives important clues as to the underlying diagnosis (see above).

Are there any associated symptoms?
Important associated symptoms include:
- Dyspnoea: pulmonary embolism, pneumonia, pneumothorax, pulmonary oedema in cardiac ischaemia, hyperventilation in anxiety.
- Cough: purulent sputum in pneumonia, haemoptysis in pulmonary embolism, frothy pink sputum in pulmonary oedema.
- Rigors: pneumonia (particularly lobar pneumonia).
- Calf swelling: has PE arisen from deep vein thrombosis?
- Palpitations: arrhythmia can cause angina or result from cardiac ischaemia, PE, or pneumonia.
- Clamminess, nausea, vomiting, and sweating are features of myocardial infarction or massive pulmonary embolism.

Are risk factors present?
Important risk factors include:
- Ischaemic heart disease: smoking, family history, cholesterol, hypertension, diabetes.
- PE: recent travel, immobility, or surgery, family history, pregnancy, malignancy.
- Pneumothorax: spontaneous (young, thin men), trauma, emphysema, asthma, malignancy, staphylococcal pneumonia, cystic fibrosis.

EXAMINING THE PATIENT WITH CHEST PAIN

The examination should focus on determining the cause of the pain and then looking for risk factors and consequences of the underlying problem. A schematic guide to examining the patient with chest pain is given in Fig. 1.1.

What is the cause of the pain?
Pay particular attention to:
- Pulse: tachycardia or arrhythmia.
- Blood pressure: discrepancy between left and right arms in aortic dissection.
- Chest wall tenderness: rib fracture, costochondritis, anxiety, shingles.
- Chest examination: pneumothorax, consolidation, pleural rub.
- Cardiac examination: fourth heart sound (PE or MI), rub (pericarditis).

Are there risk factors?
The following risk factors may be present:
- Abnormal lipids: xanthelasma, tendon xanthoma.
- Nicotine stained fingers: predisposition to ischaemic heart disease.
- Hot, oedematous, tender calf suggesting deep vein thrombosis.
- Hypertension: ischaemic heart disease.

What are the complications?
Complications may include:
- Pulse: arrhythmia, tachycardia.
- Blood pressure: shock in tension pneumothorax, massive pulmonary embolism, MI.
- Cardiac failure: pulmonary oedema and 3rd heart sound.
- Murmurs: acute mitral regurgitation and ventricular septal defect after MI; aortic regurgitation in dissecting aortic aneurysm.

INVESTIGATING THE PATIENT WITH CHEST PAIN

All patients with chest pain should have an electrocardiogram (ECG) and chest X-ray (CXR). Further investigation will be directed by findings in these tests in conjunction with the history and clinical examination. An algorithm for the investigation of the patient with chest pain is given in Fig. 1.2.

Electrocardiogram
ST depression and elevation (Fig. 1.3) on ECG are suggestive of myocardial ischaemia and acute MI, respectively. Changes suggestive of PE are shown in Fig. 1.4. Arrhythmia may also be detected on ECG.

Chest X-ray

Pneumothorax, consolidation (pneumonia, PE), widened mediastinum (aortic dissection), pulmonary oedema (myocardial ischaemia/infarction) and fractured ribs may be detected on CXR. Serial cardiac enzymes should be assessed daily for 3 days if MI is considered (Fig. 1.5).

Exercise test

An exercise test may be diagnostic when angina is suspected.

Coronary angiography

Coronary angiography allows direct visualization of the coronary arterial tree. It should be used in severe angina to determine whether angioplasty or coronary artery bypass grafting might be beneficial.

Arterial blood gases

The assessment of arterial blood gases is useful in determining the severity of PE, pneumonia, or pulmonary oedema, showing hypoxia and occasionally hypocapnia. In hyperventilation related to anxiety, the pO_2 will be elevated whilst there will be hypocapnia and a respiratory alkalosis.

Ventilation–perfusion scan

Ventilation–perfusion scan is used to diagnose PE. In some circumstances (e.g. when there is pre-existing

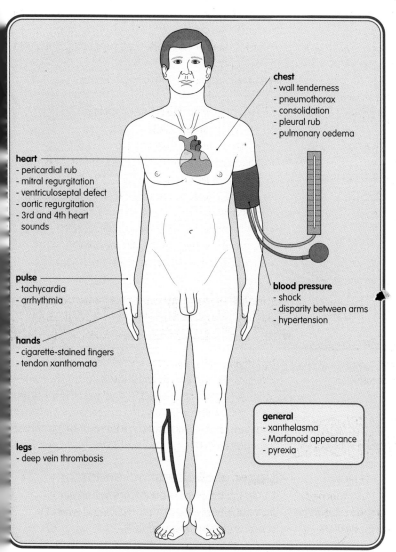

Fig. 1.1 Examining the patient with chest pain.

chest
- wall tenderness
- pneumothorax
- consolidation
- pleural rub
- pulmonary oedema

heart
- pericardial rub
- mitral regurgitation
- ventriculoseptal defect
- aortic regurgitation
- 3rd and 4th heart sounds

pulse
- tachycardia
- arrhythmia

hands
- cigarette-stained fingers
- tendon xanthomata

blood pressure
- shock
- disparity between arms
- hypertension

general
- xanthelasma
- Marfanoid appearance
- pyrexia

legs
- deep vein thrombosis

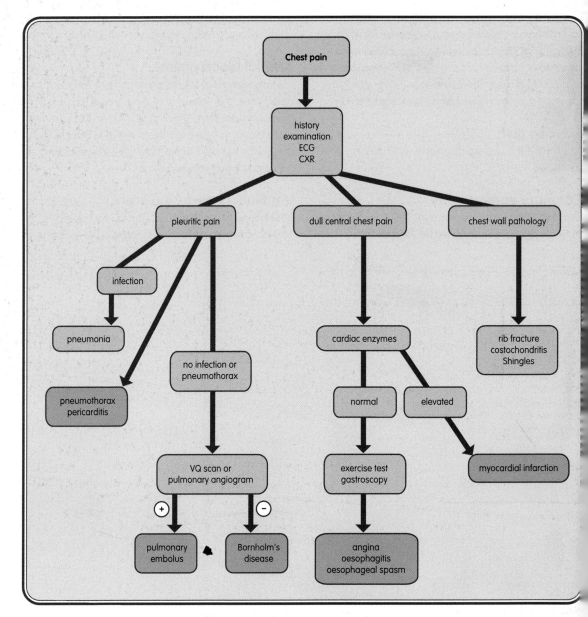

Fig. 1.2 Algorithm for the investigation of the patient with chest pain. (CXR, chest X-ray; ECG, electrocardiogram; V/Q, ventilation–perfusion.)

obstructive airways disease) interpretation of this test can be difficult, so pulmonary angiography should then be performed.

Echocardiogram

The presence of a dissecting aortic aneurysm should be confirmed by urgent echocardiography (particularly transoesophageal echocardiography) or by computed tomography scan.

Upper gastrointestinal endoscopy

Upper gastrointestinal endoscopy will confirm oesophagitis and should be considered when the cause of chest pain is unclear.

Fig. 1.3 Causes of ST elevation.

Causes of ST elevation	
Cause	**Distribution of ST elevation**
myocardial infarction	right coronary artery (inferior): aV_f, II, III left anterior descending artery (anterior): I, aV_l, V_{4-6} circumflex artery (anteroseptal): V_{1-4} (overlap between territories may be seen)
pericarditis	across all leads (saddle-shaped ST change)
Prinzmetal's angina	leads of affected coronary artery (spasm)
aortic dissection	only if coronary artery involved
left ventricular aneurysm	persistent changes following infarct

ECG changes associated with pulmonary embolus

- sinus tachycardia
- atrial arrhythmia, e.g. atrial fibrillation
- right heart strain
- right axis deviation
- right bundle branch block
- $S_1 Q_3 T_3$, i.e. deep S wave in I, Q wave in III, T wave inversion in III

Fig. 1.4 Electrocardiogram (ECG) changes associated with pulmonary embolus. Note that sinus tachycardia may be the only abnormality present.

Fig. 1.5 Cardiac enzyme elevation following myocardial infarction. (AST, aspartate aminotransferase; CK, creatine kinase; LDH, lactate dehydrogenase.)

Cardiac enzyme elevation after myocardial infarction			
Enzyme	**Begins to rise (hours after infarct)**	**Peak (hours after infarct)**	**Returns to normal (days after infarct)**
CK	6	24	2–3
AST	6–8	24–48	3–5
LDH	12–24	48–72	10–14

2. Shortness of Breath

INTRODUCTION

Shortness of breath (dyspnoea) is the subjective sensation of breathlessness which is excessive for any given level of activity. Dyspnoea may be due to any of the following:

- Pulmonary disease: disorders of the airways, lung parenchyma, pleura, respiratory muscles, or chest wall.
- Cardiac disease: where it is the result of left ventricular failure (LVF) from any cause, e.g. valvular heart disease.
- Metabolic disease, e.g. thyrotoxicosis, ketoacidosis.
- Anaemia.
- Psychogenic causes, e.g. anxiety or hyperventilation (psychogenic dyspnoea).

HISTORY IN THE PATIENT WITH BREATHLESSNESS

How breathless is the patient (severity)? Try to quantify their exercise tolerance, e.g. distance walked on the flat or on hills, whilst dressing, climbing stairs.

Orthopnoea is breathlessness on lying down. It is characteristic of heart failure but can occur with airways obstruction, or more rarely with bilateral diaphragmatic paralysis. Paroxysmal nocturnal dyspnoea is breathlessness that wakes the patient from sleep, and is generally a symptom of cardiac disease.

The onset of breathlessness will often give a clue to its aetiology:

- Acute onset may be due to a foreign body, pneumothorax, pulmonary embolism, asthma, or acute pulmonary oedema.

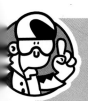

Determining the patient's exercise tolerance gives a useful marker of the progression of symptoms.

- Subacute onset is more suggestive of parenchymal disease, e.g. alveolitis, pleural effusion; pneumonia; carcinoma of the bronchus or trachea.
- Chronic onset is associated with chronic obstructive pulmonary disease (COPD), cryptogenic fibrosing alveolitis; occupational fibrotic lung disease, non-respiratory causes (e.g. LVF, anaemia, or hyperthyroidism).

In addition to the above, the following factors should be assessed when taking a history from a patient with breathlessness:

- Is the breathlessness associated with a cough? A chronic persistent cough may be due to smoking, asthma, COPD, drugs (especially angiotensin-converting enzyme [ACE] inhibitors), occupational agents, cardiac failure, or psychogenic factors.
- How long has the cough been present?
- Is the cough worse at any particular time of day?
- Are there any precipitating factors?
- If there is sputum, ask what it looks like.
- Does the patient have haemoptysis? This is coughing up blood—either frank blood or blood-tinged sputum. It needs to be distinguished from haematemesis and nasopharyngeal bleeding. (See Chapter 5 for the causes of haematemesis.)
- Ask about stridor (a harsh sound caused by turbulent airflow through a narrowed airway). Inspiratory stridor suggests extrathoracic obstruction, expiratory stridor suggests intrathoracic obstruction, and inspiratory and expiratory stridor suggests a fixed obstruction.
- Does the patient wheeze? These are whistling noises caused by turbulent airflow through narrowed intrathoracic airways. The commonest cause is asthma.
- Does the breathlessness affect the activities of daily living and quality of life?
- Occupational history, including exposure to dusts or allergies. Dyspnoea only during the working week may be suggestive of occupational lung disease.

EXAMINING THE PATIENT WITH BREATHLESSNESS

The findings on examination of common respiratory conditions are listed in Fig. 2.1, and the examination approach in the patient with breathlessness is summarized in Fig. 2.2. A more detailed description showing examination findings in respiratory disease can be found in Chapter 26.

Inspection

Note the respiratory rate from the end of the bed, or whilst feeling the pulse.

Look for cyanosis (a blue colour in the mouth and tongue due to inadequate oxygenation, i.e. 5 g reduced haemoglobin per 100 ml of blood). It is commonly associated with lung disease and cardiac disease, and hypoventilation from other causes.

Note, however, that cyanosis is an unreliable guide to the degree of hypoxaemia. Peripheral cyanosis is due to poor peripheral circulation, e.g. in cardiac failure, peripheral vascular disease, or arterial obstruction, and physiological when due to cold. Cyanosis is rarely seen in anaemic patients.

The following factors should also be looked for when assessing the patient with breathlessness:

- Anaemia.
- Clubbing: respiratory causes include carcinoma of the bronchus; pus in any part of the respiratory tract, e.g. empyema, lung abscess, bronchiectasis, cystic fibrosis; fibrosing alveolitis; chronic supperative pulmonary tuberculosis, pleural mesothelioma.

Don't forget to look at the sputum pot:
- Purulent, moderate quantity—bronchitis or pneumonia.
- Purulent, copious quantity—bronchiectasis or pneumonia.
- Pink and frothy—pulmonary oedema.
- Blood stained—causes of haemoptysis.
- Rust-coloured—pneumococcal lobar pneumonia.

- Chest movements on inspiration and expiration: an abnormality is normally found on the side of diminished movements.
- Barrel-shaped chest: emphysema.
- Kyphoscoliosis: can decrease chest size and expansion.
- Ankylosing spondylitis: can 'fix' the chest.
- Use of accessory muscles of respiration.
- Rhythm of respiration: Cheyne–Stokes respiration describes periods of fast and deep inspiration followed by periods of apnoea due to depression of the central respiratory centre in the medulla. This may occur with severe chest infections, metabolic acidosis, opiate overdose, and raised intracranial pressure.

Findings on examination of common respiratory conditions					
Condition	Movement on side of lesion	Position of trachea	Percussion	Tactile vocal fremitus	Breath sounds
pleural effusion	↓	central or deviated away from effusion if massive	↓ ('stony dull')	↓	↓ with bronchial breathing at top of effusion
pneumothorax	↓	central or deviated away	↑	↓	↓
pneumonia	↓	central or deviated towards if associated with collapse	↓	↑	bronchial breathing (absent if obstruction of bronchus)
pulmonary fibrosis	↓	central or deviated towards if upper lobe involvement	↓	↑	bronchial breathing

Fig. 2.1 Findings on examination of common respiratory conditions.

Palpation

- Feel for lymphadenopathy secondary to malignant disease or infections.
- Palpate the trachea: displacement may indicate underlying chest disease or cardiac disease.
- Check the movement of the rib cage.
- Feel for tactile vocal fremitus.
- Compare both sides anteriorly and posteriorly.

Auscultation

- Expiration: may be prolonged in COPD.
- Bronchial breathing: consolidation, cavitation, or at the top of an effusion.
- Breath sounds: diminished over an effusion, pneumothorax, and in the obese.
- Rhonchi or wheezes: partially obstructed bronchi; found in asthma, bronchitis, and occasionally LVF.
- Crepitations (sudden opening of small closed airways): pulmonary congestion (fine crepitations in early inspiration); fibrosing alveolitis (fine crepitations in late inspiration); bronchial secretions (coarse crepitations).
- Friction rub: pleural disease.

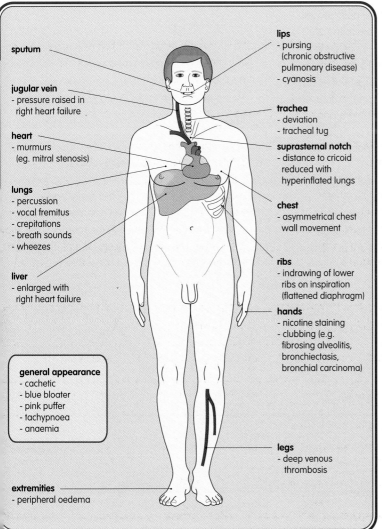

Fig. 2.2 Examining the patient with breathlessness.

sputum

jugular vein
- pressure raised in right heart failure

heart
- murmurs (eg. mitral stenosis)

lungs
- percussion
- vocal fremitus
- crepitations
- breath sounds
- wheezes

liver
- enlarged with right heart failure

general appearance
- cachetic
- blue bloater
- pink puffer
- tachypnoea
- anaemia

extremities
- peripheral oedema

lips
- pursing (chronic obstructive pulmonary disease)
- cyanosis

trachea
- deviation
- tracheal tug

suprasternal notch
- distance to cricoid reduced with hyperinflated lungs

chest
- asymmetrical chest wall movement

ribs
- indrawing of lower ribs on inspiration (flattened diaphragm)

hands
- nicotine staining
- clubbing (e.g. fibrosing alveolitis, bronchiectasis, bronchial carcinoma)

legs
- deep venous thrombosis

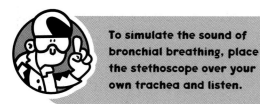

To simulate the sound of
bronchial breathing, place
the stethoscope over your
own trachea and listen.

INVESTIGATING THE PATIENT WITH BREATHLESSNESS

An algorithm for the investigation of the patient with breathlessness is given in Fig. 2.3. The following investigations should be performed:

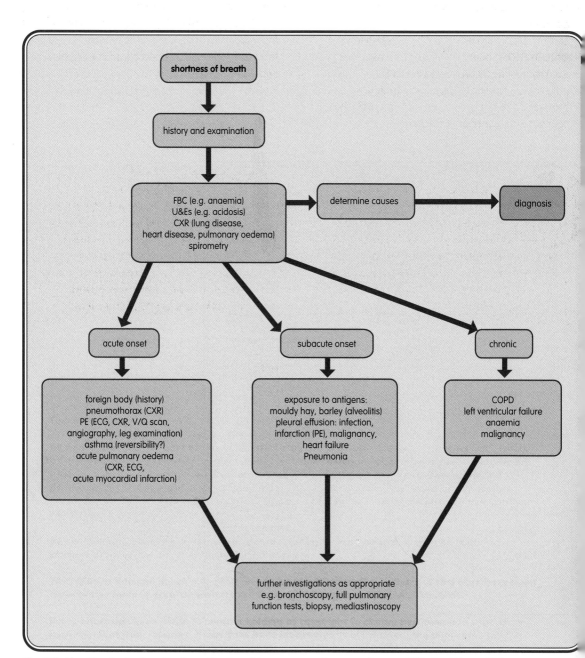

Fig. 2.3 Algorithm for the investigation of the breathless patient. Note that more than one cause of shortness of breath may be apparent. (COPD, chronic obstructive pulmonary disease; CXR, chest X-ray; ECG, electrocardiogram; FBC, full blood count; PE, pulmonary embolus; V/Q, ventilation–perfusion ratio.)

- Full blood count: anaemia leading to breathlessness, leucocytosis in pneumonia.
- Urea and electrolytes, and bicarbonate: renal failure secondary to dehydration, sepsis, or acidosis, producing breathlessness; hyponatraemia of fluid overload.
- Chest X-ray: examine methodically (see pp. 179–180).
- Electrocardiogram (ECG): $S_1 Q_3 T_3$ pattern in PE (see Fig. 1.4), p pulmonale (tall p waves >2.5 mm in lead II) in COPD with cor pulmonale; cardiac conditions leading to breathlessness, e.g. myocardial infarction with consequent pulmonary oedema.

- Arterial blood gases: pH, partial pressures of oxygen and carbon dioxide, and hydrogen ion concentration (see respiratory failure, Chapter 29, pp. 179–181).
- Spirometry: to distinguish between obstructive and restrictive lung pathology, and to test reversibility to treatments.
- Transfer factor and lung volume.
- Ventilation–perfusion scan: suspected pulmonary emboli.
- Bronchoscopy with or without transbronchial biopsy.

Metabolic acidosis leads to 'deep sighing' breathlessness (Kussmaul respiration). Causes include uraemia, diabetic ketoacidosis, salicylate ingestion, methanol ingestion, and lactic acidosis.

The classical $S_1 Q_3 T_3$ pattern on the ECG with pulmonary emboli is rare. The ECG commonly shows sinus tachycardia, but other changes include right bundle branch block, right ventricular strain, and atrial fibrillation.

3. Palpitations

INTRODUCTION

Always check what the patient means by 'palpitations' or clarify what you mean by them as the word means different things to different people. It is usually understood as an awareness of the heartbeat. The most common cause is an arrhythmia although other causes include conditions causing an increase in stroke volume (e.g. regurgitant valvular disease) or conditions causing an increase in cardiac output, often non-cardiac causes (e.g. exercise, thyrotoxicosis, anaemia, or anxiety). If an arrhythmia is suspected try to determine whether there is an underlying cause.

DIFFERENTIAL DIAGNOSIS BY DESCRIPTION OF THE RHYTHM

Regular rhythm
The differential diagnosis of regular palpitations includes the following:
- Heavy heart beats with normal rate: most often cardiac consciousness with sinus rhythm. It tends to be worse at rest, especially when lying in bed at night and during periods of stress.
- Fast heart rate: sinus tachycardia, atrial flutter with block, or ventricular tachycardia.
- Bursts of fast beats: paroxysmal atrial tachycardia. There is often a very long history dating back years with a single attack followed by a long interval before the next attack. Other causes include atrial flutter, junctional rhythm, or ventricular tachycardia.
- Slow heart rate: sinus bradycardia (look for signs of hypothyroidism), atrioventricular block.

Irregular rhythm
The differential diagnosis of irregular palpitations includes the following:
- Missed beats, 'thumps': multiple ectopics from the atrium or ventricle. The symptoms are more troublesome at rest and may disappear during exercise.

- Fast (or normal if treated): atrial flutter with variable block, atrial fibrillation (may be worse with exercise), multiple premature beats with sinus tachycardia.

HISTORY

Obtain a full description of the palpitations. Are they continuous or intermittent? Are they fast, normal rate, or slow? Are they regular or irregular? When did the palpitations start?—this can vary from a few minutes to decades. Generally, if the onset dates back years and there have been no serious complications (e.g. syncope) the palpitations are usually benign.

How often do the palpitations occur and how long do they last for? They may last for days or seconds, with intervals between episodes of a few hours to years. The patient may fear serious underlying cardiac disease, although there is usually a benign cause.

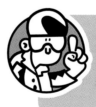

Ask the patient to tap out the heart rhythm on the desk top. This will often give a good guide to rate and rhythm.

Are there any associated features? These may be related to the underlying cause (e.g. angina, features of hyperthyroidism) or a consequence of the palpitations (e.g. faintness or dizziness). Always obtain a full drug history as medication is often the culprit.

Causal and contributory factors
Ask about smoking, alcohol, and caffeine (tea, coffee, cola) intake. These may contribute to extrasystoles. Myocardial ischaemia may lead to any supraventricular

or ventricular arrhythmia. Digoxin, which is commonly used to control atrial fibrillation, may also cause any arrhythmia, especially in the presence of hypokalaemia. Note that most antiarrhythmic agents also have a proarrhythmic effect. Ask about rheumatic heart disease as atrial fibrillation often accompanies mitral stenosis.

Non-cardiac causes of sinus tachycardia and causes of sinus bradycardia are outlined in Figs 3.1 and 3.2, respectively.

Non-cardiac causes of palpitations include the following:

- Thyrotoxicosis: may cause sinus tachycardia, paroxysmal atrial tachycardia, atrial flutter/fibrillation.
- Myxoedema: may be responsible for sinus bradycardia.
- Anxiety: a very common cause of palpitations.

CONSEQUENCES OF PALPITATIONS

Palpitations may not affect the patient or may just be a minor nuisance. If a benign arrhythmia is present, reassurance that the condition is not serious is often all that is required. Changes in rate may be more serious, compromising coronary blood supply and leading to symptoms of myocardial ischaemia or cardiac failure.

Tachycardia or bradycardia may lead to a reduction in cardiac output and cause dizziness or collapse, e.g. Stokes–Adams attacks in complete heart block.

EXAMINING THE PATIENT WITH PALPITATIONS

A guide to examining the patient with palpitations is given in Fig. 3.3. Look for signs of anaemia or hypo/hyperthyroidism. Next feel the pulse. Note the following:

- Rate: beats per minute.
- Rhythm: regular, regularly irregular (e.g. Wenckebach second degree heart block), irregularly irregular (e.g. multiple ectopic beats or atrial fibrillation).
- Volume, e.g. a collapsing pulse of hyperdynamic circulation or a slow volume pulse of shock or aortic stenosis.

If the patient is symptom free at the time of examination, the pulse may be normal.

The blood pressure will be low if the arrhythmia leads to a reduction in cardiac output. Hypertension may predispose to atrial fibrillation.

The jugulovenous pressure may be elevated if cardiac failure is present. Cannon a waves are visible with complete heart block, and a waves are absent in atrial fibrillation.

An irregularly irregular pulse (e.g. in atrial fibrillation) is irregular in rhythm and volume.

Non-cardiac causes of sinus tachycardia
• exercise • fever • anaemia • thyrotoxicosis • pregnancy • arteriovenous fistulae • anxiety • cigarettes, alcohol, caffeine • sympathomimetic drugs • heavy metals • gastro-oesophageal reflux disease

Fig. 3.1 Non-cardiac causes of sinus tachycardia.

Causes of sinus bradycardia
• athletes • hypothyroidism • obstructive jaundice • raised intracranial pressure • hypopituarism • hypothermia • cardiac causes include ischaemia, drugs (e.g. digoxin and β-blockers), inflammation, degeneration/fibrosis

Fig. 3.2 Causes of sinus bradycardia.

Feel for heaves and thrills with associated right ventricular enlargement and valvular heart disease. Assess the rate and rhythm by auscultation. The peripheral pulse rate may be slower than the apical rate in atrial fibrillation (pulse deficit). The first heart sound is of variable intensity in heart block and atrial fibrillation. Listen for cardiac murmurs, e.g. evidence of mitral valve disease predisposing to atrial fibrillation. Focus on any abnormal findings (see Chapter 4).

INVESTIGATING THE PATIENT WITH PALPITATIONS

An algorithm for the investigation of the patient with palpitations is given in Fig. 3.4. The following tests should be performed:

Blood tests
- Full blood count: anaemia.
- Urea and electrolytes: especially disturbances of potassium; less commonly, magnesium deficiency may contribute to refractory arrhythmias.
- Thyroid function tests: hypo/hyperthyroidism.
- Drug concentration if appropriate, e.g. digoxin levels.

Other tests
Electrocardiogram (ECG): mandatory for anyone with palpitations and can often reveal the precise nature of the palpitations if present.
- 24-Hour ECG: for intermittent symptoms. It should be carried out with a diary of symptoms to see if they correlate with any rhythm disturbances found.
- Echocardiogram: to exclude any underlying valvular disease.

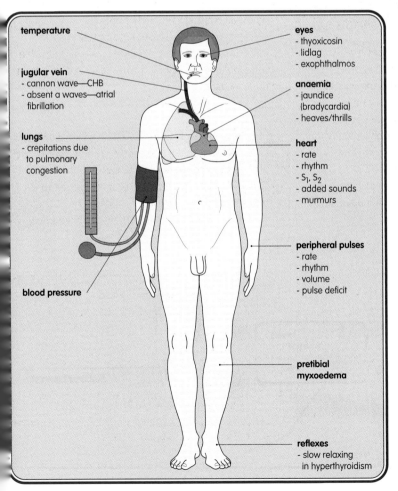

temperature

jugular vein
- cannon wave—CHB
- absent a waves—atrial fibrillation

lungs
- crepitations due to pulmonary congestion

blood pressure

eyes
- thyoxicosin
- lidlag
- exophthalmos

anaemia
- jaundice (bradycardia)
- heaves/thrills

heart
- rate
- rhythm
- S_1, S_2
- added sounds
- murmurs

peripheral pulses
- rate
- rhythm
- volume
- pulse deficit

pretibial myxoedema

reflexes
- slow relaxing in hyperthyroidism

Fig. 3.3 Examining the patient with palpitations. (CHB, complete heart block.)

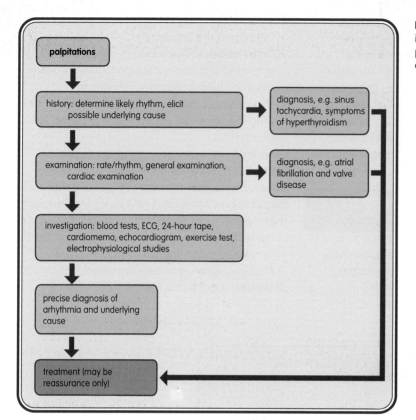

Fig. 3.4 Algorithm for the investigation of the patient with palpitations. (ECG, electrocardiogram.)

- 'Cardiomemo': if symptoms do not occur every day, a 'cardiomemo' can record the heart rhythm by phone at the press of a button.
- Exercise test: the induction of symptoms, under controlled conditions with ECG monitoring, may be appropriate.

- Electrophysiological studies: more rarely, patients may be referred for specialized studies. These can be used to induce arrhythmias, locate the origin of the arrhythmic focus, and to assess the response to drug treatment.

INTRODUCTION

Heart murmurs are due to vibrations caused by turbulent flow within the heart. The commonest causes in examinations are due to left-sided valvular heart disease and tricuspid regurgitation. Non-valvular causes include:

- Innocent 'flow' murmurs, especially in children.
- High output states, e.g. pregnancy, thyrotoxicosis, and fever.
- Congenital heart disease, e.g. atrial septal defects (ASD), ventricular septal defects (VSD), patent ductus arteriosus (PDA), and coarctation of the aorta.

DIFFERENTIAL DIAGNOSIS OF HEART MURMURS

The differential diagnosis of heart murmurs includes ejection systolic murmurs, pansystolic murmurs, diastolic murmurs, and continuous murmurs.

Ejection systolic murmurs

These usually originate in the right or left ventricular outflow tracts. They reach a crescendo in mid-systole and die down before the second heart sound.

Causes of ejection systolic murmurs in the aortic area (second right intercostal space) include the following:

- Supravalvular, e.g. supra-aortic stenosis or coarctation of the aorta.
- Valvular, e.g. aortic stenosis or aortic sclerosis.
- Subvalvular, e.g. hypertrophic obstructive cardiomyopathy.
- Hyperkinetic states.

Causes of ejection systolic murmurs in the pulmonary area (second left intercostal space) include the following:

- Supravalvular, e.g. pulmonary arterial stenosis.
- Valvular, e.g. pulmonary valve stenosis.
- Subvalvular, e.g. infundibular stenosis.
- Flow murmurs, hyperkinetic states, and left-to-right shunts, e.g. ASD.

Causes of ejection systolic murmurs at the apex include flow murmurs and aortic stenosis (radiation from the aortic area).

Pansystolic murmurs

These murmurs are of uniform intensity and are heard throughout systole, merging with the second heart sound.

Causes of pansystolic murmurs at the lower left sternal edge include tricuspid regurgitation and VSD, and those at the apex include mitral regurgitation.

Diastolic murmurs

Causes of early diastolic murmurs at the left sternal edge include aortic regurgitation and pulmonary regurgitation, and causes of mid-diastolic murmurs include tricuspid stenosis and increased flow across a non-stenotic tricuspid valve (e.g. ASD and tricuspid regurgitation).

Causes of diastolic murmurs at the apex include the following:

- Mitral stenosis.
- Carey Coombs murmur (due to thickening of mitral valve leaflets in acute rheumatic fever).
- Austin Flint murmur (due to fluttering of the anterior mitral valve cusp in aortic regurgitation by the regurgitant stream).
- Increased flow across a non-stenotic mitral valve, e.g. VSD and mitral regurgitation.
- Graham Steell murmur: pulmonary regurgitation secondary to pulmonary hypertension (also heard at left sternal edge).

Continuous murmurs

Continuous murmurs are heard during systole and diastole, such as in PDA, coronary arteriovenous fistula, ruptured aneurysm of the Sinus of Valsalva, cervical venous hum, or ASD with mitral stenosis.

Pure diastolic murmurs are ALWAYS pathological.

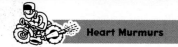
HISTORY IN THE PATIENT WITH HEART MURMURS

There are no symptoms of cardiac murmurs *per se* and so the history should focus on possible causes of the murmur or consequences of the responsible lesion. Ask about the following:

- Rheumatic fever: particularly affecting the mitral valve.
- Ischaemic heart disease, e.g. mitral regurgitation.
- Congenital heart disease.
- Hypertension: flow murmurs.
- Family history: hypertrophic cardiomyopathy is inherited as an autosomal dominant condition.
- Aortic regurgitation may be associated with rheumatoid arthritis or seronegative arthropathies, e.g. ankylosing spondylitis, Reiter's syndrome, colitic and psoriatic arthropathy, Marfan's syndrome, syphilitic aortitis, or coarctation of the aorta. If you suspect any of these, question further about joint symptoms, gastrointestinal symptoms, neurological symptoms, etc.
- Mitral regurgitation may be caused by connective tissue disorders (e.g. systemic lupus erythematosus, rheumatoid arthritis), ankylosing spondylitis, or by congenital conditions, e.g. Marfan's syndrome, Ehlers–Danlos syndrome, pseudoxanthoma elasticum, or osteogenesis imperfecta.

Consequences

The following consequences of a heart murmur may be noted:

- None: aortic valve disease and mitral regurgitation may remain asymptomatic for years.
- Fatigue and weakness: low cardiac output.
- Palpitations: especially atrial fibrillation.
- Angina: especially in aortic stenosis.
- Symptoms of right ventricular failure (secondary to pulmonary hypertension): congestion may result in anorexia, ankle and leg swelling, and hepatic pain.
- Symptoms of left ventricular failure: breathlessness on exertion, cough and haemoptysis (especially mitral stenosis), orthopnoea, and paroxysmal nocturnal dyspnoea (PND).
- Syncope due to poor cardiac output in conditions obstructing the outflow tract, e.g. severe aortic stenosis.
- Symptoms of systemic emboli, e.g. transient ischaemic attacks or stroke; often a complication in mitral stenosis.
- Symptoms of enlarged left atrium pressing on other structures (especially in mitral stenosis), e.g. recurrent laryngeal nerve leading to hoarseness (Ortner's syndrome), oesophagus leading to dysphagia, left main bronchus leading to left lung collapse.
- Symptoms of infective endocarditis.

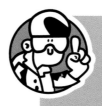

In patients with pulmonary hypertension, pulmonary oedema may be precipitated by the following:

- **Onset of uncontrolled atrial fibrillation.**
- **Chest infection.**
- **Anaesthesia.**
- **Exercise.**
- **Pregnancy.**

EXAMINING THE PATIENT WITH HEART MURMURS

Always follow the examination routine—inspection, palpation, then auscultation. Many clues can be gained about the nature of the murmur before the stethoscope is placed on the chest.

Mitral stenosis

Clinical symptoms

Dyspnoea on exertion is an early symptom, and may progress to orthopnoea and PND. Breathlessness often worsens considerably with the onset of atrial fibrillation, and is often accompanied by palpitations. Cough and haemoptysis may occur because of bronchitis, pulmonary infarction, pulmonary congestion, and bronchial vein rupture. Systemic emboli may occur in patients, particularly in atrial fibrillation. Fatigue and cold extremities are late symptoms, probably secondary to a low cardiac output. Chest pain occurs in a few people and may be due to coronary artery embolism or severe pulmonary hypertension. The patient may have coexistent coronary artery disease.

Clinical signs
The clinical signs of mitral stenosis are given in Fig. 4.1.

Differential diagnosis
The differential diagnosis of mitral stenosis includes the following:

- Inflow obstruction, e.g. hypertrophic cardiomyopathy or left atrial myxoma.
- Aortic regurgitation.
- Tricuspid stenosis.

Investigations
The electrocardiogram (ECG) may show atrial fibrillation or 'p' mitrale in sinus rhythm. There may be signs of right ventricular hypertrophy (RVH)—e.g. a dominant R wave in V_1—and right axis deviation.

The murmur of mitral stenosis is louder after exercise. Ask the patient to jog on the spot or do sit-ups on the examination couch if the murmur is soft.

The chest X-ray (CXR) shows left atrial enlargement visible as a double shadow behind the heart. Valve calcification may be seen in lateral projections. There may also be signs of pulmonary oedema, and a splayed carina.

Echocardiography can be used to assess the area of the mitral valve orifice, and the gradient across the mitral valve. It can also be used to assess left ventricular

Fig. 4.1 Mitral stenosis. (RVH, right ventricular hypertrophy.)

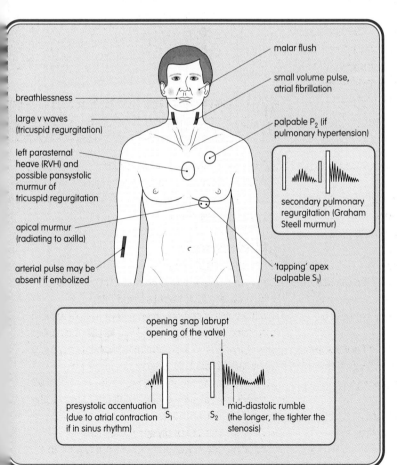

malar flush

small volume pulse, atrial fibrillation

breathlessness

large v waves (tricuspid regurgitation)

left parasternal heave (RVH) and possible pansystolic murmur of tricuspid regurgitation

palpable P_2 (if pulmonary hypertension)

secondary pulmonary regurgitation (Graham Steell murmur)

apical murmur (radiating to axilla)

arterial pulse may be absent if embolized

'tapping' apex (palpable S_1)

opening snap (abrupt opening of the valve)

presystolic accentuation (due to atrial contraction if in sinus rhythm) S_1 S_2 mid-diastolic rumble (the longer, the tighter the stenosis)

function and measure the size of the left atrium, and the right-sided heart chambers.

Cardiac catheterization is usually reserved for patients with suspected coronary artery disease but can be used to measure the pulmonary capillary wedge pressure as an indirect gauge of left atrial pressure, and the left ventricular end diastolic pressure (LVEDP), and hence the gradient across the mitral valve. The measurements should be repeated after exercise if the right-sided heart pressures are normal.

Mitral regurgitation
Clinical symptoms
Progressive exertional dyspnoea, palpitations, and fatigue are common, with symptoms of pulmonary oedema if severe. Atrial fibrillation, systemic emboli, and chest pain are less common than in mitral stenosis.

Clinical signs
The clinical signs of mitral regurgitation are given in Fig. 4.2.

Differential diagnosis
The differential diagnosis of mitral regurgitation includes the following:

- Aortic stenosis.
- Hypertrophic cardiomyopathy.
- VSD.
- Tricuspid regurgitation.

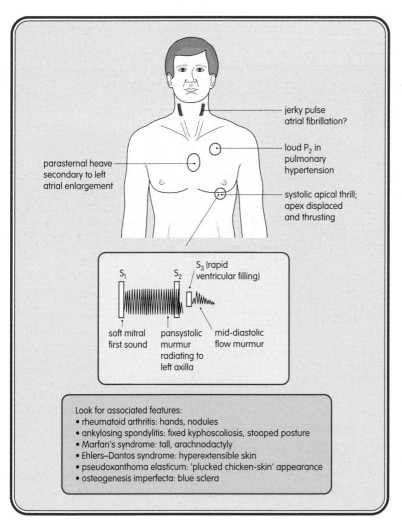

Fig. 4.2 Mitral regurgitation.

jerky pulse
atrial fibrillation?

loud P$_2$ in pulmonary hypertension

parasternal heave secondary to left atrial enlargement

systolic apical thrill; apex displaced and thrusting

S$_1$ S$_2$ S$_3$ (rapid ventricular filling)

soft mitral first sound

pansystolic murmur radiating to left axilla

mid-diastolic flow murmur

Look for associated features:
- rheumatoid arthritis: hands, nodules
- ankylosing spondylitis: fixed kyphoscoliosis, stooped posture
- Marfan's syndrome: tall, arachnodactyly
- Ehlers–Dantos syndrome: hyperextensible skin
- pseudoxanthoma elasticum: 'plucked chicken-skin' appearance
- osteogenesis imperfecta: blue sclera

Investigations

The CXR shows cardiomegaly with enlargement of the left ventricle and left atrium. In acute mitral regurgitation the heart size is normal with signs of pulmonary oedema.

The ECG may show signs of left ventricular hypertrophy (LVH), 'p' mitrale associated with left atrial hypertrophy, and occasionally atrial fibrillation.

Echocardiography may reveal a cause for the regurgitation and can be used to assess the degree of left ventricular dilatation, which is useful for following the progress of the regurgitation.

Aortic stenosis

Clinical symptoms

Initially the patient may be asymptomatic. Classically late symptoms are angina pectoris, exertional dyspnoea, and syncope. Sudden death may occur, probably secondary to ventricular dysrhythmias.

Clinical signs

Clinical signs in aortic stenosis are given in Fig. 4.3.

Investigations

The ECG shows signs of LVH with increased QRS voltages and ST/T segment changes.

The CXR usually shows a normal heart size. The ascending aorta may be prominent due to poststenotic dilatation, and the valve may be calcified.

Echocardiography may show a calcified valve and can be used to estimate the valve area. Cardiac chamber dimensions can be assessed, and doppler studies can be used to assess the gradient across the valve.

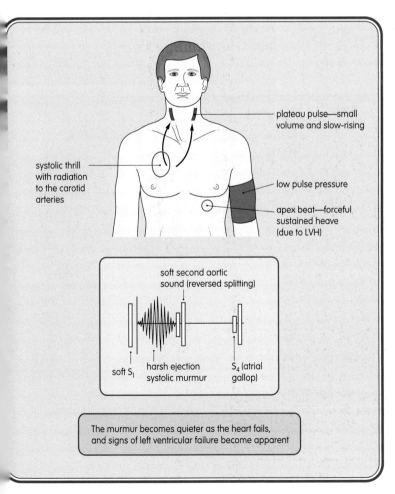

Fig. 4.3 Aortic stenosis. (LVH, left ventricular hypertrophy.)

plateau pulse—small volume and slow-rising

systolic thrill with radiation to the carotid arteries

low pulse pressure

apex beat—forceful sustained heave (due to LVH)

soft second aortic sound (reversed splitting)

soft S_1

harsh ejection systolic murmur

S_4 (atrial gallop)

The murmur becomes quieter as the heart fails, and signs of left ventricular failure become apparent

Cardiac catheterization is usually only necessary to exclude coexisting coronary disease but can determine the systolic gradient across the valve.

Aortic regurgitation
Clinical symptoms
The patient is usually asymptomatic until the ventricle fails, giving rise to symptoms of heart failure. Angina rarely occurs.

Clinical signs
Clinical signs in aortic regurgitation are given in Fig. 4.4. The pulse has a sharp rise and fall ('collapsing' or 'water hammer') with a wide pulse pressure. Other

When listening for aortic regurgitation, ask the patient to sit up and hold his or her breath in expiration.

manifestations of this are visible pulsation in the nail bed (Quincke's sign), visible arterial pulsation in the neck (Corrigan's sign), head bobbing (de Musset's sign), 'pistol shot' femoral artery sound (Traube's sign), and a diastolic murmur following distal compression of the artery (Duroziez's sign).

Differential diagnosis
The differential diagnosis of aortic regurgitation includes the following:
- Pulmonary regurgitation.
- PDA.
- VSD and aortic regurgitation.
- Ruptured aneurysm of the Sinus of Valsalva.

Investigations
The ECG shows signs of LVH and the CXR reveals cardiomegaly. Echocardiography can assess chamber size and may give a clue to the aetiology. Cardiac catheterization can be used to assess the severity of the regurgitation, assess ventricular function, and for coronary arteriography.

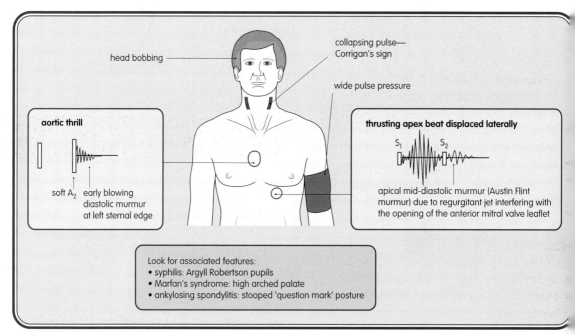

Fig. 4.4 Aortic regurgitation.

5. Cough and Haemoptysis

INTRODUCTION

Coughing is a non-specific reaction to irritation anywhere in the respiratory tract from the pharynx to the lungs, and it is the commonest manifestation of lower respiratory tract disease. Any cough that persists for over 3 weeks merits further investigation in the absence of an obvious cause.

DIFFERENTIAL DIAGNOSIS OF COUGH AND HAEMOPTYSIS

Cough

The differential diagnosis of cough includes:
- Postnasal drip: sinusitis.
- Upper respiratory tract infections, e.g. pharyngitis, laryngitis, tracheobronchitis.
- Pressure on the trachea (e.g. from a goitre): this may be associated with stridor.
- Croup and laryngitis.
- Lower respiratory tract causes: almost any lung pathology may be associated with cough, in particular asthma (suspect if there is a nocturnal cough), chronic obstructive pulmonary disease (COPD), bronchiectasis, and left ventricular failure.
- Drugs (e.g. angiotensin-converting enzyme [ACE] inhibitors) and irritants, especially occupational agents.
- Psychogenic cough.
- Non-respiratory causes, e.g. pericardial irritation, gastro-oesophageal reflux.
- Causes of haemoptysis.

Haemoptysis

Common causes of haemoptysis include the following:
- Acute infections, e.g. exacerbations of COPD.
- Bronchiectasis: can be responsible for massive haemoptysis.
- Bronchial carcinoma: secondary deposits and benign tumours can also lead to haemoptysis but are less common.
- Pulmonary tuberculosis: a common cause worldwide.
- Pulmonary embolus with infarction.

- Left ventricular failure can lead to the production of pink, frothy sputum.
- Mitral stenosis.
- Other infections, such as lobar pneumonia ('rusty' sputum) or less commonly lung abscess.
- Trauma (e.g. contusions to the chest, inhalation of foreign bodies, or after intubation).

Rare causes of haemoptysis include the following:
- Bleeding diatheses.
- Vasculitis, e.g. Goodpasture's syndrome and Wegener's granulomatosis.
- Diffuse interstitial fibrosis.
- Idiopathic pulmonary haemosiderosis.
- Arteriovenous malformations (Osler–Weber–Rendu disease [hereditary haemorrhagic telangiectasia], a favourite in exams but rare in practice).
- Eisenmenger's syndrome.
- Sarcoidosis and amyloidosis.
- Primary pulmonary hypertension.
- Cystic fibrosis.

Note that in up to 15% of cases no cause for haemoptysis is found.

HISTORY IN THE PATIENT WITH COUGH AND HAEMOPTYSIS

The nature of the cough may help in the diagnosis (Fig. 5.1). The following factors should be assessed in the patient with cough or haemoptysis:
- How long has the cough been present? A chronic cough is more commonly associated with tuberculosis, foreign bodies and asthma.

Be aware that Osler–Weber–Rendu disease occurs more often in exams than in clinical practice.

- Has the patient been in contact with any person with infection?
- How severe is the cough? Complications include worsening of bronchospasm, vomiting, rib fractures, urinary incontinence, and syncope.
- Does the patient smoke? This can often cause a cough in its own right by acting as an irritant, but may also be associated with malignancy.
- Ask about drug history, in particular treatment with ACE inhibitors. Of people on ACE inhibitors, 10–20% will have a dry, tickly cough. It is more common in women than men. The patient may find the cough tolerable once reassured that there is no serious underlying condition, and the ACE inhibitor may be continued if needed.
- Are there any occupational agents or exposure to dust which might account for the cough?
- Has there been any weight loss? Think of carcinoma or lung abscess. Ask about other features of malignancy if suspected, such as change in bowel habit.
- Has there been a history of trauma to the chest?
- Is there a family history of bleeding disorders?
- Ask about a past history of rheumatic fever— haemoptysis in mitral stenosis.
- If a diagnosis is suspected, ask more leading questions.
- Don't forget non-respiratory causes, e.g. are there any symptoms suggestive of gastro-oesophageal reflux disease?

EXAMINING THE PATIENT WITH COUGH AND HAEMOPTYSIS

A full general and respiratory examination should be carried out (Fig. 5.2, and see Chapters 2 and 27). Assess the following:

- If the patient appears breathless, assess the severity and count the respiratory rate.
- Check for anaemia: if present think of malignancy, connective tissue diseases, or chronic infection.
- If there is clubbing, suspect bronchial carcinoma, lung abscess, mesothelioma, bronchiectasis, cystic fibrosis, or fibrosing alveolitis.
- If the patient is cyanosed, there may be COPD, or Eisenmenger's syndrome.
- Examine for lymphadenopathy, caused by infections or malignancy.
- Look at the sputum pot if the cough is productive.
- Examine for a goitre. Is there retrosternal extension?
- Examine specifically for signs of bronchial carcinoma, (e.g. Horner's syndrome, paraneoplastic syndromes).
- Examine the legs for DVT, with pulmonary embolus as a cause for haemoptysis.
- Look at the skin. Punctate lesions on mucous membranes are present with Osler–Weber–Rendu disease.
- Check for facial pain in sinusitis.
- Proceed to a full respiratory examination, including auscultation for murmurs over the lung fields with

Fig. 5.1 Details regarding the nature of the cough that may be important for diagnosis.

Details of coughs that may be important for diagnosis

- If the cough is productive, look at the sputum (see Chapter 2)
- A 'brassy' cough, described as hard and metallic, may be associated with pressure on the trachea
- A cough associated with retrosternal pain, 'like a hot poker', occurs in tracheitis
- A bovine cough results from laryngeal paralysis, usually from bronchial carcinoma infiltrating the left recurrent laryngeal nerve
- Croup is a hard and hoarse cough of laryngitis
- Associations with stridor may occur with whooping cough and in the presence of laryngeal or tracheal obstruction
- Ask about other associated symptoms, e.g. a wheeze may occur with asthma or left ventricular function; there may be orthopnoea or paroxsymal nocturnal dyspnoea (see Chapter 2)
- If associated with pleuritic pain, suspect pulmonary embolus
- A hacking, irritating frequent cough occurs in pharyngitis
- Associations with haemoptysis should trigger the differential diagnosis of haemoptysis

arteriovenous malformations, bronchial breathing in lobar consolidation, fine crepitations with left ventricular failure and fibrosing alveolitis, and the coarser crepitation in bronchiectasis.

- Auscultate the heart for the murmur of mitral stenosis or a pericardial rub.
- Listen for the pleural rub of pulmonary infarction.
- In pulmonary hypertension, there will be a loud pulmonary component of the second heart sound, a right ventricular heave, a pulmonary systolic murmur, and prominent a-waves in the jugulovenous pressure.

- A localized rhonchus, not disappearing on coughing, suggests a blocked major airway from a carcinoma or a foreign body.

INVESTIGATING THE PATIENT WITH COUGH AND HAEMOPTYSIS

An algorithm for the investigation of the patient with cough and haemoptysis is given in Fig. 5.3. The

Fig. 5.2 Examining the patient with cough and haemoptysis.

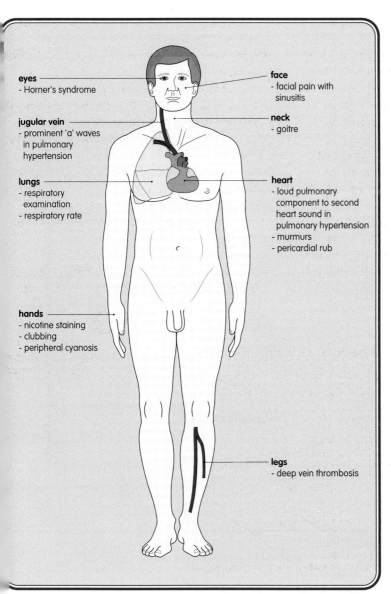

eyes
- Horner's syndrome

jugular vein
- prominent 'a' waves in pulmonary hypertension

lungs
- respiratory examination
- respiratory rate

hands
- nicotine staining
- clubbing
- peripheral cyanosis

face
- facial pain with sinusitis

neck
- goitre

heart
- loud pulmonary component to second heart sound in pulmonary hypertension
- murmurs
- pericardial rub

legs
- deep vein thrombosis

following investigations should be performed in the patient with cough or haemoptysis:

- Full blood count: anaemia with malignancies.
- Urea and electrolytes.
- Chest X-ray: this may reveal the pulmonary cause of the cough, e.g. pneumonia, a straight left heart border with mitral stenosis, infiltrative lung diseases, honeycombing or cyst formation with bronchiectasis, bilateral hilar lymphadenopathy in sarcoidosis.
- Sputum: microscopy, culture and cytology.
- Pharyngoscopy: if an upper respiratory cause is suspected.

- Ventilation/perfusion scan: if a pulmonary embolus is suspected.
- Bronchoscopy with or without biopsy.
- Specific lung function tests: if the cause has not been found after the above tests have been carried out (see Chapter 29).
- High-resolution computed tomography: to confirm the presence of interstitial disease; it is useful in confirming bronchiectasis.
- Gastroscopy or barium meal: to investigate possible gastro-oesophageal reflux disease.

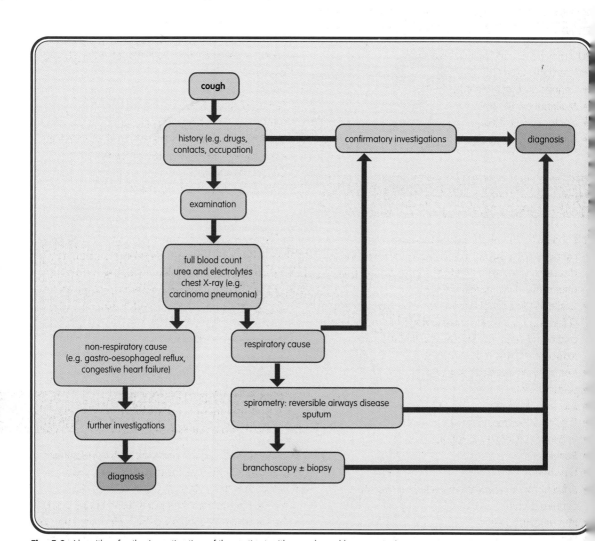

Fig. 5.3 Algorithm for the investigation of the patient with cough and haemoptysis. Confirmatory investigations include sputum and blood cultures for pneumonia, and a ventilation–perfusion scan for pulmonary emboli.

6. Pyrexia of Unknown Origin

INTRODUCTION

Most fevers are due to viral illnesses and are self limiting. Pyrexia of unknown origin (PUO) is a persistent and unexplained fever that lasts more than 3 weeks.

CAUSES

PUO may be caused by the following:
- Infections: 20–40%.
- Connective tissue disorders: 20%.
- Malignancy: 10–20%.
- Undiagnosed: 20%.
- Drugs, e.g. phenytoin: rare.

HISTORY IN THE PATIENT WITH PUO

This should be thorough. Note especially:
- Foreign travel: the incubation period of many tropical diseases may mean that the fever starts some time after arrival back home.
- Contact with animals (zoonoses), e.g. leptospirosis, Q fever, salmonellosis, cat-scratch fever, psittacoses and ornathoses, toxoplasmosis, hydatid disease, toxocariasis, meningitis, anthrax.
- Contact with infected people.
- Sexual history.
- Alcohol intake.
- Previous illnesses.
- Previous surgery or accidents.
- Rashes.
- Diarrhoea.
- A full history of medication, including over-the-counter drugs.
- Immunization history.
- Symptoms such as sweats, weight loss, and itching.
- Lumps.
- Familial disorders, e.g. familial Mediterranean fever.

Every symptom should be explored in detail. The diagnosis should be made by going over the history repeatedly to look for additional or missed clues.

EXAMINING THE PATIENT WITH PUO

The examination of a patient with PUO is shown in Fig. 6.1. It should be especially thorough and may need to be repeated several times. Particular attention should be given to:
- Teeth and throat.
- Temporal artery tenderness.
- Eye signs, e.g. conjunctival petechiae.
- Skin lesions, e.g. rashes, petechiae, and infarctions.
- Lymphadenopathy and organomegaly.
- Cardiac murmurs.
- Rectal and vaginal examinations.

The temperature and pulse should be recorded at least 4-hourly when a patient is admitted with PUO.

INVESTIGATING THE PATIENT WITH PUO

An algorithm for the investigation of the patient with PUO is given in Fig. 6.2. Investigations are best directed from the history and examination. For example, if the patient has just returned from a part of the world where malaria is endemic, thick and thin blood films should be requested. Often there will be no clue, and the best way to proceed is to ask for general non-specific screening tests, which may then suggest an area to focus on.

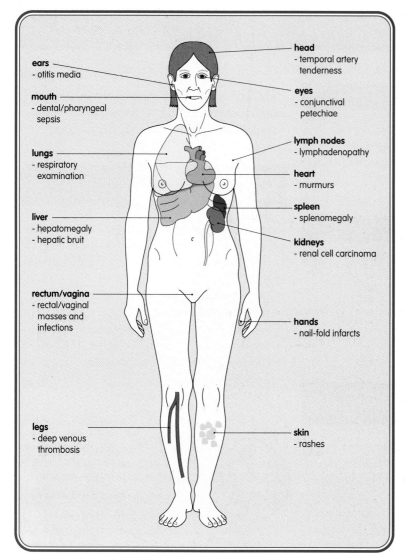

Fig. 6.1 Examining the patient with pyrexia of unknown origin (PUO).

ears
- otitis media

mouth
- dental/pharyngeal
  sepsis

lungs
- respiratory
  examination

liver
- hepatomegaly
- hepatic bruit

rectum/vagina
- rectal/vaginal
  masses and
  infections

legs
- deep venous
  thrombosis

head
- temporal artery
  tenderness

eyes
- conjunctival
  petechiae

lymph nodes
- lymphadenopathy

heart
- murmurs

spleen
- splenomegaly

kidneys
- renal cell carcinoma

hands
- nail-fold infarcts

skin
- rashes

Full blood count and differential white cell count

Full blood count and differential white cell count may yield information on the following:

- Neutrophil leucocytosis: bacterial infections, myeloproliferative disease, malignancy (e.g. hepatic metastases), collagen vascular diseases.
- Leucopenia: viral infections, lymphoma, systemic lupus erythematosus, brucellosis, disseminated tuberculosis, drugs.
- Monocytosis: subacute bacterial endocarditis, inflammatory bowel disease, Hodgkin's disease, brucellosis, tuberculosis.

- Abnormal mononuclear cells: glandular fever, cytomegalovirus infection, toxoplasmosis.
- Eosinophilia: parasitic infections (e.g. trichiasis, hydatid disease), malignancy (especially Hodgkin's disease), pulmonary eosinophilia.

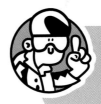

Always go over the history and examination repeatedly, even when investigations are in progress.

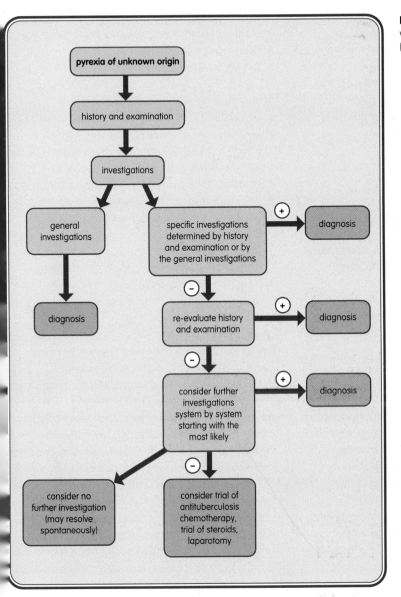

Fig. 6.2 Investigation of the patient with pyrexia of unknown origin (PUO).

Erythrocyte sedimentation rate

A very high erythrocyte sedimentation rate suggests the following:

- Multiple myeloma.
- SLE.
- Temporal arteritis.
- Polymyalgia rheumatica.
- Still's disease.
- Rheumatic fever.
- Lymphoma.
- Subacute bacterial endocarditis.

Urea and electrolytes

Assessment of urea and electrolytes may reveal renal impairment or hyponatraemia due to pneumonia.

Liver function tests

Abnormal results may lead to more detailed investigations of the liver. Note, however, that alkaline phosphatase may also be raised in metabolic bone disease, Hodgkin's disease, Still's disease, and in patients with bony metastases.

Bacteriology and serology

Microscopy and culture from every site possible:

- Urine: bacteria (infections), haematuria (may suggest subacute bacterial endocarditis or hypernephroma).
- Blood cultures: several samples are needed from different veins at different times of the day.
- Faeces' microscopy for ova, cysts and parasites.
- Vaginal and cervical swabs.
- Urethral swabs in men.
- Sputum microscopy and culture.
- Throat swab cultures.

With regard to serology, many specific tests are available, e.g. glandular fever, psittacosis, brucellosis. A second sample must be taken 2–3 weeks later to show a rising antibody titre or IgM titres may signal acute infection.

Chest X-ray

Chest X-ray should be performed to show, for example, tuberculosis, subphrenic abscess, and bilateral hilar lymphadenopathy (sarcoidosis).

Further investigations

Further investigations should be directed by the results of previous investigations. For example, if a renal problem is suspected, further tests might include an intravenous pyelogram and renal ultrasound. If a pulmonary problem is suspected, a ventilation/perfusion scan or pulmonary angiography may be useful to exclude multiple pulmonary emboli as the cause of PUO.

If there are no clues from previous investigations, the following further investigations should be considered:

- Immunoglobulins: raised immunoglobulin (IgG) suggests SLE or chronic hepatitis; raised IgM suggests viral hepatitis; raised IgA suggests Crohn's disease.
- Rheumatoid factor.
- Mantoux test for tuberculosis.
- Bone marrow aspiration.
- Lumbar puncture.

All non-essential drugs should be stopped on admission. It may be necessary to withhold other drugs at this stage, one at a time for 48 hours each.

If there is still no clue as to the cause of the fever, the system most likely to be responsible should be investigated. Thus, to investigate the abdominal system, the following investigations should be considered:

- Abdominal ultrasound, e.g. subphrenic or pelvic abscess.
- Abdominal computed tomography scan, e.g. retroperitoneal lymphadenopathy, lymphoma.
- Barium studies, e.g. malignancy or abscess.
- Liver biopsy, e.g. granulomatous diseases or brucellosis.

Very rare causes should be considered if not already investigated. These include hyperthyroidism, phaeochromocytoma, and familial Mediterranean fever.

Factitious fever is caused by the deliberate manipulation of the thermometer. This is classically said to occur in young women. The diagnosis should be suspected if other causes have been excluded, and there is no evidence of a chronic illness, no increase in pulse rate when pyrexial, or if the patient looks inappropriately well despite fever.

If all else fails, it may be necessary to carry out an exploratory laporotomy, although the postoperative complication rate is 15–20%. Consideration should also be given to treating tuberculosis with antituberculosis chemotherapy, endocarditis with antibiotics, and vasculitides with steroids.

7. Haematemesis and Melaena

INTRODUCTION

Haematemesis is the vomiting of fresh (bright red) or altered ('coffee ground') blood. Melaena is the production of black, tarry stools, and is due to bleeding from the upper gastrointestinal (GI) tract of more than 100 mL of blood. GI bleeding is an emergency, and treatment may need to be initiated before a diagnosis has been made (Chapter 32).

DIFFERENTIAL DIAGNOSIS OF HAEMATEMESIS AND MELAENA

The differential diagnosis of haematemesis and melaena includes the following:

- Peptic ulcer disease: the commonest cause, accounting for about half of major upper GI bleeds. The acute mortality rate is about 10%.
- Erosive gastritis: implicated in about 20% of upper GI bleeds, although they are an unusual cause of severe GI bleeding unless associated with other pathology.
- Mallory–Weiss tears: lacerations of the gastro-oesophageal junction accounting for about 10% of upper GI bleeds. Often due to retching after an alcohol binge.
- Oesophagitis/hiatus hernia: secondary to chronic gastro-oesophageal reflux.
- Ruptured oesophageal varices: secondary to portal hypertension accounting for 10–20% of upper GI bleeds. The acute mortality rate is up to 40%.
- Vascular abnormalities: may cause upper or lower GI bleeding. The commonest abnormalities are vascular ectasias or angiodysplasias.
- Gastric neoplasms: about 5% of upper GI bleeds.
- Rarer causes, e.g. oesophageal or stomal ulcers, oesophageal tumours, blood dyscrasias, aortoenteric fistula complicating an abdominal aortic graft, pancreatic tumour, pseudoaneurysm.

HISTORY IN THE PATIENT WITH HAEMATEMESIS AND MELAENA

The history may have to be taken after initial resuscitation procedures. It is important to determine whether the blood has been vomited or coughed. In cases of difficulty, the presence of food mixed with the blood or an acid pH is suggestive of haematemesis, although the vomitus may not be acidic in patients with carcinoma of the stomach.

Haematemesis may be due to blood swallowed from the nasopharynx or mouth.

You must ask about the following:

- Non-specific symptoms of GI blood loss: faintness, weakness, dizziness, sweating, palpitations, dyspnoea, pallor, collapse. These symptoms may precede the actual haematemesis/melaena.
- Weight loss and anorexia: carcinoma.
- Current drugs: aspirin, nonsteroidal anti-inflammatory drugs, or excessive alcohol are suggestive of gastric erosions; iron causes therapy black stools but this is not melaena.
- Symptoms of chronic blood loss: suggests gastric carcinoma if associated with anorexia and weight loss.
- Heartburn: oesophagitis.
- Intermittent epigastric pain relieved with antacids: peptic ulceration.
- Sudden severe abdominal pain: perforation.
- Dysphagia or odynophagia (pain on swallowing): oesophageal carcinoma.
- Chronic excessive alcohol intake: oesophageal varices.
- Enquiry into the causes of liver failure (Chapter 10): oesophageal varices.
- Retching especially after an alcohol binge: Mallory–Weiss tear.
- Family history: inherited bleeding disorders.
- A past history of GI bleeds and their cause.

EXAMINING THE PATIENT WITH HAEMATEMESIS AND MELAENA

The approach to examining the patient with haematemesis and melaena is given in Fig. 7.1. Step back from the patient for a few seconds. Do they look well, or pale and clammy? An initial common-sense impression affects the immediacy of subsequent management.

If haemoptysis is suspected, a full respiratory examination should be carried out.

General examination

The general examination should assess the following:

- Anaemia: mucous membranes. If clinically anaemic, this may indicate chronic blood loss.
- Jaundice: may indicate portal hypertension.
- Clubbing: inflammatory bowel disease, cirrhosis.
- Lymphadenopathy: especially Virchow's node (left supraclavicular lymph node) associated with gastric carcinoma (Troisier's sign).
- Pulse: tachycardia can be the first warning of a large GI bleed and may precede a blood pressure fall. A young and healthy patient may lose more than 500 mL of blood before a rise in heart rate or fall in blood pressure occurs.
- Blood pressure: if hypotensive, intravenous fluids should be given. The pulse and blood pressure measurements should be repeated frequently to monitor haemodynaimc trends.
- Skin: bruises, purpura (bleeding disorders); telangiectasia [Osler–Weber–Rendu disease (hereditary haemorrhagic telangiectasia— autosomal dominant)]; neurofibromata.
- Mouth: pharyngeal lesions; pigmented macules (Peutz–Jeghers syndrome).
- Cachexia.

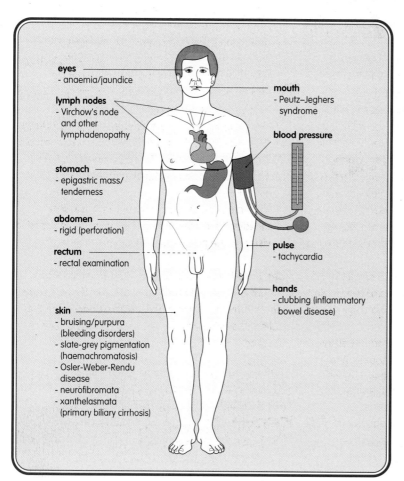

Fig. 7.1 Examining the patient with haematemesis and melaena.

eyes
- anaemia/jaundice

lymph nodes
- Virchow's node and other lymphadenopathy

stomach
- epigastric mass/ tenderness

abdomen
- rigid (perforation)

rectum
- rectal examination

skin
- bruising/purpura (bleeding disorders)
- slate-grey pigmentation (haemachromatosis)
- Osler-Weber-Rendu disease
- neurofibromata
- xanthelasmata (primary biliary cirrhosis)

mouth
- Peutz–Jeghers syndrome

blood pressure

pulse
- tachycardia

hands
- clubbing (inflammatory bowel disease)

Specific examination

This includes a search for signs related to the differential diagnosis:

- A rigid abdomen suggests perforation.
- Epigastric tenderness suggests peptic ulcer disease, oesophagitis, hiatus hernia, or gastric carcinoma.
- Epigastric mass: gastric carcinoma.
- If malignancy is suspected, examine for metastases.
- Signs of chronic liver failure (Chapter 10) including those suggesting specific diagnoses: xanthelasmata in primary biliary cirrhosis; slate-grey pigmentation in haemochromatosis; Kayser–Fleischer rings in Wilson's disease.
- A rectal examination is essential. This will confirm the presence of melaena, which may be present despite haemodynamic stability.

INVESTIGATING THE PATIENT WITH HAEMATEMESIS AND MELAENA

An algorithm for the investigation of the patient with haematemesis and melaena is given in Fig. 7.2. The following investigations should be carried out:

- A full blood count should be performed as part of the investigation. The haemoglobin may be normal in the acute phase, despite a large GI bleed, as it takes some hours for haemodilution to occur. A low haemoglobin on initial presentation suggests chronic blood loss, and the white cell count may be raised after a GI bleed. Platelet count may be reduced after an acute bleed, or increased after chronic blood loss. A very low platelet count should raise suspicion of a bleeding diathesis.
- Group and save even if there is only a small GI bleed, and the patient is haemodynamically stable. Blood should be cross-matched for more significant bleeding.
- A clotting screen should also be performed as the prothrombin time is raised in liver disease. More specific investigations may be indicated (e.g. in patients with haemophilia or von Willebrand's disease).
- Urea is raised due to the absorption of protein when blood reaches the small bowel. Chronic renal failure can be associated with GI bleeding.

- On erect chest X-ray, the presence of gas under the right hemidiaphragm indicates perforation.

Further investigations are done to confirm the site of the bleeding, and to make a definitive diagnosis:

- Fibre-optic endoscopy allows direct visualization of the pathology and can identify the source of the bleeding. It will determine the most appropriate form of medical therapy. The risk of rebleeding may be estimated, for example, Mallory–Weiss tears or erosive gastritis have a low risk of rebleeding with appropriate management, whereas oesophageal varices have a much higher risk of rebleeding. Treatment may be given endoscopically, e.g. injection of a sclerosant into a bleeding varix, or cautery of a bleeding vessel.
- Barium examinations are becoming rarer as endoscopy is becoming more widely available, though they may be useful when endoscopy is contraindicated (e.g. in patients with an unstable cervical spine).
- Abdominal ultrasound should be performed to determine whether liver cirrhosis is present, or to look for metastases if carcinoma is suspected. Abdominal computed tomography scanning may be helpful if a mass is present.
- Isotope studies require active bleeding to be present. They may be useful for continued bleeding despite a thorough search of the GI tract, and will help the surgeon if resection of the bleeding segment is considered.
- Mesenteric angiography again requires active bleeding to localize the source. It can also be used to visualize the portal venous system.

Despite extensive investigation, a small minority of patients will remain undiagnosed. If bleeding is severe laparotomy may be required, but if it is not severe the patient may attend for repeat 'top-up' transfusions as required.

Elevated blood urea with normal serum creatinine suggests gastrointestinal blood loss

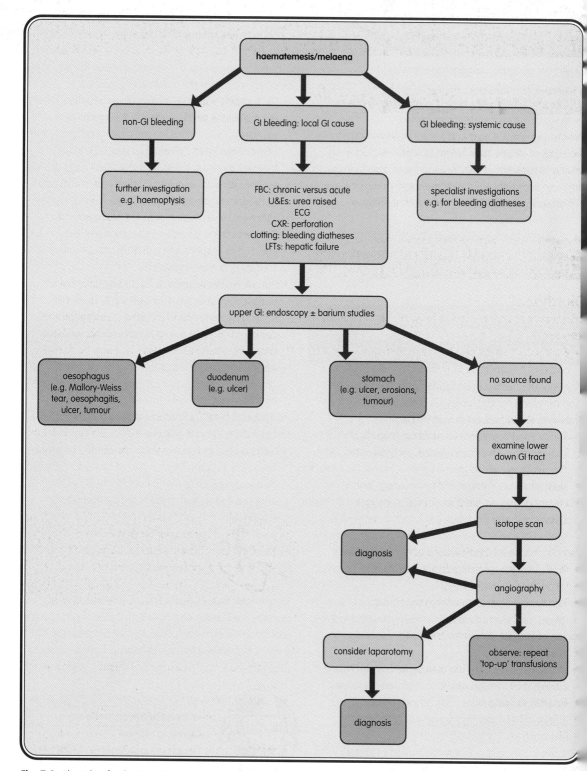

Fig. 7.2 Algorithm for the investigation of the patient with haematemesis and melaena. (ECG, electrocardiogram; CXR, chest X-ray; FBC, full blood count; GI, gastrointestinal; LFTs, liver function tests; U&Es, urea and electrolytes.)

8. Change in Bowel Habit

INTRODUCTION

Always ask about the patient's normal bowel habit as there are considerable differences between people, usually varying from three times a day to once every 3 days. It is important to note a change in bowel habit as this is more commonly associated with pathology.

DIFFERENTIAL DIAGNOSIS OF A CHANGE IN BOWEL HABIT

Diarrhoea

Infective causes of changes in bowel habit include the following:
- Bacterial: *Staphylococcus aureus* (from dairy products and meat), *Bacillus cereus* (fried rice), *Clostridium perfringens* (meat), *Escherichia coli* (meat), *Vibrio parahaemolyticus* (seafood), *Campylobacter* (poultry), *Salmonella* (meat, poultry, and dairy), and *Shigella* (faecal–oral transmission). Less common bacteria include *Yersinia enterocolitica*, *Chlamydia*, and *Neisseria gonorrhoeae*.
- Viral: rotavirus, Norwalk virus, cytomegalovirus.
- Protozoa: *Giardia lamblia*, *Cryptosporidium*, *Entamoeba histolytica*.

Osmotic causes of diarrhoea include:
- Medications, e.g. antacids and lactulose.
- Disaccharidase deficiency.
- Factitious diarrhoea, e.g. laxative abuse.

Secretory causes of diarrhoea include:
- Infections.
- Endocrine causes: VIPoma, carcinoid syndrome, Zollinger–Ellison syndrome.
- Factitious diarrhoea.
- Villous adenoma.
- Bile salt malabsorption.

Inflammatory causes of diarrhoea include:
- Ulcerative colitis.
- Crohn's disease.

- Malignancy, e.g. lymphoma.
- Radiation enteritis, e.g. following radiotherapy.

Causes of malabsorption include:
- Tropical sprue and Whipple's disease.
- Lymphatic obstruction, e.g. lymphoma, carcinoid syndrome, Kaposi's sarcoma, sarcoidosis.
- Pancreatic disease, e.g. cystic fibrosis and chronic pancreatitis.
- Bacterial overgrowth, e.g. blind loop syndrome.

Increased motility may be caused by irritable bowel syndrome and systemic disorders such as hyperthyroidism, scleroderma, and diabetes mellitus.

Chronic infections should also be considered in a patient with a change of bowel habit, e.g. giardiasis or amoebiasis.

Constipation

Ask what is meant by constipation. It usually means that the bowels are only opened infrequently, and that the faeces are hard, with pain on defaecation.

Make sure that by 'constipation' and 'diarrhoea', you and the patient mean the same thing.

Medical causes of constipation include the following:
- Low-fibre diet.
- Poor bowel habit.
- Endocrine causes: hypothyroidism and hyperparathyroidism.
- Metabolic causes: hypokalaemia, hypercalcaemia, and uraemia.
- Neurological causes: paraplegia and multiple sclerosis.

- Irritable bowel syndrome (often a mixed picture with diarrhoea and constipation).
- Medications: anticholinergic agents, opiates, diuretics, verapamil, psychotropics, and disopyramide.
- Prolonged bed rest or immobility.
- Dehydration.
- Psychogenic causes, e.g. depression, agitation.
- Others: amyloidosis and scleroderma.

Surgical causes of constipation include:
- Perianal disease, e.g. fissure, thrombosed haemorrhoids.
- Intestinal obstruction due to a mass, e.g. carcinoma of the rectum/sigmoid colon.
- Pelvic mass including pregnancy.
- Outlet delay: rectocele, rectal intussusception, rectal prolapse.
- Colonic stricture, e.g. diverticulitis and Crohn's disease.
- Hirschsprung's disease (aganglionic segment of the rectum, usually presenting in the first years of life).
- Postgastrectomy (although this usually causes diarrhoea).
- Postoperative pain.

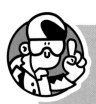

Note the features of acute gastrointestinal (GI) obstruction: absolute constipation, vomiting, pain, and abdominal distension.

HISTORY IN THE PATIENT WITH A CHANGE IN BOWEL HABIT

Ask about the following:
- Normal bowel habit (note interindividual variation).
- Onset: sudden or chronic. Infectious diarrhoea is usually of acute onset.
- Frequency of defecation.
- Stool appearance: formed, loose or watery; colour—normal, red (blood from low in the GI tract), black (melaena), yellow (mucus and slime), 'redcurrant jelly' (intussusception), putty-coloured (obstructive jaundice); volume; do the stools float? (high fat content—think of malabsorption).
- Drugs: antacids, laxatives, cimetidine, digoxin, antibiotics, alcohol.
- Tenesmus (a sense of incomplete voiding).
- Smell: offensively malodorous in malabsorption; characteristic smell of melaena.
- Foreign travel.
- Contact with diarrhoea sufferers.
- Relationship to food.
- Stress.
- Associated features, e.g. pain, fever, vomiting, weight loss.
- Symptoms of thyrotoxicosis.
- Nocturnal diarrhoea: autonomic neuropathies from diabetes mellitus.
- Sexual history: gay bowel syndrome—suspect this if multiple or unusual organisms are cultured.

EXAMINING THE PATIENT WITH A CHANGE IN BOWEL HABIT

The examination approach in the patient with a change in bowel habit is given in Fig. 8.1.

INVESTIGATING THE PATIENT WITH A CHANGE IN BOWEL HABIT

An algorithm for the investigation of the patient with change in bowel habit is given in Fig. 8.2. The following investigations should be performed in this type of patient:
- Full blood count.
- Urea and electrolytes, including calcium.
- Thyroid function tests.
- Blood glucose: diabetes.
- Liver function tests.
- Albumin: decreased in malabsorption, protein-losing enteropathies, inflammatory diseases.
- In malabsorption: anaemia—vitamin B_{12}, folate, iron; hyponatraemia in profound secretory diarrhoea; increased prothrombin time due to malabsorption of fat-soluble vitamins; hypocalcaemia.

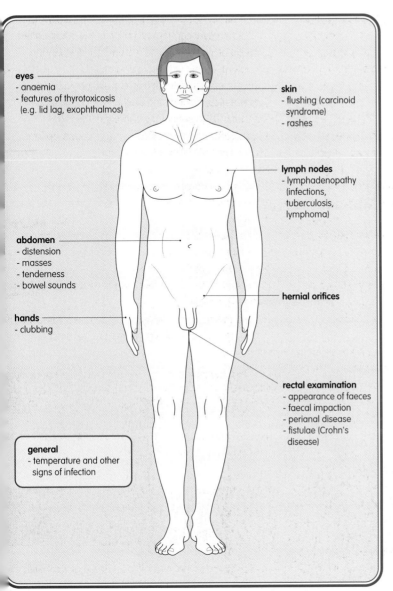

Fig. 8.1 Examining the patient with a change in bowel habit.

eyes
- anaemia
- features of thyrotoxicosis (e.g. lid lag, exophthalmos)

skin
- flushing (carcinoid syndrome)
- rashes

lymph nodes
- lymphadenopathy (infections, tuberculosis, lymphoma)

abdomen
- distension
- masses
- tenderness
- bowel sounds

hernial orifices

hands
- clubbing

rectal examination
- appearance of faeces
- faecal impaction
- perianal disease
- fistulae (Crohn's disease)

general
- temperature and other signs of infection

- Specialized tests: serum vasoactive intestinal polypeptide; serum gastrin (Zollinger–Ellison syndrome); calcitonin (medullary thyroid carcinoma); cortisol (Addison's disease); urinary 5-hydroxyindoleacetic acid (carcinoid syndrome); culture and microscopy for ova, cysts, and parasites.
- Stool: if weight >300g per 24 hours consider a secretory process; if fat content >10g per 24 hours consider malabsorption; laxative screen; leucocytes in inflammatory processes.

- Abdominal X-ray: pancreatic calcification suggests chronic pancreatitis, distended intestinal loops and fluid levels suggest obstruction, and gross dilatation of the colon suggests Hirschsprung's disease.
- Fibre-optic sigmoidoscopy with or without biopsy: inflammatory bowel disease.
- Barium enema.
- Colonoscopy: carcinoma, melanosis coli, or inflammation.
- Colonic transit study: to confirm constipation and measure the transit time.

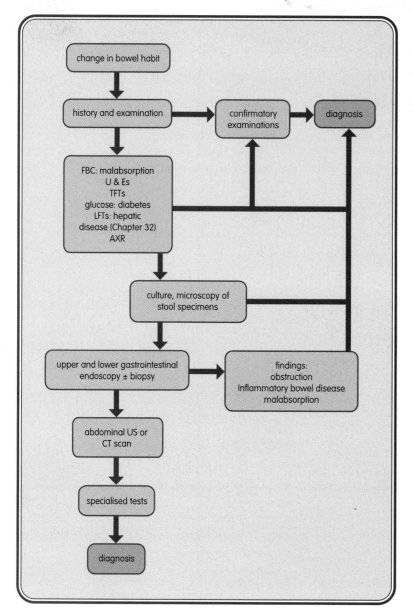

Fig. 8.2 Algorithm for the investigation of the patient with a change of bowel habit. (AXR, abdominal X-ray; CT, computed tomography; FBC, full blood count; LFT, liver function test; U&Es, urea and electrolytes; US, ultrasound; TFTs, thyroid function test.)

- Studies of pelvic floor function: defaecography and anal manometry.
- Upper GI series: Crohn's disease, lymphoma, carcinoid syndrome.
- Upper GI endoscopy with or without duodenal biopsy (malabsorption).
- Abdominal ultrasound: suspected mass.
- Abdominal CT scan: pancreatitis, tumours.

9. Weight loss

INTRODUCTION

Weight loss is due to either a decreased energy intake or increased energy output, or both. Involuntary weight loss is a common manifestation of physical or psychological illness and always warrants further investigation. It should be confirmed objectively with records of previous weights. If this is not possible, a change in clothes size gives a useful clue. Family members may be able to give a more objective history.

DIFFERENTIAL DIAGNOSIS OF WEIGHT LOSS

Distinguish deliberate from involuntary weight loss from the outset. The differential diagnosis of weight loss includes the following causes.

Psychiatric/psychological
- Anorexia nervosa: typically young Caucasian females, with disturbance of body image and fear of weight gain, weight loss of >15% body mass, and amenorrhoea.
- Depression or agitation.
- Catatonia.
- Schizophrenia.
- Laxative or diuretic abuse.
- Neglect, e.g. 'tea and toast' diet in widowhood.

Physiological
- Dieting or food fads.
- Smoking.
- Increase in exercise.

Endocrine
- Uncontrolled diabetes mellitus: often with increased appetite.
- Hyperthyroidism: weight loss despite an increased appetite.
- Adrenal insufficiency.
- Hypothyroidism: due to diminished appetite; although this more commonly presents itself with weight gain.
- Phaeochromocytoma.
- Hypopituitarism.
- Severe diabetes insipidus.

Drugs
- Anorectics.
- Amphetamines.
- Opiates.
- Laxative or diuretics.
- Tobacco smoking.
- Alcohol.

Infections
- Tuberculosis.
- Human immunodeficiency virus.
- Other chronic infections and infestations.

Chronic illnesses
- Cardiac cachexia.
- Chronic obstructive pulmonary disease.
- Disseminated carcinoma.
- Connective tissue diseases.

Gastrointestinal
- Peptic ulcer disease: pain on eating leading to decreased appetite.
- Dysphagia.
- Malabsorption: decreased absorption of nutrients and diarrhoea, e.g. inflammatory bowel disease.
- Coeliac disease.
- Liver disease.

Neurological
- Motor neurone disease.
- Myopathies.
- Poliomyelitis.

Renal
Renal pathologies leading to chronic renal failure and uraemia.

Malignancies anywhere which produce a high metabolic rate ('hungry tumours') or which lead to anorexia or dysphagia, e.g. oesophageal carcinoma, will result in weight loss.

HISTORY IN THE PATIENT WITH WEIGHT LOSS

Weight loss can be a complication of disease in any physiological system.

Try to confirm weight loss objectively with records of previous weights. Ask members of the family or friends if they have noticed weight loss. Ask about the amount of weight loss, its duration, and any accompanying symptoms such as anorexia or increased appetite.

Further factors to assess, if the cause is not apparent, include the following:

- Diet: detailed intake and any recent changes in diet history.
- Physical activity: any changes in level.
- Full drug history: including over-the-counter and illegal medicines.
- Alcohol intake: with and without associated liver disease.
- Smoking: if recent onset, this may lead to eating less; if chronic, assess its association with malignancies.
- Symptoms of chronic infection or malignancy: fever and sweats, rashes, general malaise, anorexia, change in bowel habit, floating stools (malabsorption), haemoptysis, haematemesis, haematuria, melaena (or bleeding from any other site), 'lumps and bumps', joint or muscle tenderness, contacts with infected people, dysphagia.
- Symptoms of renal insufficiency: anorexia, general malaise and lethargy, bruising, urinary symptoms (e.g. polyuria and nocturia), vomiting, hiccoughs.
- Cardiorespiratory symptoms: cardiac cachexia.
- Neurological symptoms.

Finally, the symptoms of endocrinopathies include the following:

- Diabetes: polyuria and polydipsia, weakness and fatigue, blurred vision, pruritus or thrush, nocturnal enuresis.
- Adrenal insufficiency: dizziness and collapses, weakness, nausea and diarrhoea, pigmentation.
- Thyrotoxicosis: tremor, diarrhoea, irritability, heat intolerance, palpitations.
- Phaeochromocytoma: paroxysmal (or sustained) hypertension, panic, pain (abdominal or headache), palpitations, perspiration, pallor, paroxysmal thyroid swelling (remember the 'Ps'), nausea, tremor.
- Panhypopituitarism: pallor, dizziness, loss of body hair, loss of libido, amenorrhoea, visual field defects, symptoms of hypothyroidism.

EXAMINING THE PATIENT WITH WEIGHT LOSS

General observation
The examination approach in the patient with weight loss is given in Fig. 9.1. Does the patient look like they have lost weight (loose skin, loose clothes)? Check the temperature. Does the patient look well or ill?

Hands
The hands should be examined in the patient with weight loss, and the following should be noted:

- Clubbing: malignancy, cirrhosis, inflammatory bowel disease, and infections (pus in the lungs).
- Leuconychia: liver disease.
- Koilonychia: iron-deficiency anaemia (dietary, malabsorption).
- Pigmentation: increased in Addison's disease but decreased in anaemia.

Other signs
Other signs include the following:

- Joint swelling and decreased range of movement: connective tissue diseases.
- Tremor: hyperthyroidism.
- Uraemia: yellow discoloration of the skin.
- Jaundice and other signs of liver failure, e.g. spider naevi.
- Muscle wasting.
- Goitre.

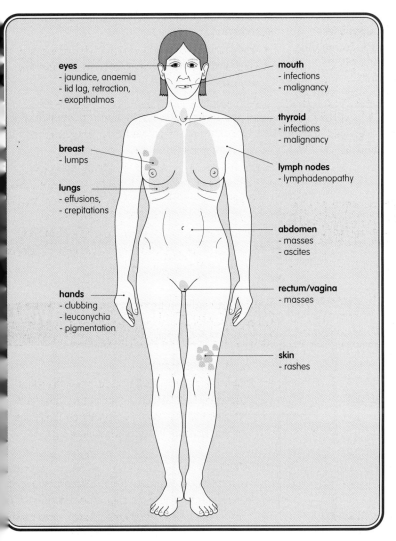

Fig. 9.1 Examining the patient with weight loss.

eyes
- jaundice, anaemia
- lid lag, retraction,
- exopthalmos

breast
- lumps

lungs
- effusions,
- crepitations

hands
- clubbing
- leuconychia
- pigmentation

mouth
- infections
- malignancy

thyroid
- infections
- malignancy

lymph nodes
- lymphadenopathy

abdomen
- masses
- ascites

rectum/vagina
- masses

skin
- rashes

- Skin rashes.
- Subacute bacterial endocarditis: splinter haemorrhages, Osler's nodes, and Janeway's lesions.
- Blood pressure: phaeochromocytoma.
- Fundi: diabetic retinopathy.
- Mouth: infections and malignancies.
- Lymphadenopathy.

Examination of individual systems

The following individual systems should be examined:
- Respiratory system: infection or malignancy. Don't forget to look out for Horner's syndrome.
- Cardiac system.
- Gastrointestinal system: including careful palpation for abdominal masses, rectal examination, and organomegaly (e.g. liver metastases).
- Breast lumps.
- Vaginal examination: pelvic malignancy.

INVESTIGATING THE PATIENT WITH WEIGHT LOSS

An algorithm for the investigation of the patient with weight loss is given in Fig. 9.2. The following investigations should be carried out:
- Full blood count: anaemia with malignancy, iron deficiency, vitamin B_{12} deficiency, or folate deficiency, with inadequate dietary intake.
- Urea and electrolytes for uraemia.

43

- Liver function tests (LFTs): liver failure or metastases, although LFTs may be normal with metastases.
- Blood glucose: diabetes, low glucose in liver failure, Addison's disease.
- Thyroid function tests.

- Chest X-ray: infection or tuberculosis, and malignancy.
- Blood cultures: infection.
- Other investigations depend on the history and examination.

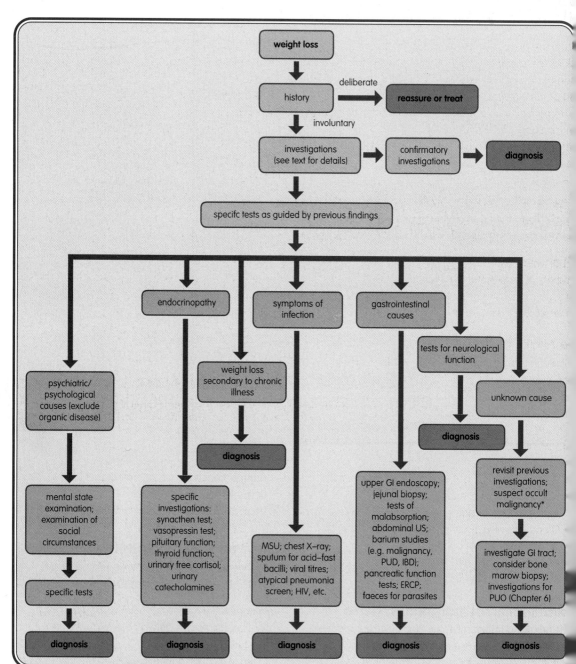

Fig. 9.2 Algorithm for the investigation of the patient with weight loss. (ECRP, endoscopic retrograde cholangiopancreatography; GI, gastrointestinal; HIV, human immunodeficiency virus; IBD, inflammatory bowel disease; MSU, mid-stream urine; PUD, peptic ulcer disease; PUO, pyrexia of unknown origin; US, ultrasound.)
* Investigate site under suspicion, e.g. endoscopy for GI tract; look for metastases.

10. Jaundice

INTRODUCTION

Jaundice (icterus) is the yellow discoloration of the skin, sclera and mucosae, which is detectable when serum bilirubin concentrations exceed approximately 50 μmol/L. Normal bilirubin metabolism is summarized in Fig. 10.1. Jaundice can arise as a result of increased red blood cell (RBC) breakdown, disordered bilirubin metabolism or reduced bilirubin excretion.

DIFFERENTIAL DIAGNOSIS OF JAUNDICE

Prehepatic

Prehepatic jaundice results from increased bilirubin production, caused by abnormal RBC breakdown (haemolysis). For more on this see Chapter 25.

Hepatic

Disordered bilirubin metabolism resulting from hepatocyte dysfunction may also cause jaundice. Hepatocellular damage can arise as a consequence of the following acute insults or chronic pathologies.

Acute hepatocellular damage

- Viral infection, e.g. hepatitis A, B, C and E; Epstein–Barr virus (EBV); cytomegalovirus (CMV).
- Non-viral infection, e.g. *Leptospira icterohaemorrhagiae*.
- Drugs, e.g. paracetamol poisoning, halothane.
- Alcohol.
- Pregnancy.
- Shock.

Chronic hepatocellular damage

- Chronic active hepatitis, e.g. autoimmune, hepatitis B.
- Cirrhosis, e.g. alcohol, chronic active hepatitis, primary biliary cirrhosis, Wilson's disease, haemochromatosis, α_1-antitrypsin deficiency.
- Metastatic carcinoma.

Posthepatic

Posthepatic jaundice is caused by reduced bilirubin excretion. This may be due to intrahepatic or extrahepatic biliary obstruction.

Extrahepatic obstruction

- Gallstones.
- Carcinoma of the head of the pancreas, ampulla of Vater or bile duct.
- Sclerosing cholangitis.
- Stricture, e.g. postendoscopic retrograde cholangiopancreatography (post-ERCP).
- Pancreatitis.
- Biliary atresia.

Intrahepatic obstruction

- Primary biliary cirrhosis.
- Alcohol.
- Viral hepatitis.
- Drugs, e.g. oral contraceptive pill.
- Pregnancy.

HISTORY IN THE PATIENT WITH JAUNDICE

The following factors should be assessed when obtaining a history in a patient with jaundice:

- Pruritis, dark urine and pale stools: underlying cholestasis.
- Duration of illness: a short history of malaise, anorexia and myalgia are suggestive of viral hepatitis. If there is a prolonged history of weight loss and anorexia in an elderly patient, carcinoma is more likely.
- Abdominal pain: the episodic, colicky, right hypochondrial pain of biliary colic will commonly be due to gallstones. A dull, persistent epigastric or central pain radiating to the back may suggest a pancreatic carcinoma.
- Fevers or rigors: cholangitis.
- Full recent drug history: particularly paracetamol, oral contraceptive pill.

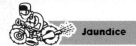

- Alcohol consumption: acute alcoholic hepatitis, cirrhosis.
- Infectious contacts: hepatitis A.
- Recent foreign travel to areas of high hepatitis risk.
- Recent surgery: halothane exposure, surgery for known malignancy, biliary stricture due to previous ERCP.

- Intravenous drug abuse, tattoos, homosexuality: increased risk of hepatitis B and C.
- Occupation: sewage workers are at an increased risk of leptospirosis.
- Family history of recurrent jaundice: inherited haemolytic anaemias and Gilbert's syndrome.

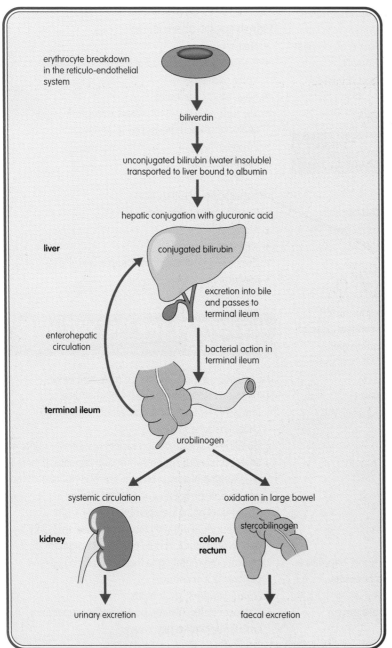

Fig. 10.1 Normal bilirubin metabolism.

EXAMINING THE PATIENT WITH JAUNDICE

There are three important groups of abnormalities that should be looked for in the jaundiced patient:

- How severe is the jaundice? Is there any evidence of encephalopathy?
- Is this an acute or chronic problem? (Are there any signs of chronic liver disease?)
- Are there any signs of specific disorders?

This approach is summarized in Fig. 10.2.

Is there evidence of encephalopathy?

The following factors suggest the presence of encephalopathy:

- Drowsiness: this will eventually progress through stupor to coma.
- Slurred speech.
- Asterixis: flapping tremor of outstretched hands.
- Seizures.
- Constructional apraxia: test by asking the patient to copy a five-pointed star.
- Hepatic fetor.

Fig. 10.2 Examining the patient with jaundice.

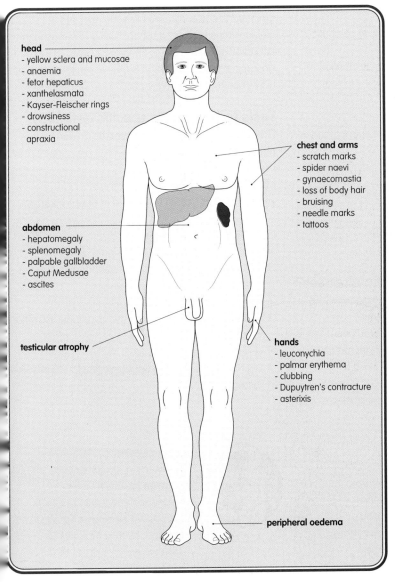

head
- yellow sclera and mucosae
- anaemia
- fetor hepaticus
- xanthelasmata
- Kayser-Fleischer rings
- drowsiness
- constructional apraxia

chest and arms
- scratch marks
- spider naevi
- gynaecomastia
- loss of body hair
- bruising
- needle marks
- tattoos

abdomen
- hepatomegaly
- splenomegaly
- palpable gallbladder
- Caput Medusae
- ascites

testicular atrophy

hands
- leuconychia
- palmar erythema
- clubbing
- Dupuytren's contracture
- asterixis

peripheral oedema

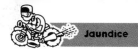
Hepatic encephalopathy can arise as a result of fulminating acute liver failure or when chronic disease decompensates. Precipitating factors include acute upper gastrointestinal bleeding, infection (particularly ascitic), high-dietary protein, drugs (e.g. diuretics, sedatives), fluid and electrolyte disturbance.

Are there any signs of chronic liver disease?

There are few clinical signs specific to acute liver disease. However, the following signs may commonly be found when liver pathology is longstanding:

- Palmar erythema.
- Leuconychia: hypoalbuminaemia.
- Clubbing.
- Dupuytren's contractures: particularly in alcoholic cirrhosis.
- Spider naevi: greater than five in the distribution of superior vena cava.
- Scratch marks: cholestasis.
- Loss of body hair.
- Gynaecomastia: elevated oestrogen, spironolactone, testicular atrophy.
- Bruising: disordered coagulation.
- Hepatomegaly: not in well-established cirrhosis.
- Splenomegaly and Caput Medusae: portal hypertension.
- Testicular atrophy: elevated oestrogen.
- Oedema: hypoalbuminaemia.

Are there any signs of specific diseases?

- Xanthelasmata: primary biliary cirrhosis.
- Kayser–Fleischer rings: Wilson's disease.
- Slate-grey pigmentation: haemochromatosis.
- Hard, irregular hepatomegaly: malignant metastases.
- Palpable gallbladder: carcinoma of head of pancreas (Courvoisier's law).
- Splenomegaly: portal hypertension, viral infection.
- Needle marks or tattoos: hepatitis B, C.

INVESTIGATING THE PATIENT WITH JAUNDICE

The investigation of jaundiced patients falls into two stages. Firstly, the type of jaundice must be determined (prehepatic, hepatic, posthepatic), then more detailed tests should be performed to determined the specific aetiology. Fig. 10.3 summarizes this approach.

Establish the type of jaundice

Quantification of urinary urobilinogen and conjugated bilirubin, along with measurement of serum liver enzymes—alanine aminotransferase, aspartate aminotransferase, alkaline phosphatase, and γ-glutamyltransferase and bilirubin will give a reasonable indication as to the type of abnormality present (Fig. 10.4). Abdominal ultrasound scan is then essential to exclude biliary obstruction.

Tests to determine specific aetiology

The following tests should be used as guided by the above initial investigations.

Haemolysis screen

The haemolysis screen is detailed in Chapter 25.

Hepatocellular screen

- Viral serology: hepatitis A, B, and C; EBV, CMV.
- Autoantibody screen: antimitochondrial antibodies, antinuclear antibodies.
- Ferritin: haemochromatosis.
- Serum caeruloplasmin and urinary copper excretion: Wilson's disease.
- α_1-antitrypsin.
- Liver biopsy: definitive diagnostic test for intrinsic liver disease.

Test for constructional apraxia by asking the patient to copy a five-pointed star without lifting the pen off the paper

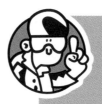

Jaundice is a common short answer question. The examiner will take you to a jaundiced patient and invite you to ask him or her some questions.

Cholestasis screen

- ERCP and percutaneous transhepatic cholangiography: detailed information regarding the biliary tree; also used to perform therapeutic manoeuvres such as stent insertion.

- Computed tomography scan: good images of the pancreas, which is often poorly visualized on an ultrasound scan.

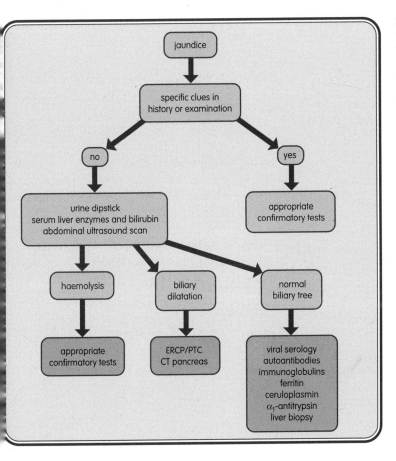

Fig. 10.3 Investigation of the patient with jaundice. (CT, computed tomography; ERCP, endoscopic retrograde cholangiopancreatography; PTC, percutaneous transhepatic cholangiography.)

	Biochemical abnormalities in different types of jaundice			
Specimen	**Test**	**Haemolysis**	**Hepatocellular**	**Cholestasis**
urine	urobilinogen	raised	normal or raised	decreased or absent
	conjugated bilirubin	absent	present	raised
faeces	stercobilinogen	raised	normal	decreased or absent
serum	bilirubin	unconjugated	unconjugated and conjugated	conjugated
	liver enzymes raised	normal	AST, ALT	alkaline phosphatase, GGT

Fig. 10.4 Biochemical abnormalities in different types of jaundice (ALT, alanine aminotransferase; AST, aspartate aminotransferase; GGT, γ-glutamyltransferase.)

11. Abdominal Pain

INTRODUCTION

Abdominal pain is a common cause for consultation (and therefore is often found in examinations). The underlying problem can often be identified by considering which structures normally lie at the site of the pain.

Be aware that there is a long list of possible differential diagnoses for abdominal pain.

DIFFERENTIAL DIAGNOSIS OF ABDOMINAL PAIN

Depending on the specific area affected, abdominal pain may result from the following causes:

Epigastric pain
- Lower oesophagus: oesophagitis, malignancy.
- Stomach: peptic ulcer, gastritis.
- Pancreas: pancreatitis, malignancy.

Right hypochondrial pain
- Biliary tree: biliary colic, cholecystitis, cholangitis.
- Liver: hepatitis, malignancy, abscess, right ventricular failure.
- Subphrenic space: abscess.

Left hypochondrial pain
- Spleen: traumatic rupture, infarction (sickle cell disease).
- Pancreas: pancreatitis, malignancy. Subphrenic space: abscess.

Central abdominal pain
- Pancreas: pancreatitis, malignancy.
- Small/large bowel: obstruction, perforation, intussusception, ischaemia, Crohn's disease, lymphoma, irritable bowel syndrome, adhesions.

- Lymph nodes: mesenteric adenitis, lymphoma.
- Abdominal aorta: ruptured aortic aneurysm.

Right iliac fossa pain
- Terminal ileum: Crohn's disease, infection (tuberculosis), Meckel's diverticulum.
- Appendix: appendicitis, carcinoid syndrome, tumour.
- Caecum/ascending colon: diverticulitis, paracolic abscess, ulcerative colitis, malignancy.
- Ovary/fallopian tubes: malignancy, ectopic pregnancy, pelvic inflammatory disease.

Left iliac fossa pain
- Sigmoid/descending colon: diverticulitis, paracolic abscess, ulcerative colitis, malignancy.
- Ovary/fallopian tubes: malignancy, ectopic pregnancy, cyst (bleeding or torsion), pelvic inflammatory disease.

Loin pain
- Kidneys:malignancy, pyelonephritis, polycystic disease.
- Ureters: colic due to stone or clot.

Suprapubic pain
- Bladder: urinary tract infection, acute urinary retention.
- Uterus/adnexae: pelvic inflammatory disease, endometriosis.

Other causes of abdominal pain
Occasionally, other medical problems can present with abdominal pain. These should be considered when some of the more common diagnoses listed above have been ruled out:
- Anxiety.
- Myocardial infarction: usually inferior myocardial infarction causing epigastric pain.
- Lower lobe pneumonia: ipsilateral hypochondrial or sometimes loin discomfort.
- Porphyria.
- Diabetic ketoacidosis.
- Addison's disease.
- Sickle cell crisis.
- Lead poisoning.
- Henoch–Schönlein purpura.

HISTORY IN THE PATIENT WITH ABDOMINAL PAIN

When a patient presents with abdominal pain, the first priority is to determine whether he or she has an 'acute abdomen' requiring urgent admission to hospital. The history should focus on the pain itself and then associated symptoms.

The pain itself

The onset, course, nature, and site of the pain must be accurately assessed.

Sudden onset of sustained severe pain is often due to perforation or rupture of a viscus, such as the bowel, spleen, or abdominal aorta.

Colicky pain is a griping pain that comes and goes. It is due to muscular spasm in a viscus wall, such as the bowel, ureters, and gallbladder. The muscles contract in an attempt to overcome obstruction caused by a stone, tumour, foreign body, strictures, strangulated hernias, or intussusception.

Gradual onset with sustained pain can be seen in inflammatory conditions, such as ulcerative colitis or Crohn's disease, infection including abscess formation, or gastroenteritis and malignancy.

The site and radiation of pain may help to determine the organ involved (as above)—pancreatic and aortic pain may radiate to the back, ureteric pain often radiates from 'loin to groin', and diaphragmatic irritation caused by subphrenic pathology such as an abscess causes referred shoulder tip pain.

Associated symptoms

The history should now assess other symptoms that may suggest the cause of pain or the consequence of the disease.

Vomiting is common. Haematemesis is seen in upper gastrointestinal bleeding from ulcers or varices, projectile vomiting is seen in pyloric stenosis, and faeculent vomiting results from severe large bowel obstruction.

Rigors suggest sepsis, e.g. abscess, cholangitis, or urinary tract infection. Rigors are particularly common with Gram-negative septicaemia.

Change in bowel habit may be an important symptom. Absolute constipation (no faeces or wind passed rectally) indicates complete bowel obstruction, whereas gastroenteritis or diverticulitis often cause diarrhoea. Constipation alternating with diarrhoea is a feature of colonic malignancy but is also seen in irritable bowel syndrome.

Rectal bleeding may indicate malignancy, inflammatory bowel disease, diverticulitis, dysentery, and angiodysplasia. Dark-red bleeding is a feature of bowel infarction.

Dysuria, haematuria, and urinary frequency indicate urinary infection. Renal stones are occasionally passed per urethra.

Vaginal discharge will often be present in pelvic inflammatory disease.

Do not forget constipation as a cause of abdominal pain in the elderly

EXAMINING THE PATIENT WITH ABDOMINAL PAIN

The first question that must be asked is 'Is the patient acutely ill?' Signs of shock and peritonism should be looked for. The examination should then focus on specific signs. Fig. 11.1 summarizes the examination approach.

Is the patient acutely ill?

Pulse and blood pressure

Tachycardia and hypotension indicate shock. Consider septicaemia (particularly Gram-negative), severe bleeding (ruptured abdominal aortic aneurysm, spleen), fluid loss (vomiting, diarrhoea, pancreatitis) and, rarely, acute addisonian crisis.

Peritonism

The patient often lies still as movement exacerbates the pain. Look for rebound tenderness and guarding (involuntary spasm of the abdominal wall on palpation). When the peritonism becomes generalized the abdomen will be rigid and bowel signs will be absent due to paralysis of peristalsis. Causes of peritonism are summarised in Fig. 11.2.

What is the underlying cause?

- Pyrexia: high temperatures indicates infection; low-grade pyrexia can be found in malignancy, bowel infarction, inflammatory bowel disease and pancreatitis.
- Jaundice: hepatitis or pancreatitis (causing periampullary oedema).
- Dehydration: rapid fluid loss.
- Cachexia: suggests a chronic pathology, particularly malignancy.
- Clubbing: inflammatory bowel disease or small bowel lymphoma.
- Lymphadenopathy: lymphoma; or may be due to metastases.
- Cullen's sign (periumbilical or central bruising) and Grey Turner's sign (bruising in the flanks): severe haemorrhagic pancreatitis, rarely leaking abdominal aortic aneurysm.

- Recent surgical scar: may indicate a source of peritoneal sepsis, such as an anastomotic leak.
- Abdominal distension: if marked, indicates bowel obstruction and is accompanied by a resonant percussion note. Occasionally, visible peristalsis may be present.
- Tenderness: it is important to consider what structures lie at the site of tenderness. As discussed, rebound tenderness indicates peritonism.
- Mass: this can be malignant or inflammatory as in Crohn's disease.
- Ascites: malignancy, peritoneal sepsis, pancreatitis.
- Bowel sounds: high-pitched (tinkling) suggests obstruction; absence indicates an ileus (paralysis of bowel) from whatever cause.
- Hernial orifices (inguinal and femoral): these must be examined, particularly if obstruction is suspected.
- Pelvic and rectal examination: pelvic inflammation, cervical excitation, ectopic pregnancy, rectal mass or bleeding, stool consistency.
- Urine dipstick: should be used to determine the presence of white blood cells (infection), RBCs (stone, tumour or infection), glucose, and ketones.

INVESTIGATING THE PATIENT WITH ABDOMINAL PAIN

All patients admitted to hospital with abdominal pain should have a full blood count (FBC) and serum

blood pressure
- shock

abdomen
- surgical scar
- distension
- Grey Turner's and Cullen's signs
- tenderness
- guarding
- mass
- ascites
- bowel sounds

pulse
- tachycardia

hands
- clubbing
- anaemia

urogenital
- hernial orifices
- rectal examination
- vaginal examination
- pregnancy test
- urine dipstick

general
- unwell
- pyrexia
- dehydration
- jaundice
- cachexia
- lymphadenopathy

Fig. 11.1 Examining the patient with abdominal pain.

Causes of peritonism	
Cause	**Examples**
infection	spread from paracolic/subphrenic abscess following surgery or paracentesis bowel perforation
chemical irritation	bile faeces gastric acid pancreatic enzymes
transmural inflammation	Crohn's disease salpingitis

Fig. 11.2 Causes of peritonism.

biochemistry performed. The use of radiology and other tests will depend on a focused differential diagnosis. The diagnostic pathway is outlined in Fig. 11.3:

- Full blood count: leucocytosis is seen in infection and occasionally inflammation and malignancy. Anaemia may be due to acute blood loss or chronic pathology such as malignancy.
- Serum amylase: very high in acute pancreatitis, but may also be raised in perforated peptic ulcer, diabetic ketoacidosis, cholecystitis, abdominal trauma, and myocardial infarction.
- Urea and electrolyte: dehydration, renal failure as a consequence of obstructive uropathy or shock.
- Serum calcium: hypercalcaemia may cause renal stones and pancreatitis; hypocalcaemia may be a consequence of pancreatitis.
- Blood glucose: hypoglycaemia will result from liver failure or Addison's disease; hyperglycaemia will be present in ketoacidosis and may complicate acute pancreatitis.

- Liver function tests: abnormal in acute hepatitis, biliary disease, and shock.
- Microscopy, culture, and sensitivity of mid-stream urine: to exclude infection.
- Abdominal X-ray: erect and supine films should be performed if the following are suspected: perforation—air beneath the diaphragm representing free gas; obstruction—dilated loops of bowel with fluid level; pancreatitis—sentinel loop due to ileus in overlying loop of small bowel; infarction—'thumb printing' representing mucosal oedema; renal stone—90% of such stones are radiopaque.
- Abdominal ultrasound scan: dilatation of biliary tree and ureters; intra-abdominal mass; ascites; abscess

Where there is difficulty in making the diagnosis, a computed tomography scan, laparoscopy/laparotomy, or diagnostic tests for the unusual causes of abdominal pain should be considered.

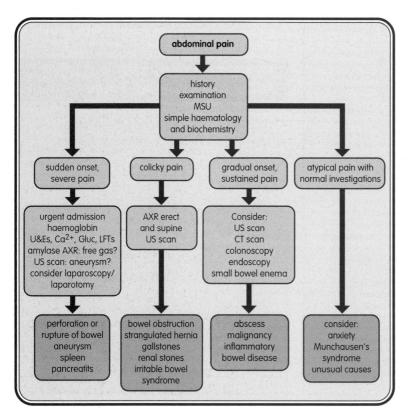

Fig. 11.3 Diagnosis in the patient with abdominal pain. (AXR, abdominal X-ray; CT, computed tomography; Gluc, glucose; LFTs, liver function tests; MSU, midstream urine; U&Es, urea and electrolytes; US, ultrasound.)

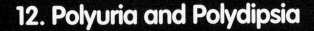

12. Polyuria and Polydipsia

INTRODUCTION

Polyuria is the passing of excessive volumes of urine. Urine output depends on fluid intake and body losses, and typically ranges from 1–3.5 L/day. Polydipsia, the ingestion of excessive volumes of fluid, is usually a consequence of polyuria.

Water is normally reabsorbed from the loop of Henle as it passes through the hyperosmolar renal medulla. Fluid in the collecting ducts enters the hyperosmolar renal medulla, with water reabsorption being controlled by antidiuretic hormone (ADH) (Fig.

12.1). The secretion of this is controlled by the hypothalamus in response to osmolality changes in the blood. A rise in osmolality leads to an increase in ADH secretion, and a fall results in a decrease in ADH secretion.

DIFFERENTIAL DIAGNOSIS OF POLYURIA

The differential diagnosis of polyuria includes the following.

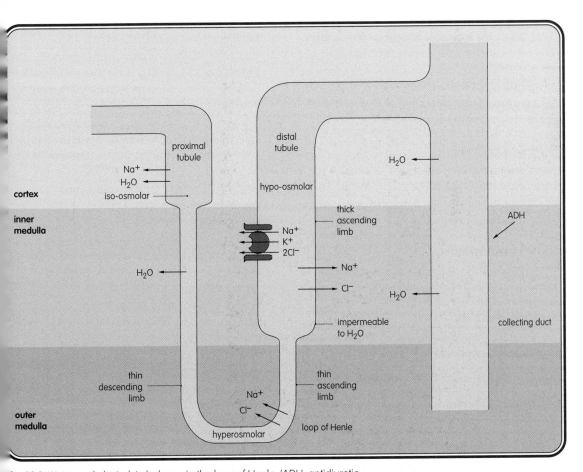

Fig. 12.1 Water and electrolyte balance in the loop of Henle. (ADH, antidiuretic hormone.)

Insufficient secretion of ADH

This type of diabetes insipidus (DI) may be secondary to lesions of the hypothalamic/pituitary axis and includes the following:

- Idiopathic: often familial and the commonest form.
- Surgery or irradiation to the pituitary gland.
- Trauma: especially head injury.
- Malignancy, e. g. craniopharyngioma, pinealoma, glioma, and secondary deposits.
- Infections, e.g. meningitis and pneumonia.
- Infiltrations, e.g. sarcoid and histiocytosis X.

Inhibition of ADH release

This leads to increased thirst and thus polydipsia. Examples include psychogenic DI and lesions affecting the thirst centre.

Inability of the kidney to respond to ADH

This is nephrogenic DI and may be congenital or acquired. The familial form is due to a primary renal tubular defect. The secondary defect may be due to an inability to maintain renal medullary hyperosmolality and includes electrolyte imbalances such as hypercalcaemia and hypokalaemia, lithium toxicity, and secondary to long standing pyelonephritis or hypdronephrosis, and renal papillary necrosis (analgesic nephropathy).

Chronic renal failure

Chronic renal failure may occur as a result of the depressed ability of the kidneys to concentrate urine. The volume of urine may therefore increase to excrete the same osmotic load.

Acute renal failure

Polyuria occurs in the diuretic phase of acute renal failure and in postobstructive uropathy.

Osmotic diuresis

Incomplete reabsorption in the tubules of substances in the glomerular filtrate leads to osmotic diuresis, i.e. increased solute per nephron. This occurs with glucose in diabetes mellitus (DM), hypercalcaemia in chronic renal failure, and in intravenous infusion with hypertonic solutions.

HISTORY IN THE PATIENT WITH POLYURIA OR POLYDIPSIA

After asking general questions, focus on suspected causes. The following should be ascertained:

- Differentiate between polyuria (an increase in urine production) and frequency (the frequent passage of small amounts of urine).
- Weight loss: think of diabetes; malignancies (especially of the brain—does the patient have headaches?); myeloma leading to renal failure; ectopic production of adrenocorticotrophic hormone (ACTH); and bony metastases.
- General features of infection: a history of recurrent infection should suggest diabetes.
- Psychiatric symptoms: especially if thirst appears to dominate the picture, patients may resent investigations, especially a water deprivation test, and may drink surreptitiously. There may be an inconsistency or variation in the severity of the symptoms, and an absence of nocturnal symptoms. There may also be other neurotic symptoms.
- Symptoms of renal failure: such as haematuria, nausea and vomiting; likely precipitating factors.
- If renal failure is suspected, consider associated systemic conditions, such as collagenoses (e.g. systemic lupus erythematosus and polyarteritis nodosa), gout, subacute bacterial endocarditis, amyloid, Wegener's granulomatosis, and Goodpasture's syndrome.
- Hypercalcaemia: produces symptoms of nausea, vomiting, constipation, abdominal pain, and, if severe, confusion and coma (Chapter 35).
- Hypokalaemia: leads to muscle weakness and paralysis (Chapter 33).
- Drug history: analgesic abuse may cause renal papillary necrosis; lithium may cause nephrogenic DI; vitamin D or milk-alkali syndrome may lead to hypercalcaemia; steroids and nephrotoxic drugs.
- History of head injury or childhood meningitis?
- History of hypertension? If so, suspect hypertensive renal disease.
- Family history; e.g. in DI, DM, and nephrogenic DI.

EXAMINING THE PATIENT WITH POLYURIA OR POLYDIPSIA

The examination approach in the patient with polyuria or polydipsia is summarized in Fig. 12.2. The general appearance of the patient should be noted, thus:

- Yellow-brown skin: renal failure.
- Skin manifestations: DM, e.g. necrobiosis lipidica diabeticorum, granuloma annulare, infections.

- Wasting: malignancy or diabetes.
- Anaemia: malignancy or chronic renal failure.
- Clubbing: bronchogenic carcinoma leading to excess ACTH or parathyroid hormone (PTH) production.
- Brown arcs on nails: chronic renal failure.
- Optic signs: band keratopathy or subconjunctival calcification in hypercalcaemia; visual defects in tumours of the hypothalamus or pituitary; fundal changes of hypertension or diabetes.

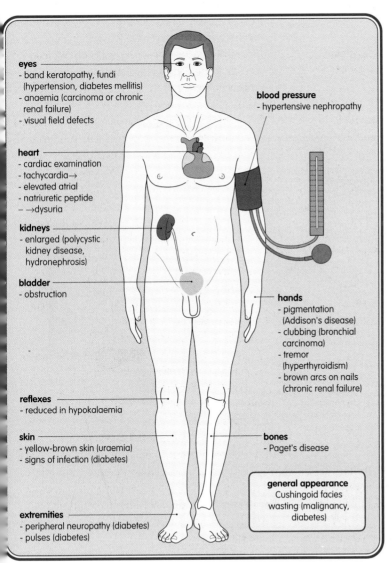

Fig. 12.2 Examining the patient with polyuria or polydipsia.

eyes
- band keratopathy, fundi (hypertension, diabetes mellitis)
- anaemia (carcinoma or chronic renal failure)
- visual field defects

blood pressure
- hypertensive nephropathy

heart
- cardiac examination
- tachycardia→
- elevated atrial
- natriuretic peptide
- →dysuria

kidneys
- enlarged (polycystic kidney disease, hydronephrosis)

bladder
- obstruction

hands
- pigmentation (Addison's disease)
- clubbing (bronchial carcinoma)
- tremor (hyperthyroidism)
- brown arcs on nails (chronic renal failure)

reflexes
- reduced in hypokalaemia

skin
- yellow-brown skin (uraemia)
- signs of infection (diabetes)

bones
- Paget's disease

general appearance
Cushingoid facies
wasting (malignancy, diabetes)

extremities
- peripheral neuropathy (diabetes)
- pulses (diabetes)

Cardiovascular system

Check for tachycardias (producing atrial natriuretic peptide) and peripheral vascular disease in DM. Also, check the blood pressure for hypertensive nephropathy.

Abdominal examination

Palpate the kidneys as they may be palpable in polycystic kidney disease or hydronephrosis. A large bladder may indicate urinary tract obstruction.

Neurological examination

The neurological examination should assess the following:
- Diabetic peripheral neuropathy.
- Hypotonia and areflexia with hypokalaemia.
- Wasting in malignancy.
- Paraneoplastic syndromes.

INVESTIGATING THE PATIENT WITH POLYURIA AND POLYDIPSIA

An algorithm for the investigation of the patient with polyuria and polydipsia is given in Fig. 12.3. The following investigations should be carried out:
- Urinalysis: specific gravity with or without osmolality.
- Urea and electrolytes: renal failure and hypokalaemia. If renal impairment is found, further investigations may include creatinine clearance, tests for systemic diseases associated with renal failure, and an ultrasound scan of the kidneys. (If hypokalaemia is found, go through the differential diagnosis—see Fig. 33.7—to look for causes. Remember simple things like drugs—is the patient on diuretics?)

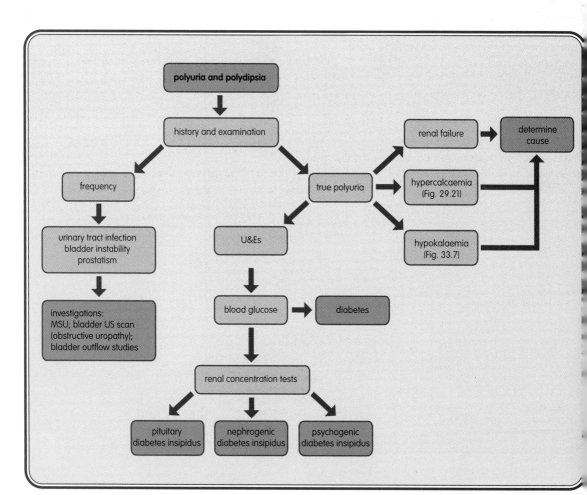

Fig. 12.3 Algorithm for the investigation of the patient with polyuria and polydipsia. (MSU, mid-stream urine; U&Es, urea and electrolytes; US, ultrasound.)

- Blood glucose: DM.
- Full blood count: anaemia with chronic renal failure, or malignancy (e.g.leukaemia), and reticuloses.
- Serum calcium corrected for plasma proteins: if raised, further tests to elucidate the cause will be required, such as PTH assay, tests of pituitary function, bone scan, myeloma screen, alkaline phosphatase, and bone X-rays for Paget's disease, thyroid function tests, Kveim test and serum angiotensin-converting enzyme for sarcoidosis, and synacthen test to exclude adrenal insufficiency.
- Chest X-ray (CXR): bilateral hilar lymphadenopathy with sarcoidosis, and bronchial neoplasm with ectopic PTH secretion. If there are any abnormalities

on the CXR it may be necessary to proceed to bronchoscopy with or without biopsy.
- Skull X-ray: brain tumour, e.g. craniopharyngioma or secondary deposits.

If either a hypothalamic or pituitary cause or renal tubular dysfunction is suspected, it may be appropriate to proceed with renal concentration tests. It is mandatory to exclude other potential causes for polyuria, as renal concentration tests may be dangerous.

The patient is told to drink nothing from 4 pm the day before attending the outpatient department. If the urine osmolality the next morning is not above 800 mmol/kg inpatient tests are required (Figs 12.4 and 12.5).

Procedure for testing outpatients with polyuria and polydipsia

- weigh the patient
- deprive of all fluids the night before the tests
- the next morning, weigh the patient every 2 hours (a decrease in weight by >3% indicates dehydration, so stop the test)
- collect urine and blood for osmolality
- if the urine osmolality fails to reach 800 mmol/kg give intramuscular DDAVP (DDAVP is synthetic vasopressin which acts in the same way as ADH)
- collect blood and urine for osmolality

Fig. 12.4 Procedure for testing outpatients with polyuria and polydipsia. (ADH, antidiuretic hormone; DDAVP, desmopressin.)

Interpretation of outpatient test results

	Fluid deprivation		i.m. DDAVP	
	plasma osmolality	urine osmolality	plasma osmolality	urine osmolality
pituitary DI	↑	→	↑	↑
psychogenic DI*	↑	↑	↑	↑
nephrogenic DI	→	→	→	→

Fig. 12.5 Interpretation of outpatient test results. (DI, diabetes insipidus; *may be some acquired resistance to ADH; ↑ increase in osmolality; → no significant change in osmolality.)

13. Haematuria and Proteinuria

INTRODUCTION

Haematuria and proteinuria are common presentations of renal disease, although both may also be due to systemic conditions. Haematuria is abnormal if there are more than 2 red blood cells per high-power field; proteinuria is defined as more than 150 mg of protein per 24-hour collection of urine. Red-coloured urine may also be due to haemoglobinuria (haemolysis), porphyria, drugs e.g. rifampicin, or even the ingestion of beetroot.

DIFFERENTIAL DIAGNOSIS OF HAEMATURIA AND PROTEINURIA

Haematuria

This is best classfied by the site of pathology.

Systemic conditions
- Clotting disorders and anticoagulants.
- Thrombocytopenia.
- Sickle cell disease.
- Endocarditis.
- Vasculitides.

Kidneys
- Glomerulonephritis and its associated conditions, e.g. Hodgkin's disease, subacute bacterial endocarditis, systematic lupus erythematosus, polyarteritis nodosa, Wegener's granulomatosis, Goodpasture's syndrome.
- Infections, e.g. pyelonephritis, tuberculosis.
- Tumours: carcinoma, nephroblastoma, angioma, adenoma, papilloma.
- Cystic disease: polycystic kidney disease, medullary sponge kidney.
- Sudden release of retained urine, e.g. postcatheterization for urinary retention.
- Drugs, e.g. sulphonamides.
- Hydronephrosis.
- Papillary necrosis.
- Hydatid disease.

When thinking of causes of haematuria, think of the site of pathology along the renal tract. At each site, tumours, calculi, and infection are possible.

Ureters
- Calculi.
- Tumours: carcinoma, papilloma).
- Trauma.

Bladder
- Cystitis: infection, chemical-induced cystitis, postradiation cystitis.
- Tumours: carcinoma, papilloma, haemangioma, sarcoma.
- Trauma.
- Calculi.
- Infections: tuberculosis.
- Schistosomiasis.

Prostate
- Prostatic carcinoma.
- Tuberculosis.

Urethra
- Calculi.
- Trauma.
- Tumours: angioma.
- Foreign bodies, e.g. urinary catheters.

Other sites
Haematuria may result from lesions in adjacent organs (by fistula formation or inflammation) such as:
- Colonic diverticulitis.
- Inflammatory bowel disease.
- Acute appendicitis in a pelvic appendix.
- Acute salpingitis.
- Pelvic inflammatory disease.
- Carcinoma of the colon or genital tract.

Proteinuria

Benign proteinuria may result from the following:

- Functional proteinuria: pyrexia, strenuous exercise, congestive cardiac failure, acute medical illnesses, pregnancy.
- Idiopathic transient proteinuria: intermittent.
- Orthostatic proteinuria: common in the under-30s; significant proteinuria when upright but normal when supine.

Other differential diagnoses include:

- Urinary tract infections.
- Vaginal mucus.
- Diabetes mellitus.
- Glomerulonephritis.
- Causes of nephrotic syndrome (Fig. 13.1).
- Myeloma: Bence Jones protein in urine (light chain dimers).
- Obstructive nephropathy.
- Analgesic abuse.

In addition to the above, tubular proteinuria, due to tubular or interstitial damage, may occur. Proteinuria results from failure of the tubules to reabsorb some of the plasma proteins that have been filtered by the normal glomerulus. The loss of protein is usually mild and may result from the following:

- Congenital disorders: Fanconi's syndrome (a proximal tubular defect), cystinosis, renal tubular acidosis.
- Heavy metal poisoning: lead, cadmium, Wilson's disease.
- Recovery phase of acute tubular necrosis.
- Chronic nephritis and pyelonephritis.
- Renal transplantation.

Finally, overflow proteinuria may occur. This is when abnormal amounts of low molecular mass proteins (filtered at the glomerulus) are neither reabsorbed nor catabolized completely by the renal tubular cells, e.g. as in acute pancreatitis (amylase). The following may be responsible:

- Multiple myeloma: Bence Jones protein.
- Haemolytic anaemia and march haemoglobinuria: haemoglobin.
- Myelomonocytic leukaemia: lysozyme.
- Myoglobinuria and crush injuries: myoglobin.

HISTORY IN THE PATIENT WITH HAEMATURIA AND PROTEINURIA

Bear the differential diagnosis in mind.

If haematuria is present in a woman, ensure that she is not menstruating.

The following factors should be determined when obtaining a history in the patient with haematuria or proteinuria:

- Ask about associated urinary symptoms, such as, frequency (urinary tract infection, bladder calculus, prostatism), hesitancy, strangury (the desire to pass something that will not pass, e.g. a calculus) and dysuria (painful micturition reflecting urethral or bladder inflammation).
- Is the haematuria worse with exercise? This suggests tumour or calculus.
- Ask about loin pain. This suggests pyelonephritis or renal calculi.
- Ask about colicky pain. This suggests a ureteric calculus.
- Has there been a history of fever, e.g. with pyelonephritis?
- Are there generalized features of carcinoma, e.g. anorexia and weight loss?
- Ask about symptoms arising from lesions in adjacent organs.
- Ask about drugs, e.g. analgesics (nephropathy) or sulphonamides.
- Is there a history of trauma?
- Is there a past history of radiotherapy?
- Does the urine contain crystals or stones?
- Are there any signs of systemic or chronic illness, e.g. recurrent infections and polyuria with diabetes mellitus?
- Has there been recent foreign travel, e.g. schistosomiasis or tuberculosis?
- Is there a family history? Are there clotting disorders—does the patient bruise easily? Is there a history of renal problems, e.g. polycystic kidney disease, sickle cell disease?

The following factors should be assessed, particularly if proteinuria is suspected:

- Ask about the appearance of the urine. Heavy proteinuria turns the urine dark and frothy. However, the urine may appear normal, and proteinuria may only be picked up on formal testing.
- Are there symptoms of urinary tract infection, e.g. frequency, dysuria, urgency, or incontinence?
- Does the patient have a vaginal or penile discharge?
- Are there signs of systemic disease, e.g. diabetes mellitus?
- Does the patient have a temperature or other signs of acute illness?
- Are there symptoms of congestive cardiac failure, e.g. shortness of breath, orthopnoea, ankle swelling?
- Ask about heavy metal exposure and other drugs, e.g. analgesic abuse.
- Is the proteinuria only present after vigorous exercise?
- Is the proteinuria absent in early morning specimens (orthostatic proteinuria)?
- Ensure the patient is not pregnant.
- Do not forget to keep the causes of nephrotic syndrome in mind (Fig. 13.1).

EXAMINING THE PATIENT WITH HAEMATURIA AND PROTEINURIA

The examination approach is summarized in Fig. 13.2.

INVESTIGATING THE PATIENT WITH HAEMATURIA AND PROTEINURIA

An algorithm for the investigation of the patient with haematuria and proteinuria is given in Fig. 13.3. Ultimately, it may be necessary to proceed to a renal biopsy, but initially urine, blood and radiological tests should be performed.

Urine
The following urinary tests should be performed:
- Albumin.
- Glucose.
- Urobilinogen: jaundice.

Ask about the appearance of the urine:
- **If the urine is blood stained at the start of micturition and clear later on, the site of pathology is likely to be the urethra or prostate.**
- **If the urine is more blood stained towards the end of micturition, the site of pathology is likely to be the bladder.**
- **If the urine is evenly blood stained throughout micturition, the site of pathology is likely to be the kidney or ureter.**

Causes of nephrotic syndrome	
Cause	**Examples**
renal disease	glomerulonephritis, renal artery stenosis, renal vein thrombosis, transplant rejection
systemic disease	amyloidosis, SLE, polyarteritis nodosa, Henoch–Schönlein purpura
metabolic disease	diabetes mellitus, hypothyroidism
neoplastic disease	lymphoma, plasma cell myeloma, carcinoma, e.g. lung, GI tract
infections	malaria, schistosomiasis, hepatitis B, infective endocarditis, cytomegalovirus, infectious mononucleosis
drugs	heavy metals, gold and mercury compounds, captopril, penicillamine, probenecid
familial disorders	congenital nephrotic syndrome, Alport's syndrome, sickle cell anaemia
allergy	bee stings, poison oak, pollen, vaccines

Fig. 13.1 Causes of nephrotic syndrome. (GI, gastrointestinal; SLE, systemic lupus erythematosus.)

- Porphyrins: porphyria.
- Microscopy: red blood cells, white blood cells, casts, crystals, protein.
- Culture: infection.
- Early morning urine: acid-fast bacilli, if tuberculosis is suspected.
- Cytology: malignancy.

Urine may be tested for protein at different times in the day. Protein is normally absent in orthostatic proteinuria first thing in the morning before getting up. (The patient is asked to void the bladder before sleep.) It may also be tested after exercise.

24-Hour collection of urine for protein

24-Hour collection of urine for protein is useful for distinguishing mild to moderate proteinuria, in which the loss is not sufficient to cause protein depletion, from severe proteinuria, in which the loss is usually 5–10 g.

Differential protein clearance

Differential protein clearance (selectivity) is occaisingly performed in patients with nephrotic syndrome. Patients with selective proteinuria (small molecular mass proteins are cleared more rapidly than large proteins) are more likely to respond to steroid therapy.

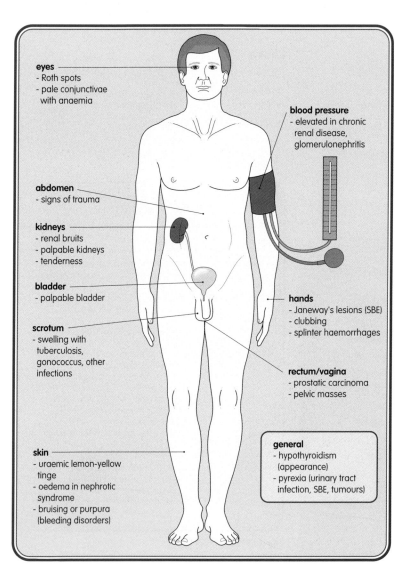

Fig. 13.2 Examining the patient with haematuria and proteinuria. (SBE, subacute bacterial endocarditis.)

eyes
- Roth spots
- pale conjunctivae with anaemia

blood pressure
- elevated in chronic renal disease, glomerulonephritis

abdomen
- signs of trauma

kidneys
- renal bruits
- palpable kidneys
- tenderness

bladder
- palpable bladder

hands
- Janeway's lesions (SBE)
- clubbing
- splinter haemorrhages

scrotum
- swelling with tuberculosis, gonococcus, other infections

rectum/vagina
- prostatic carcinoma
- pelvic masses

skin
- uraemic lemon-yellow tinge
- oedema in nephrotic syndrome
- bruising or purpura (bleeding disorders)

general
- hypothyroidism (appearance)
- pyrexia (urinary tract infection, SBE, tumours)

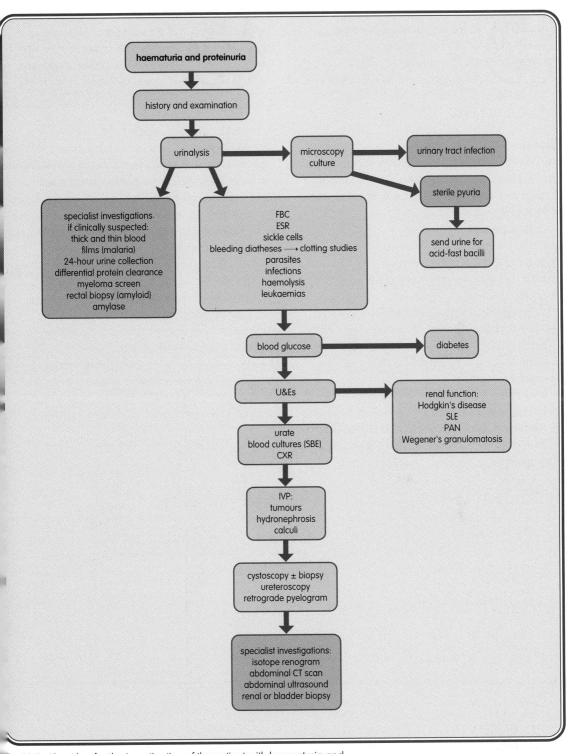

Fig. 13.3 Algorithm for the investigation of the patient with haematuria and proteinuria. (CT, computed tomography; CXR, chest X-ray; FBC, full blood count; ESR, erythrocyte sedimentation rate; IVP, intravenous pyelogram; PAN, polyarteritis nodosa; SBE, subacute bacterial endocarditis; SLE, systemic lupus erythematosus.)

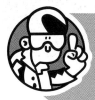

Causes of a sterile pyuria:
- Tuberculosis.
- Tumours.
- Analgesic nephropathy.

Remember, urea and electrolytes may be normal despite significant renal disease.

Blood

The following blood tests should be performed:

- Full blood count: platelet deficiency in bleeding disorders, sickle cells, parasites, leucocytosis with infections.
- Erythrocyte sedimentation rate.
- Clotting studies: bleeding diathesis.
- Blood glucose: diabetes mellitus.
- Urea and electrolytes: renal function.
- Urate: gout.
- Blood cultures: infective endocarditis.
- Specialized investigations according to clinical suspicion: thick and thin films for malaria; serum complement and autoantibodies for glomerulonephritis.
- Myeloma screen: immunoelectrophoresis; urine for Bence Jones protein.
- Hepatitis B, cytomegalovirus, and Epstein–Barr virus serology: potential causes of nephrotic syndrome.

Radiology

The following radiological tests should be performed:

- Chest X-ray: primary and secondary tumours, tuberculosis, polyarteritis.
- Abdominal X-ray: renal outline and stones. Ninety per cent of renal calculi are opaque; urate, cysteine, and xanthine stones may be radiolucent.
- Intravenous pyelogram: excretory function, stones, shape of the calyces, ureters and bladder.
- Cystoscopy: bladder lesions.
- Ureteroscopy: ureter lesions.
- Retrograde pyelogram: stones or obstructive lesions in the ureters are suspected.
- Abdominal CT scan: to visualize the kidneys, adjacent organs, and other abdominal masses.

14. Hypertension

INTRODUCTION

The level of blood pressure above which someone is 'hypertensive' is controversial and varies between different countries. However, most clinicians would consider treatment when blood pressure is persistently elevated above 160/90 mmHg. This is an arbitrary cut-off point and is influenced by age, end-organ damage, and other risk factors. Approximately 95% of all hypertensive patients have 'essential' or 'primary' hypertension and have no underlying disease. Secondary hypertension can be the result of a range of different pathological processes.

DIFFERENTIAL DIAGNOSIS OF HYPERTENSION

Essential hypertension

Essential hypertension comprises 95% of cases. There is no underlying cause.

Secondary hypertension

Secondary hypertension comprises 5% of cases. Factors leading to secondary hypertension are:

Lifestyle, e.g. obesity, high alcohol intake, lack of exercise, high salt intake.

Renal parenchymal disease, e.g. chronic pyelonephritis, glomerulonephritis, polycystic disease, tumour, tuberculosis.

Renal artery disease, e.g. atherosclerosis, fibromuscular dysplasia, vasculitis.

Obstructive uropathy, e.g. hydronephrosis due to a stone or tumour.

Congenital, e.g. coarctation of the aorta.

Drugs, e.g. combined oral contraceptive pill, non-steroidal anti-inflamatory drugs (NSAIDs).

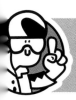

95% of patients with hypertension have no underlying disease.

- Endocrine, e.g. phaeochromocytoma, hyperaldosteronism, Cushing's syndrome.
- Raised intracranial pressure.

HISTORY IN THE PATIENT WITH HYPERTENSION

Hypertension is usually asymptomatic and is often found incidentally. The history should be approached in three parts.

Firstly, how long has the patient had hypertension and what treatments have been given so far? Secondly, how severe is the hypertension and has it resulted in complications? Finally, are there any risk factors suggesting that an underlying pathology may be present?

Presentation and history of hypertension

Important questions to address are as follows:

- How was the hypertension discovered? For example, at a routine pre-operative assessment or with malignant (accelerated) hypertension.
- For how long has the blood pressure been monitored? Unless severe, the diagnosis should not be made until blood pressure is persistently elevated for at least 6 months.
- What treatments, if any, has the patient been given so far? If blood pressure control is poor despite taking correct doses of three antihypertensive agents, the patient is said to have 'resistant hypertension'.

How severe is the hypertension and are there complications?

Mild hypertension is asymptomatic. However, when hypertension is severe or chronic and associated with complications, the following symptoms may occur:

- Headaches.
- Dyspnoea.
- Symptoms of frank cardiac failure (see p.9).
- Angina pectoris or myocardial infarction.
- Transient ischaemic attacks or stroke.
- Visual disturbance.

Is the history suggestive of an underlying cause?

Ask about the following:

- Lifestyle history, paying particular attention to alcohol and smoking (atherosclerosis).
- Precise drug history.
- Previous medical history, e.g. recurrent pyelonephritis, nephrectomy.
- Family history may suggest underlying polycystic disease.
- Symptoms of phaeochromocytoma are rare but include episodic pallor, headache, tremor, palpitations, and nausea.

EXAMINING THE PATIENT WITH HYPERTENSION

Patients with uncomplicated mild essential hypertension will have no associated clinical signs. However, when a patient is found to be hypertensive, one should search for evidence of complications or an underlying cause (Fig. 14.1).

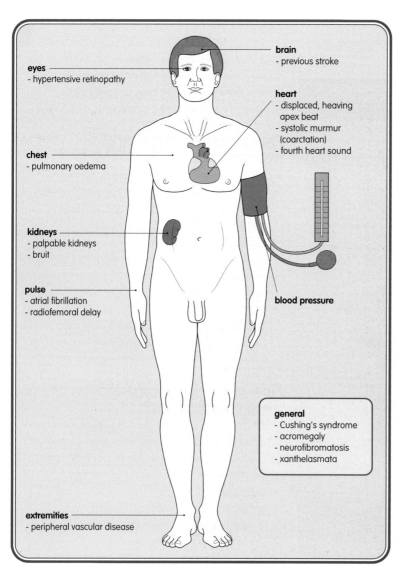

Fig. 14.1 Examining the patient with hypertension.

eyes
- hypertensive retinopathy

chest
- pulmonary oedema

kidneys
- palpable kidneys
- bruit

pulse
- atrial fibrillation
- radiofemoral delay

extremities
- peripheral vascular disease

brain
- previous stroke

heart
- displaced, heaving apex beat
- systolic murmur (coarctation)
- fourth heart sound

blood pressure

general
- Cushing's syndrome
- acromegaly
- neurofibromatosis
- xanthelasmata

Evidence of an underlying cause

- Palpable kidneys: polycystic disease, renal tumour.
- Peripheral vascular disease and xanthelasmata: renal artery stenosis.
- Renal bruit (throughout both systole and diastole): renovascular disease.
- Radiofemoral delay: coarctation of the aorta.
- Neurofibromatosis: renal artery stenosis.
- Cushing's disease.

Evidence of complications

- Atrial fibrillation.
- Displaced, thrusting apex beat indicating left ventricular hypertrophy.
- Frank cardiac failure.

- Retinopathy.
- Previous stroke.

INVESTIGATING THE PATIENT WITH HYPERTENSION

An algorithm for the investigation of the patient with hypertension is given in Fig. 14.2. At presentation all hypertensive patients should have the following tests:

- Urine dipstick: parenchymal disease, urinary tract infection, stone.
- Urea and electrolytes: renal impairment suggests underlying disease.
- Electrocardiogram: significant hypertension may result in left ventricular hypertrophy.

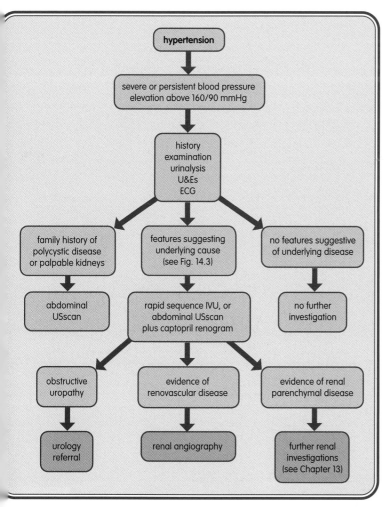

Fig. 14.2 Algorithm for the investigation of the patient with hypertension. (ECG, electrocardiogram; IVU, intravenous urogram; U&Es, urea and electrolytes.)

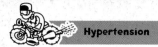
Fig. 14.3 shows those patients who should then be investigated further, using the following tests:

- 24-hour urinary vanilly mandelic acid (VMA) and catecholamine excretion: phaeochromocytoma.
- Radiological investigations: renovascular disease, renoparenchymal disease, obstructive uropathy. This should be either rapid sequence intravenous urogram, or abdominal ultrasound scan plus captopril renogram.
- Renal angiography: renal artery disease; this is a definitive test and should be performed if indicated by the radiological tests or clinical circumstances.

Indications for detailed investigation of hypertension

- recent onset or worsening of hypertension
- malignant (accelerated) hypertension
- uncontrolled hypertension despite three antihypertensive drugs
- abdominal bruit
- proteinuria, haematuria, or abnormal renal function
- hypokalaemia not otherwise explained, e.g. by diuretic therapy
- renal failure caused by angiotensin-converting enzyme (ACE) inhibitors
- young age (<30 years)
- severe generalized atherosclerosis
- unexplained pulmonary oedema

Fig. 14.3 Indications for detailed investigation of hypertension.

All hypertensive patients should have urine dipstick, urea and electrolytes, and an electrocardiogram. Only a few need any further tests.

15. Headache And Facial Pain

INTRODUCTION

Headache is one of the most common presenting symptoms. There are often few clinical signs and the history is the main diagnostic tool. Many different pathological processes can result in headache or facial pain.

DIFFERENTIAL DIAGNOSIS OF HEADACHE AND FACIAL PAIN

Headache

The differential diagnosis of headache includes the following:

- Tension headache.
- Migraine.
- Tumour: primary, secondary.
- Infection: abscess, meningitis, encephalitis, sinusitis, herpes zoster.
- Bleeding: subdural, extradural, intracerebral haematoma, subarachnoid haemorrhage.
- Vasculitic: temporal arteritis.
- Thrombosis: dural sinus thrombosis.
- Skull: fracture, tumour, Paget's disease.
- Drugs: nitrates.
- Others: benign intracranial hypertension, hydrocephalus, post-traumatic, coital cephalgia.

Facial pain

Diseases affecting the teeth, temporomandibular joint, cervical spine, sinuses, eye, ear, nose, and even heart (myocardial ischaemia) can cause pain which radiates to the face. Other causes are disease of the trigeminal nerve such as trigeminal neuralgia and postherpetic neuralgia.

HISTORY IN THE PATIENT WITH HEADACHE OR FACIAL PAIN

The onset, nature, and subsequent pattern of pain will usually provide a good shortlist of likely causes. The presence of additional symptoms and risk factors may add further weight to this list.

Solitary acute episode

This pattern is seen in infection, haemorrhage or thrombosis. (Note that it may also be the first presentation of the other causes of headache.)

Subarachnoid haemorrhage presents with a sudden onset of severe pain, 'as if someone had hit them on the back of the head'. Nausea, vomiting, neck stiffness, and photophobia result from meningeal irritation. Altered conscious level and focal neurological deficits may also occur depending on the site and size of the bleed. Fig. 15.1 lists the causes of subarachnoid haemorrhage.

Patients with *infective meningitis* present with a short history of headache, symptoms of infection (malaise, fever, and rigors) and symptoms of meningeal irritation (vomiting, photophobia, and neck pain and stiffness). However, tuberculous and malignant meningitis have a more subacute presentation which can be easily missed.

Cerebral abscess causes headaches, fits, symptoms of infection, and symptoms of raised intracranial pressure as the lesion expands (see below). The infection may have spread from a primary focus, such as the lung in bronchiectasis, middle ear, or paranasal sinuses.

Causes of subarachnoid haemorrhage

- berry aneurysm (70%)
- arteriovenous malformation (10%)
- no underlying lesion (15–20%)
- bleeding disorders
- mycotic aneurysm (endocarditis)
- tumour
- arteritis
- trauma

Fig. 15.1 Causes of subarachnoid haemorrhage. Note that berry aneurysms may be associated with coarctation of the aorta and polycystic kidney disease.

Fits, focal neurological symptoms, and symptoms of raised intracranial pressure can also result from *dural venous sinus thrombosis*. This is a rare complication of pregnancy, oral contraceptive pill use, dehydration, paranasal sinus infection, and severe intercurrent illness.

Progressive headache

A headache that comes on gradually over days or weeks and increases in severity is often a feature of a tumour, benign intracranial hypertension, or hydrocephalus. In all three the headache results from raised intracranial pressure and the has the characteristic features shown in Fig. 15.2. Temporal arteritis also presents gradually, but the nature of the headache is very different.

Cerebral tumours can be primary or secondary. The patient may have a history of malignancy elsewhere. The most common tumours to metastasize to the brain are those of the thyroid, bronchus, and breast, as well as gastric, renal and prostate tumours. In addition to headache, the patient may also develop fits and focal neurological deficits related to the site of the lesion.

Benign intracranial hypertension is most common in young women. Headache, nausea, and visual disturbance are the presenting symptoms. There is an association with obesity, empty sella turcica, and certain drugs. If left untreated, the patient may become blind due to infarction of the optic nerve.

Temporal arteritis affects predominantly in the elderly. The patient presents with a superficial headache overlying the temporal arteries. The pain may be exacerbated by brushing or combing the hair. Jaw claudication may arise as a consequence of inflammation of the branches of the external carotid artery. Visual loss may be temporary (amaurosis fugax) or permanent if the ciliary or central retinal artery are affected. Weight loss, anorexia, fever, and proximal muscle pain may also occur.

Consider temporal arteritis in any patient over 50 years old with a headache.

Episodic headache or facial pain

Migraine and cluster headaches present with episodes of pain (often severe) interspersed with long symptom-free periods. Paroxysms of pain are also a feature of trigeminal neuralgia.

Classical migraine usually starts with a prodrome lasting 5–60 minutes, characterized by a sense of ill health and visual abnormalities (fortification spectra, scotomata or teichopsia). A throbbing headache then develops, which tends to be unilateral but can become generalized. This is associated with nausea, vomiting, photophobia, and phonophobia. The attack resolves spontaneously after several hours and is often followed by sleep. In uncommon variants of migraine, headache may be accompanied by hemiplegia, ophthalmoplegia, ataxia, vertigo, or unilateral facial palsy.

Migraine is more common in women. Provoking factors include menstruation, fatigue, cheese, and red wine.

Cluster headache (migrainous neuralgia) is a severe unilateral pain centred around one eye. The pain lasts for around an hour and occurs daily for several weeks, often waking the patient from sleep. There is ipsilateral nasal congestion and the eye becomes watery. Horner's syndrome can develop and is occasionally permanent. Symptom-free periods of many months occur between attacks. Cluster headaches are more common in men and may be precipitated by alcohol.

Trigeminal neuralgia (tic douloureux) is characterized by paroxysms of lancinating pain in the distribution of the 5th cranial nerve. It is stimulated by touching 'trigger zones' on the face such as the lips, or by eating, or drinking. The pain lasts for up to 1 minute and does not occur during sleep. Spontaneous remissions can last several months. Whilst there is usually no underlying cause, trigeminal neuralgia may occasionally be secondary to multiple sclerosis (MS) in the young patient or to tumours affecting the cerebellopontine angle or 5th cranial nerve.

Symptoms of raised intracranial pressure

- headache worse on coughing, sneezing, stooping down
- headache worse in the morning
- visual disturbance due to papilloedema
- nausea and vomiting
- diplopia (false localizing 6th cranial nerve palsy)

Fig. 15.2 Symptoms of raised intracranial pressure.

Chronic headache or facial pain

Persistent pain is a feature of postherpetic neuralgia, post-traumatic headache or tension headache.

Following *shingles* of the trigeminal nerve (usually the ophthalmic division), a persistent burning pain known as postherpetic neuralgia may develop. Facial scarring is usually apparent and the pain may disturb sleep. It is uncommon in the young.

Tension headaches are the commonest cause of headaches presenting to doctors. The feeling is often described as a 'tight band around the head', being most common in the frontal and occipital regions, or as a 'pressure' behind the eyes. It is a constant pain, which tends to be worse towards the end of the day or at times of particular stress. There may be coexistent depression.

Following *head injury*, which may not necessarily be severe, a few patients develop persistent headache, similar to a tension headache. It is associated with poor memory and concentration, dizziness, irritability, and symptoms of depression. The patient may be involved in litigation related to the accident responsible.

EXAMINING THE PATIENT WITH HEADACHE OR FACIAL PAIN

The diagnosis is often clear from the history. On examination look for evidence of the pathological processes, such as raised intracranial pressure and meningism. Focal neurological deficits, if present, help to determine the site of the lesion. Fig. 15.3 summarizes the examination approach.

Signs of raised intracranial pressure
- Papilloedema: commonly, the only sign.
- False localizing sign (ipsilateral then bilateral 6th cranial nerve palsy).
- Altered level of consciousness, bradycardia, hypertension if acute or severe, which can progress to decerebrate posturing and death.

Signs of meningism
- Irritability: with a preference for a quiet, darkened room.
- Neck stiffness.

- Positive Kernig's sign: spasm and pain in hamstrings on knee extension.
- Positive Brudzinski's sign: neck flexion causes leg flexion.
- Delirium, fever, and petechial rash: may also be present in infectious meningitis.

If subarachnoid haemorrhage is suspected, look for subhyaloid (retinal) haemorrhage, bruit of an arteriovenous malformation, and a 3rd cranial nerve palsy caused by direct pressure from a posterior communicating artery aneurysm.

Signs of temporal arteritis
- Temporal artery tenderness.
- Loss of temporal artery pulsation–there may be overlying erythema.
- Optic atrophy.
- Low-grade pyrexia.

Focal neurological deficit

Focal neurological signs will help to determine the site of the lesion (see Chapter 20), and may be found in addition to other signs, such as meningism or raised intracranial pressure.

INVESTIGATING THE PATIENT WITH HEADACHE OR FACIAL PAIN

An algorithm for the investigation of the patient with headache or facial pain is given in Fig. 15.4. Investigations used in this type of patient include:
- Full blood count: normochromic normocytic anaemia suggests chronic pathology, e.g. temporal arteritis, tuberculous meningitis; leucocytosis will be seen in infection.
- Erythrocyte sedimentation rate: high in temporal arteritis but may also be raised in infection and malignancy.
- Temporal artery biopsy: temporal arteritis. This is a definitive test, but as there is often patchy vascular involvement, a negative result does not exclude the diagnosis.
- Computed tomography scan or magnetic resonance imaging of the head: presence of blood, space-

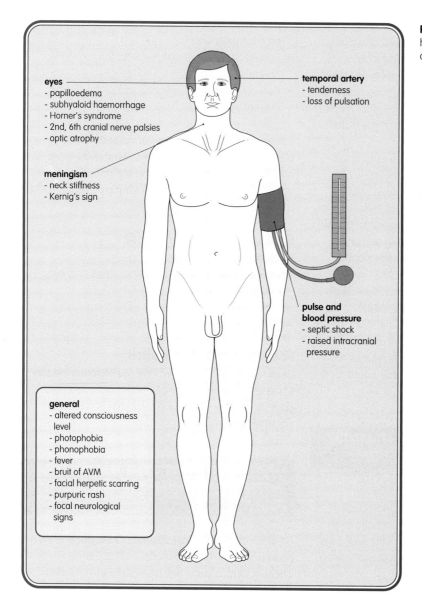

Fig. 15.3 Examining the patient with headache and facial pain. (AVM, arteriovenous malformation.)

eyes
- papilloedema
- subhyaloid haemorrhage
- Horner's syndrome
- 2nd, 6th cranial nerve palsies
- optic atrophy

meningism
- neck stiffness
- Kernig's sign

temporal artery
- tenderness
- loss of pulsation

pulse and blood pressure
- septic shock
- raised intracranial pressure

general
- altered consciousness level
- photophobia
- phonophobia
- fever
- bruit of AVM
- facial herpetic scarring
- purpuric rash
- focal neurological signs

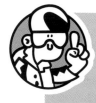

When meningitis is suspected clinically, treat with antibiotics first and then complete investigations. Patients can die awaiting confirmation of the diagnosis.

occupying lesion (tumour, abscess), or hydrocephalus. Contrast enhancement should be used if tumour is suspected.

- Lumbar puncture: this should never be performed when raised intracranial pressure is a possibility, as it causes coning. Cerebrospinal fluid (CSF) examination is invaluable in the diagnosis of meningitis. CSF should be sent to the laboratory for assessment of glucose and protein, microscopy, culture, and cytology.
- Cerebral angiography: should be performed if

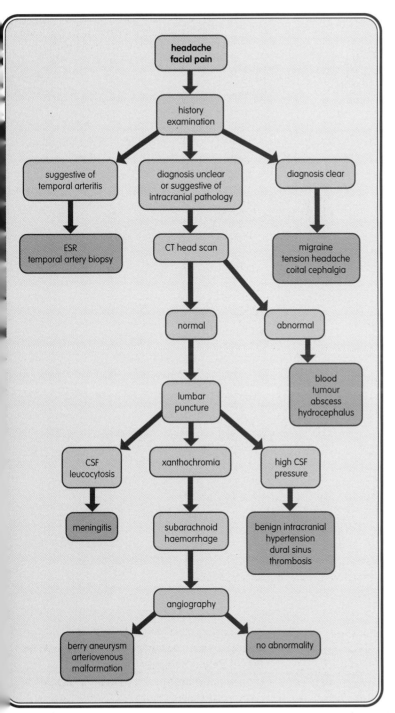

Fig. 15.4 Algorithm for the investigation of the patient with headache or facial pain. (CSF, cerebrospinal fluid; CT, computed tomography; ESR, erythrocyte sedimentation rate.)

surgery is considered in subarachnoid haemorrhage. It identifies and localizes berry aneurysms and arteriovenous malformations.
Visual fields: these should be serially measured in patients with benign intracranial hypertension, which carries a serious risk of optic nerve infarction.
• Electroencephalography: herpes simplex encephalitis shows characteristic features.

75

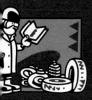

16. Joint Disease

DIFFERENTIAL DIAGNOSIS OF JOINT DISEASE

Possible causes of joint disease are extensive although in practice the common conditions include the following:
- Rheumatoid arthritis (RA).
- Osteoarthritis (OA).
- Gout.
- Seronegative arthritides: ankylosing spondylitis, Reiter's syndrome, and psoriatic arthritis.
- Septic arthritis.

The causes of a single, hot, red joint is a favourite question. They are as follows:
- **Septic arthritis, possibly secondary to rheumatoid arthritis, osteoarthritis, osteomyelitis, or injury.**
- **Trauma.**
- **Gout.**
- **Pseudogout.**
- **Haemarthrosis.**
- **Gonococcal arthritis.**
- **Rheumatoid arthritis.**

Arthritis may also be a feature of connective tissue diseases, especially systemic lupus erythematosus (SLE) and polyarteritis nodosa (PAN).

Less common causes include the following:
- Enteropathic arthropathies, e.g. inflammatory bowel disease, Whipple's disease.
- Behçet's syndrome.
- Leukaemia and lymphoma.
- Metastases: bronchial, breast, thyroid, kidney, and prostate carcinomas.
- Hypertrophic pulmonary osteoarthropathy: bronchial carcinoma.
- Viral, bacterial, and fungal infections.

- Endocrine causes: acromegaly, myxoedema, hyperparathyroidism, idiopathic hyperparathyroidism.
- Metabolic diseases: Wilson's disease, haemochromatosis, chondrocalcinosis, ochronosis, pyrophosphate arthropathy.
- Others: familial Mediterranean fever, sarcoidosis, amyloidosis, sickle cell disease, Wegener's granulomatosis.

HISTORY IN THE PATIENT WITH JOINT DISEASE

The different types of joint disease have many features in common, and examination will provide further additional important clues to the aetiology. Ask about the following:
- Onset: rapid or slowly progressive.
- Persistent or relapsing.
- Early morning stiffness: classically RA is worse first thing in the morning and OA is worse at the end of the day, although there is considerable overlap.
- Weakness: with or without wasting of muscles.
- Distribution of the affected joints (see below).
- Patient's age: RA classically affects women aged 25–55 years, and OA usually occurs in the over 40s.
- Any history of trauma.
- Recent infection, e.g. viral illness and reactive arthritis, septic arthritis, or neutropenia.
- Features associated with different arthropathies: inflammation of the eye (RA and seronegative arthropathies), shortness of breath (fibrosis or aortic regurgitation in RA, and ankylosing spondylitis), parasthesiae (entrapment neuropathies), gastrointestinal symptoms (enteropathic arthropathies), and rarer causes of arthropathies, e.g. endocrine causes.
- In patients with chronic arthritis it is important to explore the extent of loss of function. How limited are the activities of daily living?
- Chronic arthritis can lead to feelings of helplessness and depression. Assessment of these features is also an important part of the history.

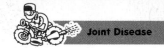
EXAMINING THE PATIENT WITH JOINT DISEASE

Rheumatoid arthritis

RA is a systemic connective tissue disorder, the joints being one of many body parts affected. Look for the following (see Fig. 36.1):

- Symmetrical deforming arthropathy.
- Swelling of the proximal interphalangeal (PIP) and metacarpophalangeal (MCP) joints.
- Wasting of the small muscles of the hand.
- Nodules on the elbows and extensor tendons.
- Ulnar deviation of the fingers: subluxation and dislocation at the MCP joints.
- Swan neck deformity: hyperextension of the PIP joints and flexion of the MCP and terminal interphalangeal (TIP) joints.
- Boutonnière deformity: flexion of the PIP joints and extension of the TIP and MCP joints.
- 'Z' thumb.
- Trigger finger.
- Palmar erythema.
- Iatrogenic Cushing's disease: steroids used in treatment.
- Swollen or deformed knees.
- Cervical spine disease.
- Anaemia.
- Arteritic lesions: nail-fold infarcts, chronic leg ulceration, and purpuric rash.

You must also carry out a general examination. In particular, look for the following:

- Eye signs: keratoconjunctivitis sicca, keratitis, episcleritis, scleromalacia perforans, cataracts due to chloroquine or steroids.
- Dry mucous membranes: Sjögren's syndrome.
- Chest signs: pleural effusion, fibrosing alveolitis.
- Neurological signs: peripheral neuropathy, mononeuritis multiplex, entrapment neuropathy.

Determine how the joint disease affects the patient's daily acivities, e.g. holding a pan, making a cup of tea.

- Vasculitic leg ulceration.
- Felty's syndrome: splenomegaly, neutropenia.
- Cardiac signs: pericarditis, myocarditis, conduction defects, and valvular incompetence.
- Secondary amyloidosis.
- Other autoimmune disorders.

Osteoarthritis

In the hands in OA look for the following (see Fig. 36.4):

- Heberden's nodes: swelling of the TIP joints.
- Bouchard's nodes: swelling of the PIP joints.
- Subluxation of the first metacarpal: square hand appearance.
- Crepitus of affected joints.
- Wasting and weakness of the quadriceps and glutei.
- Positive Trendelenburg's sign: this is a downward tilting of the pelvis when the patient stands on the affected leg.
- Joint effusions.
- Locking of the joints due to loose bodies.
- Loss of function.

The causes of joint pain can be remembered by the mnemonic SOFTER TISSUE: sepsis, osteoarthritis, fractures, tendon/muscle, epiphyseal, referred, tumour, ischaemia, seropositive arthritides, seronegative arthritides, urate, extra-articular rheumatism, e.g. polymyalgia.

Gout

Look for the following:

- Asymmetrical swelling of the small joints of the hand and feet.
- Tophi: look especially on the helix of the ear and tendon sheaths.
- Look for associations: hyperlipidaemia (xanthalasmata and corneal arcus), hypertension, signs associated with diabetes mellitus.

Seronegative arthritides

Ankylosing spondylitis

Ask the patient to sit or stand up. Look for the following:

- Loss of lumbar lordosis and a fixed kyphosis.
- A stooped 'question mark' posture.
- Rigid spine.
- Reduced chest expansion.
- Prominent abdomen.

Also examine for complications and extra-articular manifestations:

- Eyes: iritis.
- Cardiovascular system: aortitis (listen for aortic regurgitation and conduction defects.
- Chest: apical fibrosis.
- Neurological: atlantoaxial dislocation leading to paraplegia or sciatica.
- Secondary amyloidosis: feel for organomegaly.

Reiter's syndrome

This is a triad of urethritis, conjunctivitis, and seronegative arthritis. It follows non-specific urethritis or occasionally dysentery. Look for the following:

- Large joint mono- or oligoarthritis.
- Iritis.
- Keratoderma blenorrhagica (brown, aseptic abscesses on the soles and palms).
- Mouth ulcers.
- Circinate balanitis.
- Enthesopathy (plantar fasciitis or Achilles tendonitis).
- Aortic incompetence.

Psoriatic arthritis

Look for the following:

- Asymmetrical arthropathy.
- Usually involvement of the TIP joints.
- Pitting of the fingernails and onycholysis.
- Thickened nails.
- Psoriatic plaques: look particularly at the elbows, extensor aspects of limbs, scalp, behind the ears, and the navel.
- Other forms of psoriatic arthropathy: arthritis mutilans, a RA-like picture, asymmetrical mono- or oligoarthropathy, ankylosing spondylitis.

Septic arthritis

This must be recognized and treated promptly because of potential destruction of the joint and widespread

infection. It usually presents as a monoarthritis. The affected joint is swollen, painful, hot, and red.

INVESTIGATING THE PATIENT WITH JOINT DISEASE

An algorithm for the investigation of patients with joint disease is provided in Fig. 16.1. The following investigations should be performed:

- Full blood count: anaemia; raised white cell count occasionally in RA, leucopenia and thrombocytopenia in SLE, eosinophilia in PAN, neutropenia in Felty's syndrome.

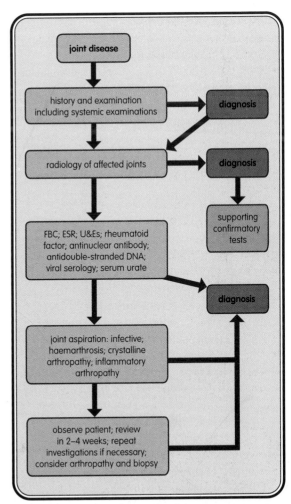

Fig. 16.1 Algorithm for the investigation of the patient with joint disease. (ESR, erythrocyte sedimentation rate; FBC, full blood count; U&Es, urea and electrolytes.)

- Erythrocyte sedimentation rate: non-specific but raised in the presence of inflammation (therefore often high in RA but less so in OA).
- Rheumatoid factor: positive in about 75% of patients with RA. It may also be positive in SLE, mixed connective tissue diseases, scleroderma, and Sjögren's syndrome.
- Antinuclear antibodies: positive in 30% of patients with RA and in 80% of patients with SLE.
- Antidouble-stranded DNA antibodies: high titres in SLE.
- Other autoantibodies according to clinical suspicion, e.g. anti-Ro and anti-La antibodies in Sjögren's syndrome, and anti-Scl70 antibodies in scleroderma.
- Viral serology: if a viral cause for the arthropathy is suspected, e.g. rubella, mumps, infectious mononucleosis, coxsackie virus, and hepatitis B virus.
- Urea and electrolytes: associated renal involvement.
- Liver function tests: liver involvement or drug treatment.
- Creatine phosphokinase: myositis.
- Serum urate: usually high in gout but beware of false positives and false negatives.

Joint aspiration should be performed. Examine the following:

- Appearance: purulence indicates infection, frank blood indicates haemarthrosis or traumatic tap.

- Microscopy for bacteria and crystals: monosodium urate indicates gout, calcium pyrophosphate indicates pseudogout.
- White cell count: high in inflammatory arthropathies.
- Culture: gonococci, tubercle bacillus, or fungi when indicated.

A chest X-ray should be performed to look for associated diseases or complications of RA:

- Pleural effusion.
- Diffuse fibrosing alveolitis.
- Rheumatoid nodules or cavities.
- Cricoarytenoid arthritis.
- Obliterative bronchiolitis.
- Rheumatoid pneumoconiosis: Caplan's syndrome.

An X-ray of the affected joints may indicate the following:

- RA: soft tissue thickening, juxta-articular osteoporosis, loss of joint space, bony erosions, subluxation.
- OA: loss of joint space, subchondral sclerosis and cysts, marginal osteophytes.
- Gout: soft tissue swelling and punched-out lesions in juxta-articular bone.
- Ankylosing spondylitis: 'bamboo spine' (squaring of the vertebrae and obliteration of sacroiliac joints); also found in Reiter's syndrome and Crohn's disease.

An X-ray of the cervical spine should also be used to look for displacement of the odontoid peg.

Finally, arthroscopy allows direct visualization inside the joint space, and can be used for biopsy and the removal of foreign bodies.

Anaemia in rheumatoid arthritis may be due to the following:
- **Normochromic normocytic anaemia of chronic disease.**
- **Microcytic anaemia from chronic blood loss secondary to drug treatment.**
- **Bone marrow suppression from treatment, e.g. gold or penicillamine.**
- **Megaloblastic anaemia from impaired folate release or pernicious anaemia.**
- **Felty's syndrome.**

In pseudogout, crystals are positively birefringent in plane-polarized light. Remember this by the 'P' s. In gout, the crystals are negatively birefringent.

17. Skin Rashes

Pigmented lesions

- Freckles (ephelides): flat, brown spots.
- Lentigo: similar to freckles but darker and not affected by sunlight.
- Seborrhoeic keratosis: benign, beige/brown plaques, 3–20 mm in diameter, with a velvety or warty surface.
- Naevus: moles.
- Blue naevus: small, slightly elevated, blue-black lesions.
- Atypical (dysplastic) naevus: over 5 mm across, ill-defined, irregular border, irregularly distributed pigmentation with erythema and accentuated skin markings.
- Melanoma: flat or raised pigmented lesion with possibly a recent change in appearance. It has varying colours and typically irregular borders.

Scaly lesions

- Psoriasis: silvery, scaled, well-demarcated plaques on skin, usually over the extensor surfaces. It can be pustular and involve the nails.
- Dermatitis and eczema: a pruritic, exudative, or lichenified eruption on the face, neck, upper trunk, wrists, and hands, and in the antecubital and popliteal fossae.
- Xerosis: dry skin.
- Lichen simplex chronicus: chronic itching associated with pigmented, lichenified, skin lesions. Lichenified lesions exhibit exaggerated skin lines overlying thickened, well-circumscribed, scaly plaques.
- Tinea corporis: ring-shaped lesion with an advancing scaly border and central clearing or scaly patches with a distinct border.
- Tinea versicolor: pale or hyperpigmented macules, or velvety, tan, pink, whitish, or brown macules that scale with scraping.
- Secondary syphilis.
- Pityriasis rosea: oval, fawn-coloured, scaly eruption following the cleavage lines of the trunk. It is commonly preceded by a herald patch.

- Discoid lupus erythematosus: red, asymptomatic, localized plaques, usually on the face and often in a 'butterfly' distribution. There is scaling, follicular plugging, atrophy, and telangiectasia of involved areas.
- Exfoliative dermatitis: scaling and erythema over a large area of the body.
- Actinic keratoses: small, pink patches that feel like bits off sandpaper when the finger is drawn over them. They are premalignant.
- Bowen's disease (intraepidermal squamous cell carcinoma): small, well-demarcated, slightly raised, pink-to-red, scaly plaques.
- Extramammary Paget's disease: this resembles chronic eczema and may involve apocrine areas such as the genitals.
- Intertrigo: fissuring, erythema, and sodden epidermis, with superficial denudation in the body folds.

Vesicular lesions

- Herpes simplex: recurrent, small, grouped vesicles on an erythematous base, especially around the oral and genital areas.
- Herpes zoster: vesicular lesions in a dermatomal distribution.
- Pompholyx: pruritic 'tapioca' vesicles or bullae on the palms, soles, and sides of fingers.
- Dermatophytid (allergy or sensitivity to fungi): pruritic, grouped, vesicular lesions involving the sides and flexor aspects of the fingers and palms.
- Dermatitis herpetiformis: pruritic papulovesicular lesions mainly on the elbows, knees, buttocks, posterior neck, and scalp. It is associated with gluten-sensitive enteropathy.
- Miliaria (heat rash): superficial, aggregated, small vesicles, papules, or pustules on covered areas of the skin.
- Scabies: pruritic vesicles and pustules especially on the sides of the. Red papules or nodules on the penile glans and shaft are pathognomonic.
- Photosensitivity.

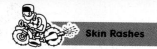

Weepy or encrusted lesions

- Impetigo: vesiculopustular lesions with thick, golden-crusted exudate associated with group A β-haemolytic streptococci or coagulase-positive *Staphylococcus aureus*, or bullous lesions associated with *S. aureus*.
- Acute-contact allergic dermatitis: erythema and oedema, with pruritus, often followed by vesicles and bullae in an area of contact with a suspected agent. They may later weep, crust, and become infected.
- Any vesicular dermatitis.

Pustular lesions

- Acne vulgaris: the most common skin condition, characterized by open and closed comedones. It varies from purely comedonal to pustular inflammatory acne to cysts to nodules.
- Acne rosacea: erythema and telangiectasia and a tendency to flush easily. May have an acneiform component, or hyperplasia of the soft tissue of the nose (rhinophyma).
- Folliculitis: pustules in the hair follicles.
- Candidiasis: superficial, denuded, beefy-red areas with or without satellite vesicopustules. Whitish, curd-like concretions on the oral and vaginal mucous membranes.
- Miliaria.
- Any vesicular dermatitis.

Figurate erythema

Figurate erythema lesions look like rings or arcs.
- Urticaria: eruptions of evanescent wheals or hives.
- Erythema multiforme: symmetrical erythematous lesions on the extensor surfaces, palms, soles, or mucous membranes, which may be macular, papular, urticarial, bullous, or purpuric. May be target lesions with clear centres and concentric erythematous rings.
- Erythema migrans: a red expansion around an initial papule with an advancing border, which is usually raised, warm, and red. The centre may clear or become indurated, vesicular, or necrotic.
- Cellulitis: a hot, red, diffuse, spreading infection of the skin.
- Erysipelas: oedematous, spreading, circumscribed, hot, erythematous area, with or without vesicle or bulla formation, frequently involving the face.

- Erysipeloid: purplish erythema, most often of a finger or the back of the hand, which gradually extends. Caused by *Erysipelothrix insidiosa*, it is often seen in fishermen and meat handlers.

Bullous lesions

- Impetigo: superficial bacterial infection caused by group A β-haemolytic streptococci or *S. aureus*.
- Pemphigus: relapsing crops of bullae appearing on normal skin, often preceded by mucous membrane bullae, erosions, and ulcerations. There may be superficial detachment of the skin after pressure or trauma (Nikolsky's sign).
- Bullous pemphigoid: tense blisters in flexural areas. They may be preceded by urticarial or oedematous lesions.
- Porphyria cutanea tarda.
- Erythema multiforme: 'target' lesions, i.e. symmetrically distributed, circular lesions, often with a central blister.
- Toxic epidermal necrolysis: usually secondary to drugs, e.g. sulphonamides, penicillins, and anticonvulsants.

Papular lesions

- Hyperkeratotic: warts, corns, seborrhoeic keratoses.
- Purple: lichen planus – pruritic, violaceous, flat-topped papules with fine white streaks and a symmetrical distribution, commonly seen along linear scratch marks on the anterior wrists, sacral region, penis, legs, and mucous membranes; drug eruptions; Kaposi's sarcoma – malignant skin lesions with dark plaques or nodules on cutaneous or mucosal surfaces, common in people with human immunodeficiency virus infection.
- Flesh-coloured and umbilicated: molluscum contagiosum – a viral infection causing single or multiple, rounded, dome-shaped, waxy papules, 2–5 mm in diameter, which are umbilicated and contain a caseous plug.
- Pearly: basal cell carcinoma – most commonly papules or nodules with a central scab or erosion; intradermal naevi.
- Small, red, and inflammatory: acne, miliaria, candidiasis, intertrigo, scabies, folliculitis.

Nodular, cystic lesions

- Erythema nodosum: painful red nodules without ulceration on the anterior aspects of the legs; they may regress over weeks to resemble contusions.
- Furuncle (boils): painful inflammatory swellings of a hair follicle forming an abscess, caused by *S. aureus*.
- Cystic acne.
- Follicular (epidermal) inclusion cyst.

Photodermatoses

Painful erythema, oedema, and vesiculation on sun-exposed surfaces, usually the face, neck, hands, and V of the chest. Causes include drugs (e.g. amiodarone, phenothiazines, sulphonamides, and related drugs), polymorphic light eruption, and systemic lupus erythematosus (SLE).

Maculopapular lesions

Viral causes, and secondary syphilis.

Erosive lesions

- Any vesicular dermatitis.
- Impetigo.
- Lichen planus.
- Erythema multiforme.
- Oral erosions.

Ulcerated lesions

- Decubiti: bed sores or pressure sores.
- Herpes simplex.
- Skin cancers.
- Parasitic infections.
- Syphilis: chancre.
- Vasculitis.
- Stasis.
- Arterial disease.

HISTORY IN THE PATIENT WITH SKIN RASHES

The following long list of factors should be assessed when taking a history in the patient with skin rashes:
- Rash: onset, duration.
- Aggravating factors: physical or chemical agents; cold (cold urticaria or cryoglobulinaemia); heat (worsens seborrhoeic conditions and superficial skin conditions).
- Precipitants: stress may lead to alopecia or eczema.
- Site of origin: contact dermatitis and pityriasis rosea (herald patch).
- Rate of progression.
- Timing of change in skin lesions, particularly for moles.
- Character: any alteration or progression in lesions.
- Hair and nails.
- Family history: eczema, psoriasis, inherited skin disorders.
- Infective agents: foreign travel (tropical infections), pets (papular urticaria or animal scabies).
- Farm animals: orf (poxvirus), ringworm.
- Occupation.
- Chemical exposure: ay home or work, acting as antigens or direct irritants.
- Drugs taken: over-the-counter drugs, steroids may make the rash better (as in dermatitis) or worse (as in acne). How are the drugs being used?
- Foods: nuts and shellfish.
- Washing powder or soap.
- Contacts: family and friends.
- Light exposure: herpes simplex, SLE, and vitiligo.
- Hobbies: sportsmen are more prone to viral or fungal infections.
- General state of health and past medical history.
- Patient's explanation for rash.

Systemic symptoms should be assessed, and may take the following forms:
- Itching (Fig. 17.1): atopy or urticaria (e.g. scabies which is worse in bed), eczema, dermatitis herpetiformis, lichen planus, flexural psoriasis.
- Pain: inflammatory conditions, skin tumours.

Finally, the mode of spread is significant and may take the form of an annular appearance (e.g. erythema annulare, erythema multiforme, and fungal infections) or irregular spread (e.g. pyoderma gangrenosum or malignancy).

EXAMINING THE PATIENT WITH SKIN RASHES

Always examine the entire skin and look in the mouth, e.g. with lichen planus, herpes simplex and zoster, and

Drug eruptions may mimic any inflammatory skin condition. They usually start abruptly and are a widespread, symmetrical, erythematous eruption. Constitutional symptoms such as malaise, arthralgia, headache, and fever may be present.

In the patient presenting with subcutaneous nodules, think of the following:
- Rheumatoid nodules.
- Rheumatic fever.
- Polyarteritis.
- Xanthelasmata.
- Tuberous sclerosis.
- Neurofibromatosis.
- Sarcoidosis.
- Granuloma annulare.

infective exanthemata. Rashes may change with time and become characteristic or diagnostic of common dermatoses, such as the infectious exanthemata. Look at the distribution of lesions:
- If widespread and symmetrical, suspect systemic disease.
- If only areas exposed to the sun are involved, suspect light sensitivity.
- Patterns involving a dermatome distribution suggest herpes zoster.
- Dermatitis involving the hands, face, axillae, ears, and eyelids suggests contact dermatitis.
- Dermatitis involving the axillae, groins, scalp, the central chest and back, eyebrows, ears, and beard suggests seborrheic dermatitis.

- Dermatitis involving the popliteal and cubital fossae, and the face suggests atopic dermatitis.

Describe the lesion:
- Bizarrely shaped lesions suggest the cause is an external agent, e.g. caustic liquid, a self-induced injury.
- Fungal infections are characterized by slow growth, a smooth outline, an active edge with a healing centre, and asymmetry.

Terms and characteristics of dermatological lesions are given in Fig. 17.2.

Fig. 17.1 Possible causes of generalized and localized itching.

Possible causes of generalized and localized itching	
Generalized itching	**Localized itching**
• uraemia	• scabies and other mite infestations
• cholestasis	• contact eczema
• iron–deficiency anaemia	• dermatitis herpetiformis (associated with coeliac disease)
• lymphoma	• urticaria ('nettle rash')
• hypo- and hyperthyroidism	• lichen planus
• pregnancy	• prickly heat
• carcinoma	• winter itch
• multiple sclerosis	• aquagenic pruritus
• syphilis	• old age
• intestinal parasites	
• morphine ingestion	
• allergies, e.g. atopic eczema	
• diabetes mellitus	

INVESTIGATING THE PATIENT WITH SKIN RASHES

The history and examination may be enough to determine the diagnosis. If the patient is not unwell it may be possible to examine for skin changes over time to allow for the development of possible characteristic lesions. The following investigations should be performed:

- Blood tests: full blood count, urea and electrolytes, bacterial and viral titres with immunological tests for tropical diseases if appropriate, and blood cultures.
- Skin scrapings and nail clippings: fungi.
- Examination of the skin under Wood's light.
- Examination of brushings of household pets: mites.
- Culture of fluid-containing lesions.
- Skin biopsy.
- Biopsy of lesions in lymph nodes or other organs.
- Investigations for associated systemic diseases or malignancy.

Terms and characteristics of dermatological lesions	
Term	**Characteristics**
alopecia	hair loss
atrophy	loss of skin thickness
blister or bulla	vesicle >1 cm diameter
cyst	epithelium-lined cavity containing fluid or semi-solid material
erythema	area of reddened skin which blanches with pressure
fissure	crack in epidermis
indurated	hard and thickened
Köebner's phenomenon	skin lesions at sites of external injury
lichenification	thickened skin with exaggerated skin markings
macule	circumscribed change in the skin colour up to 1 cm diameter
nodule	solid skin lesion up to 1 cm diameter
papule	raised palpable spot up to 1 cm diameter
patch	macule >1 cm across
plaque	coalesced papules
purpura	area of reddened skin caused by haemorrhages which does not blanch with pressure
pustule	circumscribed, pus-filled lesion
scale	flake of hard skin
scar	connective tissue replacement following loss of dermal tissue
ulcer	irregularly shaped break in surface continuity of epithelium
vesicle	fluid-filled lesion <1 cm diameter
wheal	raised, palpable lesion with paler centres

Fig. 17.2 Terms and characteristics of dermatological lesions.

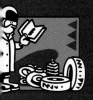

18. Loss of Consciousness

INTRODUCTION

Loss of consciousness may be transient (syncope) or ongoing (coma). Many patients are admitted to hospital with 'collapse ? cause'. Patients use the word 'collapse' to describe a variety of situations and it is essential to determine whether or not the patient has actually lost consciousness.

DIFFERENTIAL DIAGNOSIS OF LOSS OF CONSCIOUSNESS

Syncope ('blackout')

Syncope is caused by a transient loss of consciousness and motor tone due to a reduction in cerebral perfusion. There is spontaneous recovery, and it is often recurrent. Causes and forms of syncope include:

- Vasovagal attack: simple faint.
- Postural hypotension.
- Vertebrobasilar insufficiency.
- Cardiac: Stokes–Adams attacks, arrhythmias, hypertrophy obstructive cardiomyopathy (HOCM), aortic stenosis.
- Epilepsy.
  Transient ischaemic attacks: posterior cerebral circulation.
- Micturition syncope.
- Cough syncope.
- Carotid sinus syncope: increased carotid sinus sensitivity in the elderly due to atherosclerosis.

Coma

In coma, the patient remains unconscious and is unrousable. Coma can be caused by the following:
- Vascular: intracranial haemorrhage, cerebral infarction.
- Epilepsy: status epilepticus.
- Shock: anaphylaxis, sepsis, acute blood or fluid loss, cardiogenic, addisonian.
- Drugs overdose: narcotics, barbiturates, benzodiazepines.
- Alcohol: acute intoxication.

- Metabolic: hypoglycaemia, hepatic encephalopathy, uraemia, porphyria.
- Trauma, particularly closed head injury.
- Infection: meningitis, encephalitis, malaria.
- Respiratory: hypercapnia.
- Electrolyte: hyponatraemia, hyper- or hypocalcaemia.
- Endocrine: hypopituitarism, hypothyroidism.

HISTORY IN THE PATIENT WITH LOSS OF CONSCIOUSNESS

When a patient presents in coma, relatives or the GP should be contacted to gain information regarding previous medical history, prodromal illness, known alcohol or drug abuse, and whether the events leading to the coma were witnessed by anyone.

In syncope, the history should focus on the following details.

Presyncope
- What was the patient doing at the time?
- Were there any symptoms before the patient lost consciousness?
- In postural hypotension the patient may have stood up suddenly.
- If the patient had just turned his or her head, consider vertebrobasilar insufficiency.
- Prior to an epileptic fit, there is often an aura.
- In arrhythmia, the patient can be aware of palpitations, chest pain, or dyspnoea before blacking out.
- In Stokes–Adams attacks there is usually no warning.
- Exertional syncope is seen in aortic stenosis and HOCM.
- Occasionally, cough or micturition may cause syncope.

The attack itself
- What happened during the episode itself? This is where the history of a witness is vitally important.
- Seizures associated with tongue biting and urinary incontinence indicate epilepsy. (Note that if a patient remains propped upright in other forms of syncope, a secondary fit may occur).

- In Stokes–Adams attacks the patient is typically seen to go deathly pale with flushing on recovery. The length of time that the patient remained unconscious should be recorded.

Postsyncope

- How quickly did the patient recover?
- Was there any injury? Syncope is generally followed by rapid recovery. However, in epilepsy, there is usually postictal sleepiness.
- It is also very important to ask whether patients hurt themselves during the episode. If there is significant injury consider cardiac syncope (lack of warning).

Risk factors

- Is there a previous history of epilepsy, cardiac disease, cerebrovascular disease, or obstructive airways disease?
- Is the patient a diabetic on insulin?
- Is the patient a health-care worker with access to insulin?

- Is there a history of drug abuse or depression?
- Has there been recent travel to a malarial area?
- Has there been any trauma to the head?

EXAMINING THE PATIENT WITH LOSS OF CONSCIOUSNESS

The examination should be in three parts, in the order given below:
- How ill is the patient?
- Is there any evidence of the underlying cause?
- Has the patient been injured as a consequence?

Fig. 18.1 summarizes the examination approach.

How ill is the patient?

In an unconscious patient, the first priority is to establish that there is a patent **A**irway and effective **B**reathing and **C**irculation (i.e. ABC). A rapid

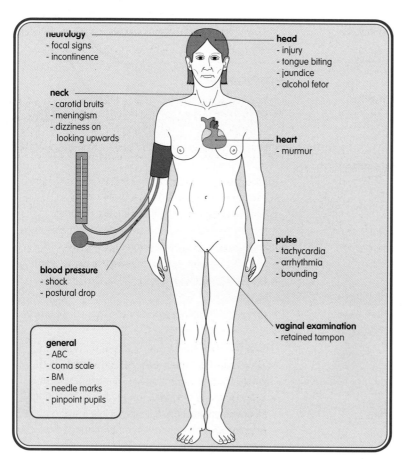

neurology
- focal signs
- incontinence

neck
- carotid bruits
- meningism
- dizziness on
  looking upwards

blood pressure
- shock
- postural drop

general
- ABC
- coma scale
- BM
- needle marks
- pinpoint pupils

head
- injury
- tongue biting
- jaundice
- alcohol fetor

heart
- murmur

pulse
- tachycardia
- arrhythmia
- bounding

vaginal examination
- retained tampon

Fig. 18.1 Examining the patient with loss of consciousness. (ABC, the Airway–Breathing–Circulation first-aid mnemonic; BM, stick test for blood sugar.)

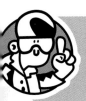

Always try to obtain a history from a witness, even if the patient has regained consciousness.

A blood sugar test should be performed urgently in all unconscious patients to exclude hypoglycaemia.

assessment of the Glasgow coma scale should then be made as shown in Fig. 18.2.

Is the patient shocked? Check the blood pressure and pulse.

Are there any clues as to the underlying cause?

The following signs may indicate the underlying cause:

- Tongue injury or incontinence (urinary or faecal): epilepsy.
- Drop in blood pressure on standing: postural hypotension.
- Dizziness on looking upwards: vertebrobasilar insufficiency.
- Rapid or irregular pulse or murmur: cardiac cause.
- Evidence of head injury skull fracture, haematoma, blood or cerebrospinal fluid in ears.
- Needle marks or pinpoint pupils: narcotic overdose.
- Smell of alcohol.

- Meningism: meningitis, subarachnoid haemorrhage.
- Focal neurology: intracranial cause such as haemorrhage or infarction.
- Jaundice: hepatic encephalopathy.
- Trousseau's and Chvostek's signs: hypocalcaemia.
- Papilloedema, bounding pulse, asterixis and warm peripheries: hypercapnia.
- Tampons in vagina: toxic shock syndrome.
- Carotid bruits: these are found in atherosclerosis and suggest a possible source of emboli in transient ischaemic attacks or stroke.

Has the patient been injured?

If conscious, the patient will be able to describe any injury resulting from the episode. If not, look for bruising or deformities due to fractures. In particular, look for evidence of head injury.

INVESTIGATING THE PATIENT WITH LOSS OF CONSCIOUSNESS

Investigation will be guided by findings in the history and clinical examination. The following investigations are useful in the different clinical scenarios (Figs 18.3 and 18.4):

- Full blood count: anaemia in severe haemorrhage or haemolysis (malaria); leucocytosis in sepsis.
- Urea and electrolytes: hypo- or hypernatraemia.
- Calcium: hypocalcaemia.
- Glucose: hypoglycaemia.
- Liver function tests: liver failure.
- Thyroid function tests: hypothyroidism.
- Electrocardiogram: arrhythmia, left ventricular hypertrophy in aortic stenosis and HOCM.
- Arterial blood gases: hypercapnia.
- Chest X-ray: pulmonary disease, aspiration pneumonia.
- Drugs screen: urine and blood.

The Glasgow coma scale		
Category	**Response**	**Score**
best verbal response	orientated	5
	confused conversation	4
	inappropriate speech	3
	incomprehensible words	2
	no speech	1
best motor response	obeys commands	5
	localizes to pain	4
	flexes to pain	3
	extends to pain	2
	no response	1
eye opening	spontaneous	4
	to speech	3
	to pain	2
	no eye opening	1

Fig. 18.2 The Glasgow coma scale, used for assessing loss consciousness in a patient.

- Electroencephalogram: epilepsy (including subclinical status epilepticus), herpes simplex encephalitis.
- Computed tomography head scan: intracranial pathology.
- Carotid dopplers: carotid atheroma.

- 24-hour tape: arrhythmia.
- ECG: source of emboli, aortic stenosis, HOCM.
- Lumbar puncture: meningitis, subarachnoid haemorrhage.
- Septic screen, including blood cultures and mid-stream urine.

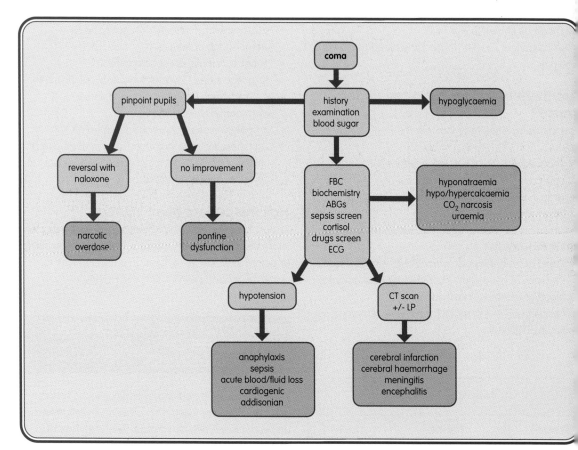

Fig. 18.3 Diagnosis in the patient with coma. (ABGs, arterial blood gases; CT, computed tomography; ECG, electrocardiogram; FBC, full blood count; LP, lumbar puncture.)

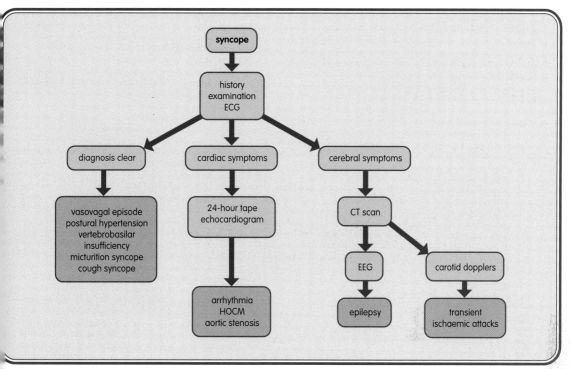

Fig. 18.4 Diagnosis in the patient with syncope. (CT, computed tomography; ECG, electrocardiogram; EEG, electroencephalogram; HOCM, hypertrophic obstructive cardiomyopathy.)

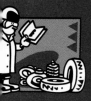
INTRODUCTION

Confusion can be acute or subacute (delirium), or chronic and progressive (dementia). Confusion is very common, particularly in the elderly and is often exacerbated by admission to hospital.

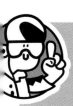

When a patient presents with confusion, try to establish whether it is a longstanding problem which is getting worse or whether it has arisen 'out of the blue' by talking to the family or carers.

DIFFERENTIAL DIAGNOSIS OF CONFUSION

Delirium

Delirium may be caused by the following:
Infection (almost any!): urinary tract infection, pneumonia, malaria, encephalitis, meningitis.
Drug intoxication: opiates, anxiolytics, steroids, tricyclics, anticonvulsants, cannabis.
Drug withdrawal: benzodiazepines, alcohol.
Metabolic: liver, kidney, respiratory or cardiac failure, hyper- or hyponatraemia, hypoglycaemia, hypercalcaemia.
Vitamin deficiency: Wernicke–Korsakoff syndrome (thiamine deficiency).
Cerebral pathology: abscess, tumour, haemorrhage, infarction, trauma (subdural haematoma).

Dementia

Among the following, Alzheimer's disease and multi-infarct dementia are the most common causes of dementia:
Degenerative diseases: Alzheimer's disease, Pick's disease, Huntington's chorea, Creutzfeldt–Jakob disease (CJD), Parkinson's disease, multisystem atrophy.
- Vascular disease: multi-infarct dementia, vasculitis, subdural haematoma.
- Tumour: particularly frontal lobe; can be primary or secondary tumours, or due to paraneoplastic phenomenon.
- Demyelination: multiple sclerosis (MS).
- Infection: human immunodeficiency virus (HIV), syphilis, subacute sclerosing panencephalitis, tuberculosis, meningitis.
- Endocrine: hypothyroidism.
- Vitamin deficiency: vitaminB_{12}, folate, thiamine, niacin (pellagra).
- Drugs: sedatives.
- Metabolic: uraemia, hepatic failure, or Wilson's disease, following prolonged hypoglycaemia or hypoxia.
- Toxic: alcohol, lead, carbon monoxide.
- Normal pressure hydrocephalus.

It is important to remember that deaf people are not necessarily confused and that depression can sometimes mimic dementia ('pseudodementia').

HISTORY IN THE CONFUSED PATIENT

The first step is to establish whether the patient has delirium or dementia. A good account from relatives, carers, or close friends is almost always the only way of getting a true picture of the pattern of disease. The history should then focus on possible underlying causes.

Pattern of confusion

Delirium develops over hours or days. It is characterized by clouding of consciousness, which fluctuates in severity, being worse at night with lucid periods in the day. It can be accompanied by poor recent memory, disorientation, and hallucinations. As a result, the patient may be agitated, uncooperative, and sometimes paranoid.

If delirium develops at around 2 days following hospital admission, consider delirium tremens due to alcohol withdrawal.

Dementia usually has a gradual onset over months or years. It is characterized by a global deterioration in higher cerebral functions, tends to be progressive, and is often exacerbated when the patient is removed from familiar surroundings, such as by admission to hospital. Multi-infarct dementia characteristically progresses in a stepwise fashion.

A more rapid onset is seen in CJD and hydrocephalus. Here, the patient gradually loses memory and intellect, and has increasing difficulty in performing even simple tasks around the house. Change in personality may be a prominent feature. Unlike delirium, there is never a change in consciousness level.

Possible underlying causes

The following should be assessed, as they may reveal an underlying cause:
- Age: dementia becomes increasingly common after the age of 60 years. In younger patients, a thorough search for a treatable underlying cause should be made.
- Symptoms of focal infection (Chapter 6).
- Symptoms of raised intracranial pressure (Chapter 15).
- Risk factors for, or known, vascular disease (Chapter 22).
- Dietary history: vitamin deficiency.
- Alcohol history: whilst chronic alcohol abuse can cause dementia in its own right, it may also be associated with folate and thiamine deficiency.

- Previous head injury: subdural haematoma.
- Drug history: particular attention should be given to sedatives, anticonvulsants, and steroids.
- Other neurological symptoms: cerebrovascular disease, MS, cerebral tumour or abscess.
- Previous medical history of any disease may be relevant: longstanding renal disease (uraemia), malignancy (cerebral metastases, hypercalcaemia or paraneoplastic) or diabetes (insulin overdose).
- Family history: Wilson's disease (autosomal recessive); Huntington's chorea (autosomal dominant).

EXAMINING THE CONFUSED PATIENT

Since the causes of confusion are so varied, a thorough clinical examination is mandatory. This approach is summarized in Fig. 19.1. Particular attention should be given to the following:
- Consciousness: the level of consciousness should be recorded using the Glasgow coma scale (Fig. 18.2).
- Mental state: repeated assessments using the same test is useful in determining objectively whether there is deterioration, and its rate and response to treatment.
- Cyanosis: hypoxia is a common cause of confusion in patients in hospital.
- Focal neurological deficit and the pattern of signs may give important clues as to the diagnosis (Chapters 20 and 22): fundoscopy should be performed looking for papilloedema (raised intracranial pressure), optic atrophy (demyelination) or subhyaloid haemorrhages (subarachnoid haemorrhage). Parkinsonism may be present in Parkinson's disease and multisystem atrophy. Myoclonus, extrapyramidal signs and aphasia are features of CJD.
- Signs of focal infection: look for neck stiffness, consolidation in the chest, abdominal tenderness or otitis media on otoscopy, carefully (Chapter 6).
- Signs of chronic liver disease: hepatic encephalopathy can cause confusion. Chronic liver disease may also indicate chronic alcohol abuse or rare disorders such as Wilson's disease.

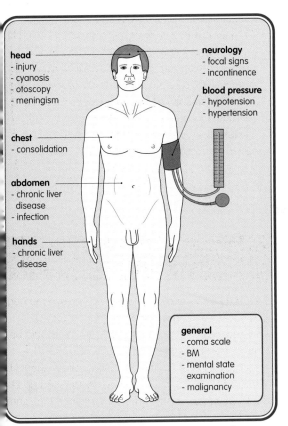

head
- injury
- cyanosis
- otoscopy
- meningism

neurology
- focal signs
- incontinence

blood pressure
- hypotension
- hypertension

chest
- consolidation

abdomen
- chronic liver
  disease
- infection

hands
- chronic liver
  disease

general
- coma scale
- BM
- mental state
  examination
- malignancy

Fig. 19.1 Examining the confused patient. (BM, stick examination for blood sugar.)

- Blood pressure: hypotension may be due to overwhelming infection or cardiac failure. Hypertension is a risk factor for cerebrovascular events and can also be caused by raised intracranial pressure.
- Evidence of head injury: subdural haematoma.
- Primary malignancy: this includes breast cancer and melanoma.
- BM stix: hypoglycaemia.

INVESTIGATING THE CONFUSED PATIENT

An algorithm for diagnosing the confused patient is given in Fig. 19.2.

Blood

- Full blood count: reactive blood picture in malignancy, infection, or inflammation; anaemia with raised mean corpuscular volume (MCV) in vitaminB_{12} or folate deficiency.
- Erythrocyte sedimentation rate: raised in malignancy, infection, inflammation.
- Urea and electrolytes (U&Es): hypo- or hypernatraemia and renal failure.
- Liver function tests: abnormal in liver disease, raised γ-glutamyl transferase in excess alcohol consumption.
- Thyroid function tests: low T_4 in hypothyroidism.
- Serum calcium: hypocalcaemia.
- Serum glucose: hypoglycaemia.
- Serum vitaminB_{12} and red blood cell folate: deficiency.
- Syphilis serology.
- Arterial blood gases for hypoxia.

Urine

Midstream urine should be obtained for microscopy, culture and sensitivity in urinary tract infection.

Radiology

Chest X-ray may show pneumonia, cardiac failure, or malignancy. Computed tomography scan or magnetic resonance imaging of the head should be performed to diagnose tumour, infarction, haematoma, hydrocephalus, and abscess.

Other tests

Consider the following when clinically indicated:
- Thick and thin films: malaria.
- HIV serology.
- Urine: toxicology screen.
- Red cell transketolase for thiamine deficiency.
- Serum copper and caeruloplasmin (reduced) and 24-hour urinary copper excretion (increased): Wilson's disease.
- Electroencephalogram: typical changes of herpes simplex encephalitis.
- Lumbar puncture and cerebrospinal fluid examination: protein, glucose, microscopy, culture, and oligoclonal bands.

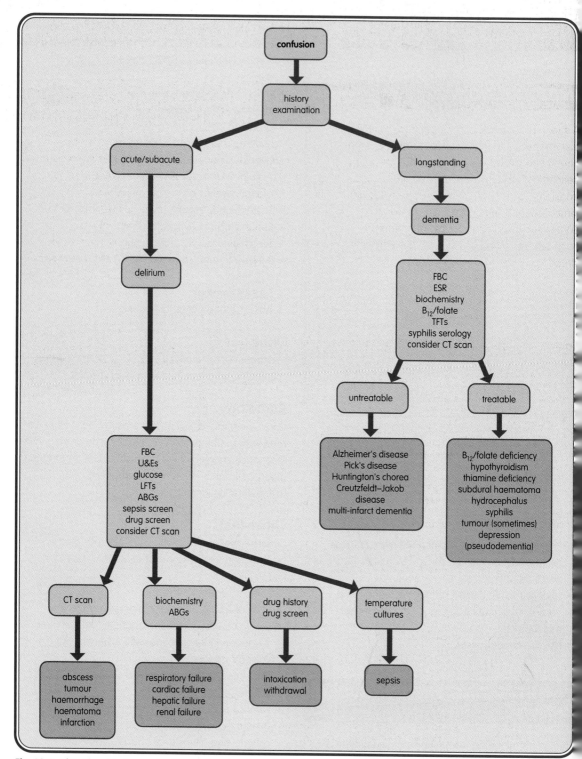

Fig. 19.2 Algorithm for diagnosing the confused patient. (ABGs, arterial blood gases; CT, computed tomography; ESR, erythrocyte sedimentation rate; FBC, full blood count; LFTs, liver function tests; TFTs, thyroid function tests; U&Es, urea and electrolytes.)

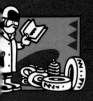

20. Acute Neurological Deficit

INTRODUCTION

A stroke is a neurological deficit due to vascular disturbance which develops over minutes (sometimes hours) and persists for at least 24 hours. Identical deficits lasting less than 24 hours are termed transient ischaemic attacks (TIAs). Cerebral infarction (embolism or thrombosis) accounts for 80% of strokes; 20% of strokes are caused by intracerebral haemorrhage. Fig. 20.1 outlines the principal types of stroke.

DIFFERENTIAL DIAGNOSIS OF STROKE

The diagnosis is often clear from the history and examination, but the following pathologies can also produce a clinical picture that is identical to stroke and should be considered in atypical presentations:
- Subdural haematoma: elderly, alcoholics.
- Cerebral abscess: consider if patient has bronchiectasis or murmer (infective endocarditis).
- Epilepsy: Todd's paralysis following jacksonian seizure.

Types of stroke	
Cause	**Aetiology**
haemorrhagic	hypertension aneurysm (particularly Charcot–Bouchard microaneurysms; also berry and mycotic aneurysms) arteriovenous malformation tumours bleeding tendency (thrombocytopenia, coagulation defects, anticoagulants) drugs (amphetamines, Ecstacy)
infarction	hypertension intracranial arterial atheroma inflammatory vasculopathy (temporal arteritis, SLE, PAN, neurosyphilis) prolonged hypotension (cardiac arrest) prothrombotic haematological disorders (hyperviscosity, antiphospholipid syndrome) drugs (amphetamines, Ecstacy) embolism
sources of embolus	carotid or vertebral atheroma cardiac: • atrial fibrillation with left atrial thrombosis • endocarditis • ventricular thrombus due to myocardial infarction or ventricular aneurysm • atrial myxoma paradoxical: • venous thrombus can reach the cerebral circulation via a patent foramen ovale or an atrial septal defect (rare)

Fig. 20.1 Causes of stroke. (PAN, polyarteritis nodosa; SLE, systemic lupus erythematosus.)

- Hemiplegic migraine: typical features of migraine also present, resolving within 24 hours.
- Demyelination: rare.
- Drugs, e.g. overdose with tricyclic antidepressants: history of depression, younger patients.
- Hypoglycaemia.

In a pontine stroke, the eyes may be deviated towards the paralysed side. In a hemispheric lesion, the eyes will deviate away from the paralysed side.

HISTORY IN THE STROKE PATIENT

The history should focus on three distinct areas. Firstly, does the story fit with the diagnosis of stroke? Secondly, where is the anatomical site of the lesion. Finally, are any risk factors present?

How has the deficit developed?

The key feature in stroke is that the symptoms develop rapidly over a few minutes or less commonly hours, but once the deficit is complete it remains stable and usually improves. Any neurological deterioration due to vascular disease is in a stepwise fashion. If there is gradual deterioration, consider one of the above differential diagnoses or hydrocephalus secondary to the stroke (oedema or blood preventing free drainage of cerebrospinal fluid (CSF)). Improvement can be complete but there is often some residual deficit.

Where is the lesion?

Any intracranial artery can be involved in stroke. The symptoms and signs will reflect which artery and therefore which part of the brain has been involved. This is summarized in Fig. 20.2.

Are there any risk factors for stroke?

Fig. 20.3 shows the main risk factors for stroke and are predominantly the same as for vascular disease elsewhere (Chapter 1).

EXAMINING THE STROKE PATIENT

Clinical examination gives information regarding three important areas in the stroke patient. What are the neurological abnormalities and do they fit with the diagnosis of stroke? Is there any evidence of an underlying cause? Have any complications arisen as a result of the stroke?

Fig. 20.4 summarizes this examination approach.

Has the patient had a stroke?

A thorough neurological examination should be performed, including a coma scale. Does the pattern of neurological deficit fit with disruption of the cerebral vascular supply (Fig. 20.2)?

Determining the likely site of the lesion helps to focus the search for an underlying cause, e.g. carotid bruits in an anterior or middle cerebral artery stroke.

Is there any evidence of an underlying cause?

There are many causes and risk factors for stroke. However, pay particular attention to the following:

- Carotid bruits: carotid atheroma.
- Murmurs: endocarditis, valvular disease, atrial septal defect.
- Pulse: atrial fibrillation.
- Blood pressure: hypertension can be the cause or result of stroke; prolonged hypotension can also cause stroke.
- Diminished peripheral pulses: peripheral vascular disease.
- Xanthelasmata, xanthomata: underlying hyperlipidaemia.
- Temporal artery tenderness: giant cell arteritis.
- Nicotine-stained fingers from heavy smoking.

Have any complications developed?

Complications are common following stroke and are related to the size of cerebral damage and the degree of neurological deficit. The more common problems along with prophylactic measures to avoid them are outlined in Fig. 20.5.

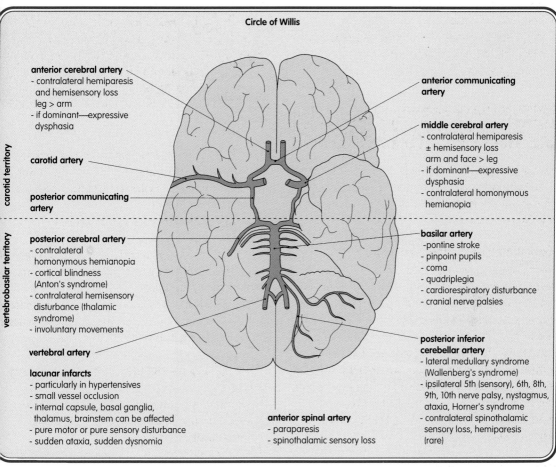

Circle of Willis

anterior cerebral artery
- contralateral hemiparesis and hemisensory loss leg > arm
- if dominant—expressive dysphasia

carotid artery

posterior communicating artery

carotid territory

posterior cerebral artery
- contralateral homonymous hemianopia
- cortical blindness (Anton's syndrome)
- contralateral hemisensory disturbance (thalamic syndrome)
- involuntary movements

vertebral artery

vertebrobasilar territory

lacunar infarcts
- particularly in hypertensives
- small vessel occlusion
- internal capsule, basal ganglia, thalamus, brainstem can be affected
- pure motor or pure sensory disturbance
- sudden ataxia, sudden dysnomia

anterior communicating artery

middle cerebral artery
- contralateral hemiparesis ± hemisensory loss arm and face > leg
- if dominant—expressive dysphasia
- contralateral homonymous hemianopia

basilar artery
- pontine stroke
- pinpoint pupils
- coma
- quadriplegia
- cardiorespiratory disturbance
- cranial nerve palsies

posterior inferior cerebellar artery
- lateral medullary syndrome (Wallenberg's syndrome)
- ipsilateral 5th (sensory), 6th, 8th, 9th, 10th nerve palsy, nystagmus, ataxia, Horner's syndrome
- contralateral spinothalamic sensory loss, hemiparesis (rare)

anterior spinal artery
- paraparesis
- spinothalamic sensory loss

Fig. 20.2 Symptoms and signs associated with different strokes. Note that haemorrhagic strokes have symptoms and signs determined by the site of the bleed. Patients may also develop headache, loss of consciousness and vomiting as a result of raised intracranial pressure.

Risk factors for stroke

- hypertension
- diabetes mellitus
- hypercholesterolaemia
- obesity
- alcohol
- oral contraceptive pill
- established vascular disease (carotid bruit, peripheral vascular disease)
- previous stroke or transient ischaemic attack
- smoking

Fig. 20.3 Risk factors for stroke.

INVESTIGATING THE STROKE PATIENT

The purpose of investigation in these patients is to exclude treatable pathologies and to guide management to prevent further strokes. In atypical presentations, investigation will clearly be important in making the correct diagnosis.

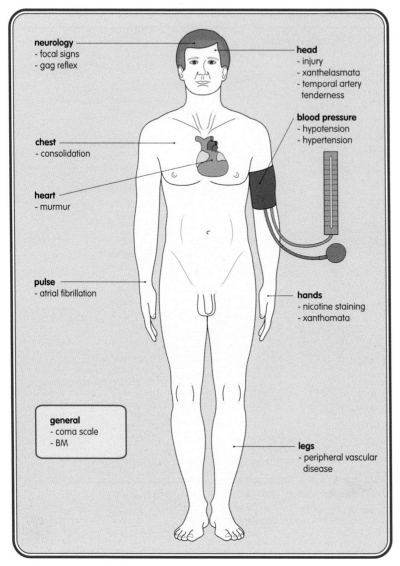

Fig. 20.4 Examining the stroke patient. (BM, stick blood sugar test)

neurology
- focal signs
- gag reflex

head
- injury
- xanthelasmata
- temporal artery tenderness

blood pressure
- hypotension
- hypertension

chest
- consolidation

heart
- murmur

pulse
- atrial fibrillation

hands
- nicotine staining
- xanthomata

general
- coma scale
- BM

legs
- peripheral vascular disease

An algorithm for investigating the patient with stroke is given in Fig. 20.6.

The following tests should be performed for all patients:

- Full blood count: polycythaemia may cause a stroke; a reactive picture may indicate inflammation, e.g. temporal arteritis.
- Erythrocyte sedimentation rate: elevated in inflammation, infection, and malignancy.
- Urea and electrolytes: renal impairment may be due to, or the cause of, hypertension.
- Blood glucose: diabetes and severe hypoglycaemia are both associated with stroke.
- Fasting lipids: hypercholesterolaemia is an important, treatable, risk factor for stroke.
- Clotting screen: to exclude coagulopathy or assess degree of anticoagulation (if the patient is receiving warfarin or heparin).
- Electrocardiogram: atrial fibrillation, recent myocardial infarction, ventricular aneurysm.
- Chest X–ray: to exclude malignancy and aspiration

The following further investigations should be performed where appropriate:

- Syphilis serology: neurosyphilis.

Complications of stroke and measures to prevent them	
Complications	**Prophylactic measures**
cerebral oedema	particularly in haemorrhagic stroke and usually non-preventable (avoid overenthusiastic rehydration)
pressure sores	careful nursing with regular turning
pneumonia	patient should be kept nil by mouth until the gag reflex returns to prevent aspiration
contractures and spasticity	regular skilled physiotherapy
malnutrition	feeding via nasogastric tube or, later, gastrostomy
depression	provision of adequate social and practical support
epilepsy	none

Fig. 20.5 Complications of stroke and measures to prevent them.

- Blood cultures: infective endocarditis.
- Computed tomography head scan: in all young patients (i.e. those less than 60 years of age); where the history is atypical; to exclude haemorrhage; where the patient may need anticoagulation; where cerebellar haemorrhage may be a possibility (needs urgent surgery); to exclude acute hydrocephalus where there is continued deterioration.
- Carotid dopplers: if bruits or recurrent carotid territory infarction.
- Carotid angiography: carotid territory infarction, in which endarterectomy or angioplasty would be considered.
- Echocardiogram: cardiac source of embolus.
- Autoantibodies: anticardiolipin antibodies (antiphospholipid syndrome) and anti double-stranded DNA (cerebral lupus), particularly in younger patients.
- 24-hour electrocardiogram monitoring: paroxysmal atrial fibrillation.

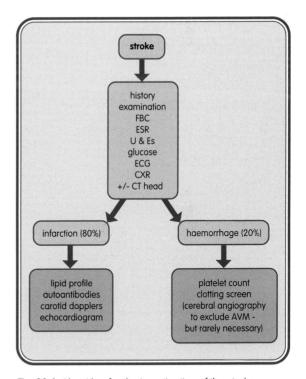

Fig. 20.6 Algorithm for the investigation of the stroke patient. Note that performing a lumbar puncture in patients with haemorrhagic stroke can precipitate coning. (AVM, arteriovenous malformation; CT, computed tomography; CXR, chest X-ray; ECG, electrocardiogram; ESR, erythrocyte sedimentation rate; FBC, full blood count; Gluc, glucose; U&Es, urea and electrolytes.)

INTRODUCTION

Splenomegaly is often a focus of short case examinations since many of its causes are chronic. Lymphadenopathy may be localized or generalized.

DIFFERENTIAL DIAGNOSIS OF LYMPHADENOPATHY AND SPLENOMEGALY

Localized lymphadenopathy

Consider which structures have lymphatic drainage to the nodes affected and examine these carefully for the following:

- Local infection: bacterial (e.g. otitis media, tuberculosis) or viral.
- Metastases: local malignancy.
- Lymphoma: Hodgkin's disease or non-Hodgkin's lymphoma.

Generalized lymphadenopathy

- Infection: particularly viral (Epstein–Barr virus [EBV], cytomegalo virus [CMV], human immunodeficiency virus [HIV], rubella), but also bacterial (tuberculosis [TB], syphilis, brucellosis) and protozoal (toxoplasmosis).
- Lymphoproliferative: Hodgkin's disease or non-Hodgkin's lymphoma, chronic lymphocytic leukaemia, acute lymphoblastic leukaemia.
- Connective tissue disorders: systemic lupus erythematosus, rheumatoid arthritis.
- Infiltration: sarcoidosis.
- Drugs: phenytoin ('pseudolymphoma').
- Endocrine: thyrotoxicosis (rare).

Splenomegaly

In general, different diseases cause different degrees of splenomegaly, as follows.

Massive splenomegaly is caused by:
- Chronic myeloid leukaemia.
- Myelofibrosis.
- Malaria: rarely.
- Kala azar: rarely.

Moderate splenomegaly is caused by all of the above plus:
- Portal hypertension.
- Lymphoproliferative disorders (see above).
- Acute leukaemias.

Just palpable splenomegaly is caused by all of the above plus:
- Infection: infectious mononucleosis, infectious hepatitis, subacute bacterial endocarditis, TB, brucellosis, schistosomiasis.
- Haemolytic anaemias (Chapter 25).
- Immune thrombocytopenias.
- Connective tissue disease: SLE, rheumatoid arthritis.
- Infiltration: amyloid, sarcoid
- Storage disorders: Gaucher's disease.
- Myeloproliferative disorders: polycythaemia rubra vera, essential thrombocythaemia.
- Megaloblastic anaemias (Chapter 25).

HISTORY IN THE PATIENT WITH LYMPHADENOPATHY OR SPLENOMEGALY

It is often not possible to make a diagnosis on the basis of the history in these patients. However, important clues in the history can help to focus the clinical examination and further investigations.

Localized lymphadenopathy
Rate of node enlargement

Lymphadenopathy associated with infection often develops quickly and may be painful. When due to lymphoma or malignancy, the rate of enlargement tends to be slower and can wax and wane in the case of lymphoma.

Sometimes the lymphadenopathy will not be noticed until it becomes large and causes disfigurement or rubs against clothes.

Symptoms in local structures

Has the patient noticed pain, erythema or a mass in

any of the structures draining into the affected node, e.g. cellulitis in inguinal lymphadenopathy or a breast mass in axillary lymphadenopathy?

Systemic symptoms
In lymphoma the patient may experience 'B symptoms' (fever, night sweats, weight loss) and these indicate a poorer prognosis (see p.371).

Generalized lymphadenopathy
A full systemic enquiry is essential in these patients as most of the causes of generalized lymphadeopathy can affect multiple systems. Special attention should be paid to the following:
- Malaise, anorexia and general debility: common but non-specific.
- 'B symptoms': haematological malignancy.
- Skin rash: rubella, SLE and sarcoidosis.
- Arthragia and arthropathy: SLE, rheumatoid arthritis, syphilis (Charcot's joints).
- Infectious contacts: rubella, TB and EBV.
- Risk factors for HIV infection (Chapter 38).
- Drug history: to exclude phenytoin or beryllium as a cause.
- Symptoms of thyrotoxicosis: heat intolerance, weight loss, increased appetite, diarrhoea, irritability.

Splenomegaly
Previous medical history
Is the patient known to have a pre-existing illness that can cause splenomegaly, e.g. chronic liver disease resulting in portal hypertension, connective tissue disease, thalassaemia (haemolysis), Gaucher's disease, or damaged cardiac valves (rheumatic fever or prosthetic valve) with subacute bacterial endocarditis?

Recent travel abroad or infectious contacts
Consider infectious mononucleosis, TB, schistosomiasis, and malaria.

Systemic symptoms
Systemic symptoms suggestive of an underlying cause include arthralgia, rash, and 'B symptoms' (as above).

Symptoms of haematological disturbance
Anaemia may be present due to marrow infiltration, chronic disease, haemolysis, vitamin deficiency, or hypersplenism (Chapter 25). Leucopenia causing

recurrent infections may result from marrow infiltration, hypersplenism, or infection. Thrombocytopenia may be due to immune platelet destruction, marrow infiltration, or hypersplenism (Chapter 23).

EXAMINING THE PATIENT WITH LYMPHADENOPATHY AND SPLENOMEGALY

When lymphadenopathy or splenomegaly are present, a full clinical examination of the lymphatic system should be made. The examination should then focus on possible underlying causes. Fig. 21.1 summarizes this examination approach.

Which lymph nodes are affected? Is there splenomegaly?
Firstly, the extent, sites, sizes, consistency, tenderness, and fixation of enlarged lymph nodes should be

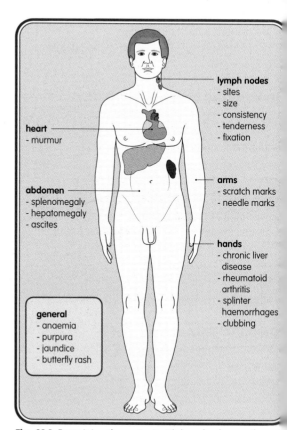

Fig. 21.1 Examining the patient with lymphadenopathy and splenomegaly.

documented. Normal reactive nodes are generally less than 1 cm in diameter, feel soft, are not fixed, and can be tender. Lymphomatous nodes are often larger and feel rubbery, but are not fixed. Lymph nodes infiltrated by carcinoma feel hard and may be fixed to surrounding tissue. Cervical, occipital, supraclavicular, axillary, and inguinal areas should be palpated carefully.

If splenomegaly is present, the size (in cm) from the left costal margin must be recorded.

It is important to distinguish the left kidney from the spleen when palpating a mass in the left hypochondrium and the differences between the two are commonly asked for in examinations (Fig. 21.2).

Is there evidence of an underlying cause?

Anaemia and purpura may be present as described above. Jaundice may result from chronic liver disease, haemolysis, or infective hepatitis. Cachexia heralds underlying malignancy.

Fig. 21.3 summarizes clinical findings that may point to particular diagnoses. Evidence of chronic liver disease, rheumatoid arthritis, and SLE should also be looked for as described in Chapters 10 and 16. Needle marks may indicate previous exposure to HIV and hepatitis B or C, or provide a source of bacteria in infective endocarditis.

Characteristic clinical features which distinguish between the spleen and left kidney	
Spleen	**Left kidney**
no palpable upper border	palpable upper border
not bimanually palpable (not ballottable)	bimanually palpable (ballottable)
notch on medial border	no notch
moves inferomedially on inspiration	moves inferiorly on inspiration
dull to percussion	resonant to percussion (overlying bowel)
occasionally friction rub present	no friction rub

Fig. 21.2 Characteristic clinical features which distinguish between the spleen and left kidney.

Additional clinical features of some conditions presenting with splenomegaly	
Disease	**Clinical features**
portal hypertension	Caput Medusae, venous hum, ascites
infectious mononucleosis	palatal petechiae, tonsillar enlargement, jaundice, tender hepatomegaly, rash
bacterial endocarditis	clubbing, splinter haemorrhages, Osler's nodes, Janeway's lesions, Roth's spots, changing murmurs, haematuria, pyrexia
sarcoidosis	pulmonary infiltrates, lupus pernio, erythema nodosum, scar infiltration, uveitis, conjunctivitis, arthritis, restrictive cardiomyopathy, peripheral neuropathy, pulmonary infiltrates
AA amyloid	hepatomegaly, renal involvement causing nephrotic syndrome (see Chapter 13)
Gaucher's disease	adult type: hepatomegaly, pathological fractures, pigmentation childhood type: mental retardation, spasticity

Fig. 21.3 Additional clinical features of some conditions presenting with splenomegaly.

Localized lymphadenopathy

Examine those structures with lymphatic drainage to the affected nodes. Erythema, increased temperature, and tenderness suggest infection, whilst a hard, non-tender mass may indicate malignancy. When there is isolated cervical lymphadenopathy, a formal ear, nose, and throat examination should also be performed since oropharyngeal malignancies commonly metastasize to these nodes.

Splenomegaly and generalized lymphadenopathy

Where there is both splenomegaly and generalized lymphadenopathy consider lymphoproliferative disorders, infection, connective tissue disease, and sarcoidosis.

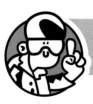

A commonly asked examination question is to palpate a mass in the left hypochondrium. Make sure you can distinguish the left kidney from the enlarged spleen.

INVESTIGATING THE PATIENT WITH LYMPHADENOPATHY AND SPLENOMEGALY

An algorithm for diagnosis of the patient with lymphadenopathy and splenomegaly is given in Fig. 21.4.

Haematology

- A full blood count may show anaemia, leucopenia, thrombocytopenia, or a combination of these.
- Blood film can provide diagnostic information (Fig. 21.5).
- Erythrocyte sedimentation rate will be elevated in infection, malignancy, and inflammation.
- Bone marrow examination includes aspiration, trephine, and cytogenetic analysis. It is indicated if the blood count or film suggest haematological abnormalities, and it is useful in the diagnosis of leukaemias, myeloproliferative disorders, immune thrombocytopenias, and pancytopenia. Occasionally it is helpful in storage diseases, lymphoma, and carcinoma, where there is marrow infiltration.

Biochemistry

- Liver function tests: transaminases will be abnormal in infective hepatitis and sometimes in EBV and CMV; elevation in alkaline phosphatase and γ-glutamyl transpeptidase will occur when the porta hepatis is obstructed by enlarged lymph nodes; unconjugated hyperbilirubinaemia will be present in haemolysis; an elevated lactate dehydrogenase indicates a poor prognosis in lymphoma.
- Serum calcium: raised in malignancy, sarcoidosis, and sometimes lymphoma.
- Serum uric acid: raised when there is rapid cell turnover such as in malignancy.
- Thyroid function tests: thyrotoxicosis.

Infection screen

- Monospot test: EBV.
- Serology: EBV, CMV, HIV (Chapter 38), rubella, hepatitis, toxoplasmosis, and brucellosis.
- Blood cultures: repeated if infective endocarditis is suspected.
- Sputum culture: TB.

Autoantibody screen

This is useful in the detection of connective tissue disorders (Chapter 16).

Imaging

- Chest X-ray: bilateral hilar lymphadenopathy (caused by lymphoma, sarcoidosis, and TB).
- Abdominal ultrasound scan: will confirm the presence of splenomegaly.
- Computed tomography scan of the chest, abdomen and pelvis: gives clear staging information in

A palpable spleen is at least twice its normal size.

malignancy and particularly lymphoma where retroperitoneal lymphadenopathy may often be missed by ultrasound scan.

Histology

The definitive diagnosis of lymphadenopathy is often made on excision biopsy of an affected node.

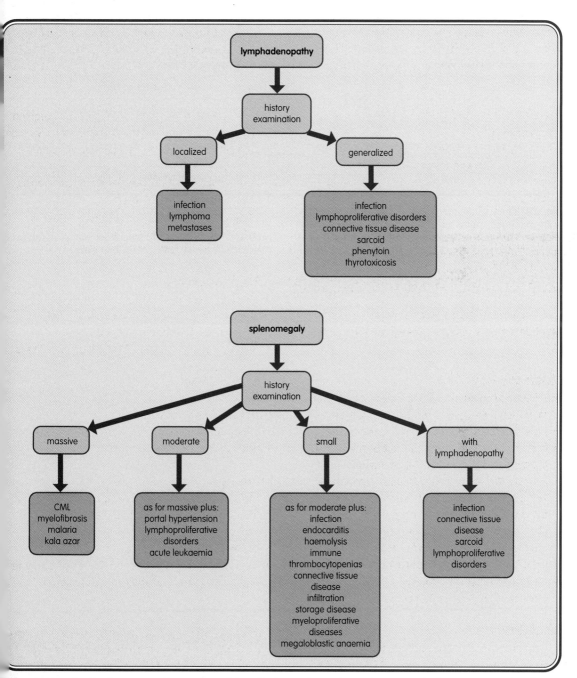

ŋ. 21.4 Algorithm for diagnosis in the patient with lymphadenopathy and ·lenomegaly. (CML, chronic myeloid leukaemia.)

Blood film abnormalities in conditions presenting with lymphadenopathy and splenomegaly	
Disease	**Blood film**
acute leukaemia	circulating blasts (Auer rods in AML)
chronic lymphocytic leukaemia	lymphocytosis, smear cells
chronic myeloid leukaemia	leucocytosis due to spectrum of myeloid cells
myelofibrosis	tear drop poikilocytes, leucoerythroblastic blood film
lymphoma	often normal (occasionally mild eosinophilia in Hodgkin's disease)
haemolysis	reticulocytosis (polychromasia), microspherocytosis, erythroblasts
EBV, infectious hepatitis, toxoplasmosis	atypical lymphocytes
malaria (thick and thin films)	parasitaemia, thrombocytopenia, haemolysis

Fig. 21.5 Blood film abnormalities in conditions presenting with lymphadenopathy and splenomegaly. Many of these disorders may also be associated with a normocytic normochromic anaemia. A leucoerythroblastic film will be seen wherever there is heavy bone marrow involvement. Autoimmune haemolytic anaemia may also arise in lymphoma and chronic lymphocytic leukaemia. (AML, acute myeloid leukaemia; EBV, Epstein–Barr virus.)

22. Sensory and Motor Neurological Deficits

INTRODUCTION

Muscle weakness or abnormal sensation can result from disease occurring anywhere along the pathway from the skin or muscle to the brain and back. Such pathological processes are outlined below.

DIFFERENTIAL DIAGNOSIS OF SENSORY AND/OR MOTOR NEUROLOGICAL DEFICITS

Muscle
- Drugs: steroids, penicillamine, and procainamide.
- Dystrophy: Duchenne, Becker's, limb girdle, and facioscapulohumeral.
- Endocrine: Cushing's syndrome, thyrotoxicosis, myxoedema, and hyperparathyroidism.
- Infection: bacterial (*Clostridium welchii*), viral (influenza), and parasitic (trichinosis).
- Inflammation: polymyositis, dermatomyositis, and sarcoidosis.
- Metabolic: periodic paralyses, McArdle's disease, and mitochondrial myopathy.
- Myotonia: myotonia dystrophica and myotonia congenita (Thomsen's disease).
- Toxin: alcohol.
- Tumour: sarcoma and paraneoplastic syndrome.

Neuromuscular junction
- Myasthenia gravis.
- Lambert–Eaton syndrome.
- *Clostridium botulinum* infection.

Peripheral nerves
Mononeuropathy
In mononeuropathy, only one peripheral nerve is involved. Consider:
- Trauma.
- Entrapment: carpal tunnel syndrome and meralgia paraesthetica.
- Stretching: ulnar nerve lesion if there is an increased carrying angle at the elbow.
- Tumour: neurofibromatosis.

Mononeuritis multiplex
In mononeuritis multiplex, two or more individual nerves are affected. The differential diagnosis includes the following:
- Connective tissue disease: polyarteritis nodosa (PAN), systemic lupus erythematosus (SLE), and rheumatoid arthritis (RA).
- Infection: leprosy, herpes zoster, and human immunodeficiency virus (HIV).
- Inflammation: sarcoid.
- Metabolic: diabetes mellitus (DM) and amyloid.
- Tumour: infiltration, paraneoplastic syndrome, and neurofibromatosis.

Peripheral neuropathy
Peripheral neuropathy is polyneuropathy causing a symmetrical deficit that is most marked distally. The differential diagnosis includes the following:
- Connective tissue disease: PAN, SLE, and RA.
- Drugs: nitrofurantoin, metronidazole, and vincristine.
- Infection: leprosy, HIV, syphilis, and diphtheria.
- Inflammation: Guillain–Barré syndrome.
- Inherited: Charcot–Marie–Tooth disease and Refsum's disease.
- Metabolic: diabetes, renal failure, porphyria, and amyloid.
- Toxins: alcohol and lead.
- Tumour: paraneoplastic syndrome and paraproteinaemias.
- Vitamin deficiency: thiamine (B_1), niacin (B_6), and vitamin B_{12}.

Brachial or lumbar plexus
- Compression: cervical rib.
- Idiopathic: neuralgic amyotrophy.
- Metabolic: DM.
- Trauma: birth injury (Erb's and Klumpke's palsies) and motorbike accidents.
- Tumour: malignant infiltration.

Spinal nerve root
Spinal nerve roots may be disrupted by the following:
- Infection, e.g. pyogenic meningitis and syphilis.
- Prolapsed intervertebral disc.

- Spinal stenosis.
- Spondylosis.
- Tumour.
- Vertebral fracture dislocation.

Anterior horn cell

The anterior horn cell may be damaged by the following:
- Motor neurone disease.
- Poliomyelitis.

The spinal cord

- Degeneration: osteoarthritis.
- Infection: abscess, HIV, tuberculosis (Pott's disease).
- Inflammation: multiple sclerosis (MS), sarcoidosis, rheumatoid arthritis (atlantoaxial subluxation).
- Metabolic: Paget's disease.
- Trauma: including radiotherapy and prolapsed intervertebral disc.
- Tumour: metastases, neurofibroma, meningioma, glioma, and ependymoma.
- Vascular: anterior spinal artery occlusion, dissecting aortic aneurysm, arteriovenous malformation, and vasculitis (PAN).
- Vitamin deficiency: subacute combined degeneration of the cord (vitamin B_{12}).
- Others: syringomyelia, spina bifida, and motor neuron disease.

The cerebellum

- Endocrine: hypothyroidism.
- Hereditary: Friedreich's ataxia and ataxia telangiectasia.
- Infection: abscess and postencephalitis.
- Inflammation: multiple sclerosis.
- Toxic: alcohol, lead, and phenytoin.
- Trauma: 'punch-drunk' syndrome.
- Tumour: metastases, acoustic neuroma, haemangioblastoma (von Hippel–Lindau disease), and paraneoplastic degeneration.
- Vascular: infarction, haematoma, and arteriovenous malformation (AVM).

The cerebral hemispheres

- Degenerative disease: see Chapter 19.
- Hydrocephalus: primary or secondary.
- Infection: abscess, meningitis, encephalitis, HIV, malaria, rabies, tuberculosis, and syphilis.

- Inflammation: sarcoid, SLE, and MS.
- Metabolic: phenylketonuria and Wilson's disease (basal ganglia).
- Toxic: alcohol.
- Trauma.
- Tumour: primary or secondary.
- Vascular: infarction, haemorrhage or haematoma, AVM, and aneurysm.
- Vitamin deficiency: thiamine, niacin, and B_{12}.

Other disorders causing cerebral disturbance, such as carbon dioxide narcosis and hepatic encephalopathy, are discussed in Chapters 15, 18, 19, and 20.

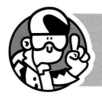

Anxiety can often present with bizarre neurological symptoms.

HISTORY IN THE PATIENT WITH SENSORY AND/OR MOTOR NEUROLOGICAL DEFICITS

It is often a daunting prospect to be faced with a patient with neurological symptoms or signs. However, despite the vast number of potential underlying pathologies, a lesion at a particular point in the pathway between brain and muscle or skin will always produce the same clinical signs regardless of the cause. There are five important aspects to consider in the history.

Onset

Sudden onset usually indicates a vascular problem such as infarction, haemorrhage or haematoma. Lesions due to trauma, MS, abscess, acute prolapsed disc, and myelitis can also develop rapidly. An insidiou onset is more typical of cervical spondylosis, motor neurone disease, neoplasm, myopathy, and syringomyelia.

Precipitants

Trauma may result in muscular and neurological deficits. Acute myasthenia can be precipitated by intercurrent illness (particularly infection), or drugs (aminoglycosides or penicillamine). MS may relapse during the puerperium and symptoms may be exacerbated by exertion, hot weather, or after a hot bath.

Development

Many lesions cause gradually progressive, unremitting disease, including tumour, motor neurone disease, hereditary ataxias, and degenerative brain diseases. Intermittent deficits can be due to transient ischaemic attacks, epilepsy, migraine, and myasthenia gravis. MS is characterized by the development of different lesions which are dissociated in time and site. Symptoms and signs due to trauma or vascular events may slowly improve with time or remain static following the initial event.

Pattern of deficit

Fig. 22.1 summarizes characteristic symptoms and signs which arise as a consequence of a lesion at a specific site. If the neurological abnormalities do not fit a specific pattern, consider MS, motor neurone disease, or paraneoplastic neuropathy.

Evidence of cause

The following factors provide evidence of cause:
- Family history: hereditary ataxias, phenylketonuria, neurofibromatosis.
- Drug history, e.g. phenytoin (cerebellar signs), vincristine (peripheral neuropathy), penicillamine (myasthenia).
- Dietary history: intake of vitamins B_1, B_6 and B_{12}.
- Alcohol history.
- Pre-existing illness, e.g. diabetes, hypertension (cerebrovascular disease), rheumatoid arthritis, or malignancy.
- History of trauma.

EXAMINING THE PATIENT WITH SENSORY AND/OR MOTOR NEUROLOGICAL DEFICITS

When assessing a patient in clinic or hospital, a full neurological examination should be performed (see Chapter 27). However, in medical school examinations you will only be expected to assess a specific part of

Symptoms and signs associated with different anatomical lesions					
Site of anatomical lesion	Symptoms	Specific signs	Muscle	Reflexes	Sensation
muscle	weakness (particularly climbing stairs, getting out of chair) pain (inflammation)	myotonia in myotonia dystrophia calf pseudohypertrophy and Gowers' sign in Duchenne muscular dystrophy	wasting (usually proximal) tone normal or reduced power reduced	normal reduced or absent in severe muscle disease only plantars downgoing	normal
neuromuscular junction	diplopia choking on food altered voice proximal limb weakness	fatiguable weakness on looking upwards or counting to 10	wasting only if severe tone normal power reduction with fatigue	normal	normal
peripheral nerve	muscle weakness sensory disturbance can be purely sensory, purely motor, or mixed	mononeuropathy and mononeuritis multiplex —signs in distribution of affected nerves polyneuropathy—signs symmetrical and distal (glove and stocking)	wasting fasciculation reduced tone reduced power	reduced or absent	deficit of all modalities (glove and stocking distribution)

Fig. 22.1 Symptoms and signs associated with different anatomical lesions (continued over page).

Symptoms and signs associated with different anatomical lesions [cont.]					
Site of anatomical lesion	**Symptoms**	**Specific signs**	**Muscle**	**Reflexes**	**Sensation**
brachial or lumbar plexus	muscle weakness sensory disturbance		wasting fasciculation reduced tone reduced power in distribution affected nerves		deficit in distribution affected nerves
anterior spinal root	muscle weakness		wasting fasciculation reduced tone reduced power in distribution affected root	reduced or absent	normal
posterior spinal root	pain in skin and muscle supplied by that root		normal	reduced or absent	deficit in distribution affected root
anterior horn cell	muscle weakness		wasting fasciculation reduced tone reduced power in distribution affected nerve	reduced or absent	normal
spinal cord	pain at site of lesion worse on coughing, sneezing, at night urinary/bowel disturbance leg weakness sensory disturbance		at level of lesion: wasting, fasciculation, reduced tone, reduced power below lesion: spasticity, increased tone, reduced power	at level of lesion: reduced or absent below lesion: increased, upgoing plantars	below lesion ipsilateral posterior column loss (proprioception, vibration sense) contralateral spinothalamic loss (pain and temperature)
cerebellum	unsteadiness tremor altered speech falls poor coordination	wide-based gait fall to side of lesion intention tremor past-pointing dysdiadochokinesis nystagmus staccato speech	reduced tone no wasting normal power	pendular	normal
cerebral hemispheres	determined by site of lesion (see Chapters 15, 19, and 20) limb weakness seizure altered speech disturbed higher functions	parietal drift dysphasia dysarthria visual disturbance	increased tone clasp-knife rigidity wasting only if disuse reduced power in pyramidal distribution (flexors stronger than extensors in arms, extensors stronger than flexors in legs)	brisk plantars upgoing	deficit determined by site of lesion

Fig. 22.1 (cont.) Symptoms and signs associated with different anatomical lesions.

the system, such as the eyes, face, legs, arms, or gait. The most common neurological short cases are peripheral neuropathy (usually due to DM), Parkinson's disease, stroke, and MS, but be prepared for anything!.

The clinical examination should aim to answer three questions. Firstly, where is the anatomical site of the lesion or lesions? Secondly, is there anything to suggest the underlying pathological process? Finally, what disability does the patient have as a consequence of their neurological deficit?

Where is the lesion?

From the moment you meet the patient, watch like a hawk. How does the patient shake your hand? Can they lift their arm up? Can they let go of your hand (myotonia)? Watch how they undress or get on to the bed. Any severe deficit will often become apparent before you even lay hands on the patient. Examine the area of interest very carefully.

Fig. 22.1 should help you identify where the anatomical lesion is likely to be on the basis of those neurological abnormalities present.

What is the underlying cause?

Once the site of the lesion is identified, think of the differential diagnosis as outlined at the beginning of this chapter. Are there any clues around the patient? Look for diabetic drinks (for peripheral neuropathy or amyotrophy).

If the patient is young, looks well, and is sitting in a wheelchair, MS is the most likely diagnosis. An elderly patient with a hemiparesis is most likely to have had a stroke. Is there a blood pressure chart?

Look at the patient's face for myotonic facies (myotonia dystrophica), Cushing's syndrome (proximal myopathy), or hypothyroidism (myopathy or cerebellar dysfunction). Does the patient have neurofibromatosis (spinal cord or peripheral nerve lesions) or connective tissue disease, such as rheumatoid arthritis (entrapment mononeuropathy, mononeuritis multiplex, or peripheral neuropathy)? Is there a cervical rib?

What disability does the neurological deficit cause?

The most important thing for the patient is not locating the anatomical site of the lesion but what that lesion prevents them from doing.

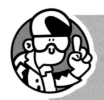

There are two of most parts of the nervous system, so don't forget to compare one side with the other!

This is an important part of the examination and is often missed.

Think what tasks the affected part of the body normally performs, and ask the patient to show you how they manage, such as doing up buttons (for peripheral neuropathy), brushing hair, or standing out of a chair (for proximal myopathy). Watching the patient walk can give useful information (Fig. 22.2).

INVESTIGATING THE PATIENT WITH SENSORY AND/OR MOTOR NEUROLOGICAL DEFICITS

The pathway of investigation is very much determined by findings on the history and clinical examination. The following tests may be useful but each patient will require only those relevant to their presentation:

- Full blood count and erythrocyte sedimentation rate: reactive picture in inflammation, infection, and neoplasm, and raised mean corpuscular volume in vitamin B_{12} deficiency and alcohol abuse.
- Urea and electrolytes: raised urea and creatinine in renal failure, potassium high or low in periodic paralyses.
- Serum calcium: raised in hyperparathyroidism.
- Serum glucose: raised in DM.
- Liver function tests: raised γ-glutamyltransferase in alcohol abuse, raised alkaline phosphatase in Paget's disease, and deranged transamines in metastases, infection, and Wilson's disease.
- Thyroid function tests: hyper- or hypothyroidism.
- Creatine kinase: markedly raised in muscle inflammation and muscular dystrophies.
- Autoantibodies: RA, SLE, and PAN.
- Serology: HIV, herpes, and syphilis where appropriate.
- Immunoglobulins: paraproteinaemias.
- Lumbar puncture: microscopy (infection and malignancy), culture and sensitivity (infection), glucose (reduced in bacterial and tuberculous

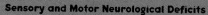
Abnormalities of gait	
Lesion	**Gait**
hemiplegia	foot is plantar flexed; leg is stiff and dragged through a semicircle
spastic paraplegia	legs stiff; walk in 'scissor fashion', like 'walking through mud'
proximal myopathy	waddling gait; trunk moves to swing legs forward; difficulty in climbing stairs or standing out of a chair
Parkinsonism	stooped posture, hesitation in starting, shuffling, festinant, difficulty in turning, poor arm swing and may freeze
cerebellar dysfunction	broad based, ataxic with a tendency to fall to the side of the lesion; unable to walk heel to toe
dorsal column disease	stamping; wide based with patient looking at the ground as unable to sense where foot is; clumsy and slaps feet to ground
foot drop	stepping; legs lifted high off the ground as no dorsiflexion of the foot
musculoskeletal disease	limping; patient avoids weightbearing on affected side due to pain

Fig. 22.2 Abnormalities of gait.

meningitis), protein (markedly raised in tuberculous meningitis, acoustic neuroma, Guillain–Barré syndrome, Behçet's syndrome, and Froin's syndrome), oligoclonal bands (raised in MS and also in SLE, syphilis, sarcoidosis, and Behçet's syndrome), and xanthochromia (yellow cerebrospinal fluid due to haemoglobin breakdown products) indicating recent subarachnoid haemorrhage.

- Electroencephalogram: may indicate structural cerebral pathology and is characteristic in herpes simplex encephalitis.
- Electromyogram: primary muscle disease (typical changes in myotonia and myasthenia); it also shows denervation but not its cause.
- Nerve conduction studies demonstrate peripheral neuropathies.

- Radiology: plain radiographs may demonstrate degenerative and destructive bone lesions and fractures; computed tomography (CT) scanning and magnetic resonance imaging (MRI) of the brain and spine are extremely useful in diagnosing and localizing central lesions; myelography can be useful in demonstrating compressive cord lesions but this technique has been largely superseded by CT scans and MRI.
- Visual evoked potentials: demonstrate previous retrobulbar neuritis in MS.
- Biopsy: if the diagnosis is in doubt, despite history, examination, and non-invasive procedures. Muscle, nerve, and brain biopsies can be performed to give a definitive histological diagnosis.

23. Bleeding and Bruising

INTRODUCTION

Bruising and bleeding arise when there is abnormal haemostasis. Haemostasis is dependent on normal platelet number and function, an intact coagulation pathway, and normal vessel walls.

DIFFERENTIAL DIAGNOSIS OF BLEEDING AND BRUISING

Platelet abnormalities
Platelets may be reduced in number or function.

Thrombocytopenia
- Reduced production: bone marrow failure, drugs (cotrimoxazole), postchemotherapy or postradiotherapy, human immunodeficiency virus (HIV).
- Increased consumption: disseminated intravascular coagulation, thrombotic thrombocytopenic purpura, autoimmune disease, systematic lupus erythematosis (SLE).
- Abnormal distribution: splenic pooling in splenomegaly.
- Dilutional: massive transfusion.

Platelet dysfunction
- Hereditary: Glanzmann's thrombasthenia.
- Acquired: aspirin, heparin, uraemia.

Coagulation abnormalities
Coagulopathies may be due to vitamin K deficiency or specific factor deficiency.

Factor deficiency
Hereditary: haemophilia A (factor VIII), haemophilia B (factor IX), von Willebrand's factor.
Acquired: liver disease.

Vitamin K deficiency
Factors II, VII, IX and X are dependent on vitamin K. Deficiency may be caused by:

- Malabsorption: bowel pathology such as coeliac disease or biliary obstruction (vitamin K is fat-soluble).
- Antagonist drugs: coumarins (warfarin).

Vessel wall abnormalities
Vessel wall abnormalities may be inherited or acquired.

Hereditary
Hereditary haemorrhagic telangiectasia.

Acquired
- Trauma.
- Physiological: senile purpura.
- Drugs: corticosteroids.
- Infections: meningococcal septicaemia.
- Vitamin deficiency: scurvy (vitamin C).
- Connective tissue disease: pseudoxanthoma elasticum, Ehlers–Danlos syndrome.
- Endocrine: Cushing's syndrome.

HISTORY IN THE PATIENT WITH BLEEDING AND BRUISING

The history should focus on three areas. Firstly, what is the pattern and extent of the bleeding and bruising? Secondly, are there any clues as to the possible underlying cause? Finally, have complications occurred?

What is the pattern and extent of bleeding and bruising?
As a general rule:
- Platelet abnormalities (low number or dysfunction) cause skin or mucosal purpura and haemorrhage, with prolonged bleeding following trauma or surgery.
- Vessel wall abnormalities cause petechiae and ecchymoses due to bleeding from small vessels, mostly in the skin, but occasionally in mucous membranes.
- Coagulopathies cause haemarthroses, muscle

haematomas, postoperative or traumatic bleeding, and mucosal bleeding (von Willebrand's disease).

What is the underlying cause?

- bleeding and bruising: 'normal' and related to recent trauma, or due to an underlying haemostatic abnormality.
- Age: senile purpura seen mostly on the upper limbs.
- Abdominal symptoms: coeliac disease, gallstones, liver disease.
- Drug history: aspirin, heparin, warfarin, steroids, previous chemotherapy.
- Family history: haemophilia, hereditary haemorrhagic telangiectasia.
- Symptoms of meningitis: meningococcal sepsis.
- Hyperextensibility of the skin or joints: Ehlers–Danlos syndrome, pseudoxanthoma elasticum.
- Poor diet: scurvy (ecchymoses predominantly on the lower limbs).
- Known acquired immune deficiency syndrome or risk factors for HIV infection.

Have complications occurred?

- Symptoms of anaemia (Chapter 25).
- Symptoms of shock.
- Muscle pain or mass.
- Joint pain or deformity.

EXAMINING THE PATIENT WITH BLEEDING AND BRUISING

The examination should be approached in a similar manner to the history. Fig. 23.1 summarizes the examination approach.

What is the pattern and extent of bleeding and bruising?

The sites and types of lesions should be documented (see above). 'Purpura' includes petechiae (small pinpoint bleeds into the skin) and ecchymoses (small bruises).

How severe has the bleeding been?

Shock should be looked for urgently in the sick patient by measuring pulse and blood pressure; signs of anaemia should also be sought (Chapter 25). Finally, look for joint deformities or a mass in muscle.

Are there signs suggestive of specific diseases?

- Signs of liver disease (Chapter 10).
- Splenomegaly (whatever cause): platelet pooling.
- Cushingoid appearance: steroid therapy, endocrinopathy.
- Hereditary haemorrhagic telangiectasia: characteristic petechiae on the tongue and lips.
- Meningism (Chapter 15).
- Scurvy: corkscrew hairs with hyperkeratosis of the follicles, perifollicular haemorrhages, gum hypertrophy, poor wound healing.
- Ehlers–Danlos syndrome: hyperextensible skin and joints, 'fish-mouth' wounds, pseudotumours over the elbows and knees.

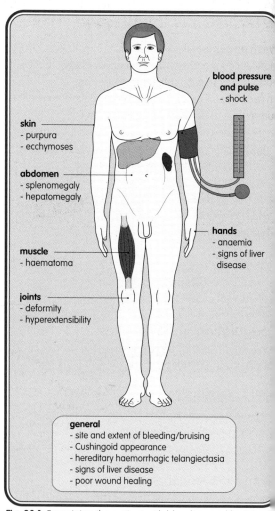

blood pressure and pulse
- shock

skin
- purpura
- ecchymoses

abdomen
- splenomegaly
- hepatomegaly

hands
- anaemia
- signs of liver disease

muscle
- haematoma

joints
- deformity
- hyperextensibility

general
- site and extent of bleeding/bruising
- Cushingoid appearance
- hereditary haemorrhagic telangiectasia
- signs of liver disease
- poor wound healing

Fig. 23.1 Examining the patient with bleeding and bruising.

Thrombocytopenic purpura and vasculitic purpura may look identical but the lesions in the latter are usually raised and may be tender.

- Pseudoxanthoma elasticum: loose skin in neck, axillae, anticubital fossae and groins, 'chicken skin', blue sclera, angioid streaks in the retina, hyperextensible joints.

INVESTIGATING THE PATIENT WITH BLEEDING AND BRUISING

When an abnormality of haemostasis is suspected, a platelet count and simple coagulation assays should be performed. More specific tests to diagnose the underlying cause can then be considered. Fig. 23.2 summarizes the normal coagulation pathway.

An algorithm for investigating the patient with bleeding and bruising is given in Fig. 23.3.

Platelet count
If thrombocytopenia is present, request a blood film (exclude artefactual result due to platelet clumping, look for acute leukaemia or disseminated intravascular coagulation) and bone marrow aspirate (increased megakaryocytes in consumptive thrombocytopenia e.g. idiopathic thrombocytopenic purpura or reduced megakaryocytes in bone marrow failure).

Prothrombin time
Prothrombin time measures the extrinsic system (VII) and common pathway (X, V, prothrombin, and fibrinogen). It is prolonged in liver disease and warfarin therapy, and is generally expressed as international normalized ratio (INR).

Activated partial thromboplastin time or kaolin–cephalin clotting time
This measures the intrinsic system (XII, XI, IX, and VIII) and common pathway (X, V, prothrombin, and fibrinogen). It is prolonged in heparin therapy, factor

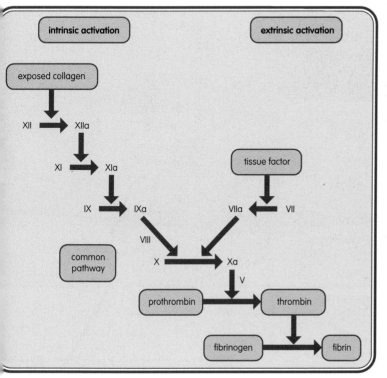

Fig. 23.2 The normal coagulation pathway.

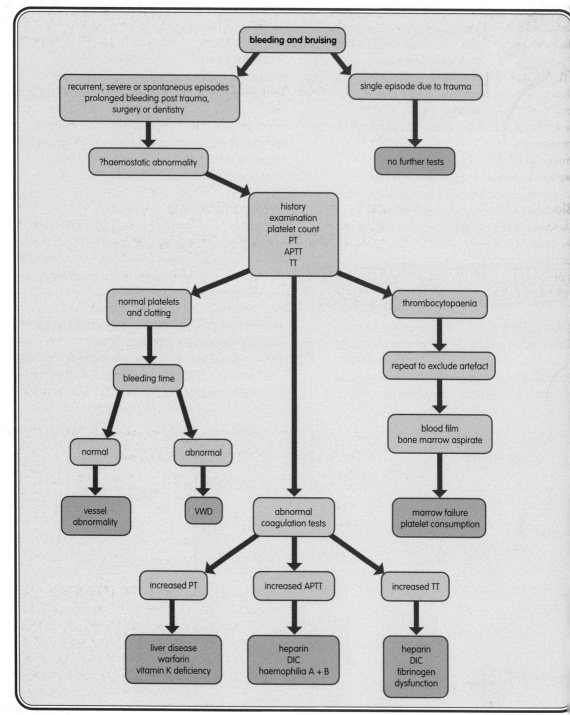

Fig. 23.3 Algorithm for investigating the patient with bruising or bleeding. (APTT, activated partial thromboplastin time; DIC, disseminated intravascular coagulation; PT, prothrombin time; TT, thrombin time; VWD, von Willebrand's disease.)

deficiency such as factor VIII (haemophilia A) and factor IX (haemophilia B, Christmas disease) and disseminated intravascular coagulation.

Thrombin time

Thrombin time measures the activity of thrombin and fibrinogen in the common pathway. It is prolonged in fibrinogen deficiency (disseminated intravascular coagulation) or fibrinogen dysfunction. Prolonged thrombin time may also result from heparin therapy (inhibition of thrombin activity).

Bleeding time (rarely performed)

Bleeding time measures platelet function. It is only performed if platelet count, coagulation screening tests (as above), blood film, and bone marrow are normal. It is prolonged in aspirin therapy, uraemia, and von Willebrand's disease.

Fibrin degradation products and D-dimers

Fibrin degradation products and D-dimers will be elevated in disseminated intravascular coagulation.

Other tests

Other specific tests are also available with haematological advice. These include specific factor assays, von Willebrand's factor, and ristocetin-induced platelet aggregation.

Tests for other diseases given in the differential diagnosis list should be performed as indicated from the history, examination, and basic laboratory tests.

24. Vertigo and Dizziness

INTRODUCTION

True vertigo is the false perception (illusion) of movement, usually rotational, of a patient or of his or her surroundings. This is often accompanied by vomiting, sweating, and pallor. It results from either disease in the labyrinth (most common cause), the 8th cranial nerve, or its connections in the brainstem.

Dizziness or unsteadiness without vertigo can result from a variety of unrelated disorders. These are discussed in more detail in their appropriate chapters.

DIFFERENTIAL DIAGNOSIS IN THE PATIENT WITH VERTIGO OR DIZZINESS

Vertigo

The differential diagnosis in the patient with vertigo includes labyrinth disorders, 8th cranial nerve disease, or brainstem lesions.

Labyrinth disorders
- Middle ear disease, e.g. otitis media.
- Ménière's disease.
- Benign positional vertigo.
- Labyrinthitis.
- Traumatic vertigo.
- Perilymphatic fistula.
- Syphilitic labyrinthitis.

8th cranial nerve disease
- Vestibular neuronitis.
- Acoustic neuroma.
- Ramsay Hunt syndrome: herpes zoster of the geniculate ganglion.
- Ototoxic drugs: aminoglycosides such as gentamicin.

Brainstem lesions
- Multiple sclerosis: demyelination.
- Vertebrobasilar ischaemia: transient ischaemic attack.
- Stoke: lateral medullary syndrome (infraction of interior cerebellar artery).

When a patient presents with 'vertigo' or 'dizziness', it is vital to establish whether true vertigo is present or not, as these symptoms result from different pathologies.

- Vertebrobasilar insufficiency.
- Migraine.
- Encephalitis.
- Tumour.
- Syringobulbia.
- Alcohol abuse.

Note that vertigo may also be a feature of temporal lobe pathology.

Dizziness
- Low cardiac output (Chapter 18).
- Hyperventilation, anxiety.
- Anaemia.
- Hypoglycaemia.
- Phaeochromocytoma.
- Postural hypotension due to drugs, e.g. overenthusiastic antihypertensive regimes, antidepressants, tranquilizers.
- Visual disturbance.
- Cerebrovascular disease.
- Pyrexia.

HISTORY IN THE PATIENT WITH VERTIGO

The diagnosis in patients with vertigo is largely made on the history. It is important to ellicit the time course of the vertigo and the likely site of the lesion by asking about other auditory and neurological symptoms. Typical features of specific diseases are shown in Fig. 24.1.

Characteristic features of diseases causing vertigo					
Disease	**Cause**	**Length of vertigo**	**Aural symptoms**	**Neurological symptoms**	**Natural history**
Ménière's disease	excess endolymphatic fluid (hydrops)	1–8 hours often preceded by sensation of fullness in the ear	fluctuating but progressive deafness tinnitus	none	episodic attacks unilateral at first becomes bilateral in 25% ceases when deafness complete
vestibular neuronitis	possibly viral	days to weeks explosive onset	none	none	spontaneously resolves in weeks
benign positional vertigo	degeneration of utricular neuroendothelium can follow head injury and vestibular neuronitis	seconds precipitated by changes in head position	none	none	episodic attacks spontaneous resolution over weeks to months
perilymphatic fistula	rupture of round window membrane often due to barotrauma can be spontaneous	months to years	deafness and tinnitus	none	often resolves with bed rest can be surgically repaired
vertebrobasilar insufficiency	'nipping' of vertebral arteries by osteophytic cervical vertebrae	seconds precipitated by neck extension or rotation	none	dysarthria diplopia visual loss syncope	episodic attacks
acoustic neuroma	schwannoma of vestibular nerve	gradual onset progressive	unilateral deafness and tinnitus	5th and 7th cranial nerve palsies ipsilateral cerebellar signs	symptoms progress until surgical removal
central lesions	tumour demyelination vascular migraine	develops gradually unremitting	often spared	usually present and dependent on site of lesion	symptoms progress until underlying cause treated

Fig. 24.1 Characteristic features of diseases causing vertigo.

Pattern of vertigo

The following should be established:

- Onset: peripheral lesions generally cause acute severe symptoms; central lesions tend to cause a gradual onset with less severe vertigo.
- Duration of vertigo .
- Recurrent episodes or a single attack?
- Relation to head position.

Aural symptoms

The presence of aural symptoms suggests that the lesion is peripheral, involving the labyrinth or 8th cranial nerve:

- Ear pain.
- Ear discharge.
- Deafness (fluctuating or progressive).
- Tinnitus.

Neurological symptoms

The following symptoms suggest central pathology or acoustic neuroma.

- Facial weakness.
- Dysarthria.
- Dysphagia.
- Diplopia.
- Loss of consciousness.
- Seizures.
- Weakness, altered sensation, poor limb coordination.

History suggestive of an underlying caus

- Recent viral illness causes vestibular neuronitis.
- Previous head injury may lead to labyrinth concussion, benign positional vertigo.

- Previous otological surgery.
- Drug history, e.g. aminoglycosides.
- Risk factors for vascular disease: hypertension, high cholesterol, smoking, family history.
- Recent flying or diving, e.g. barotrauma—perilymphatic fistula.

EXAMINING THE PATIENT WITH VERTIGO

he clinical examination is often normal. The following pecific abnormalities should be looked for carefully:

- Nystagmus: horizontal and away (fast phase) from the side of the lesion. Occasionally, brainstem lesions may also cause vertical nystagmus.
- Romberg's sign: positive if the patient is more unsteady on standing when the eyes are closed compared with when they are open; in vestibular disorders. The patient will tend to fall to the side of the lesion.
- Hallpike's manoeuvre: the patient is asked to lay down quickly with their head tilted to one side; in benign positional vertigo there will be a latent period of a few seconds followed by nystagmus.

Focal neurological signs: if present, these suggest a central lesion, acoustic neuroma, or Ramsay Hunt syndrome. Pay particular attention to assessment of the 8th cranial nerve, gait, and cerebellar signs.

Eyes: papilloedema (tumour with raised intracranial pressure), optic atrophy (demyelination), and ophthalmoplegia (cranial nerve defect, demyelination).

Ears: otoscopy may reveal otitis media or a herpetic rash. Herpetic lesions may also be found on careful examination of the surrounding skin.

Lying and standing blood pressures: postural hypotension.

j. 24.2 summarizes the examination approach.

INVESTIGATING THE PATIENT WITH VERTIGO

Audiometry: to distinguish between conductive and sensorineural deafness.

Caloric tests: normally, running cold and then warm

water into the external auditory meatus causes contralateral and then ipsilateral nystagmus, respectively; where there is pathology in the ipsilateral labyrinth, 8th cranial nerve, or brainstem, this normal response will be reduced or absent.

- Electronystagmography: a more accurate assessment of the presence and type of nystagmus.
- Imaging: high-resolution computed tomography scanning and magnetic resonance imaging are useful tools when a central lesion or acoustic neuroma are suspected.

An algorithm for approaching the diagnosis in the patient with vertigo is given in Fig. 24.3.

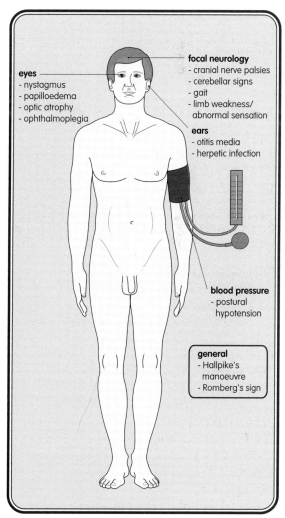

Fig. 24.2 Examining the patient with vertigo.

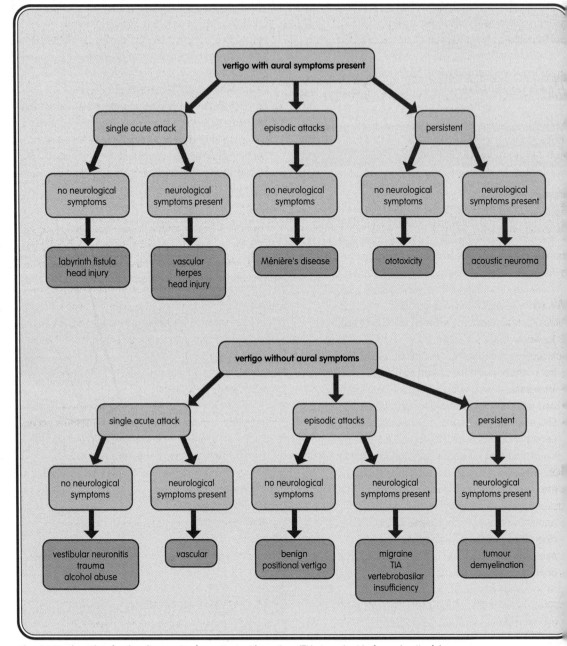

Fig. 24.3 Algorithm for the diagnosis of a patient with vertigo. (TIA, transient ischaemic attack.)

25. Anaemia

A patient is anaemic when the haemoglobin concentration in the blood is less than 13.5 g/dL in men and 11.5 g/dL in women.

DIFFERENTIAL DIAGNOSIS OF ANAEMIA

The size of the red blood cells gives important clues as to the likely underlying abnormality.

Microcytic red blood cells

Microcytic RBCs have a mean cell volume of less than 80 fL; where fL stands for femtolitre (= 10^{-15} L). Causes include:

- Iron-deficiency anaemia (Fig. 25.1).
- Thalassaemia.
- Anaemia of chronic disease (Fig. 25.2).
- Sideroblastic anaemia.
- Lead poisoning.

Normocytic red blood cells

Normocytic RBCs have a mean cell volume of 80–95 fL. Causes include:

- Anaemia of chronic disease (Fig. 25.2).
- Haemolysis (Fig. 25.3).
- Acute blood loss.
- Bone marrow hypoplasia.

Macrocytic red blood cells

Macrocytic RBCs have a mean cell volume of more than 95 fL. Causes include:

- Megaloblastic anaemia: folate deficiency (Fig. 25.4), vitamin B_{12} deficiency (Fig. 25.5).
- Normoblastic anaemia: alcohol, liver disease, hypothyroidism, pregnancy, reticulocytosis.

HISTORY IN THE ANAEMIC PATIENT

It is important to establish first how symptomatic the patient is of their anaemia. The history should then focus on whether any complications of anaemia are present and whether there are any clues as to the likely underlying diagnosis.

Symptoms of anaemia

When anaemia develops over a long time, the haemoglobin can be very low before symptoms occur. Anaemia is tolerated less well in the elderly. The following symptoms may present:

- Asymptomatic: particularly if the anaemia develops over a long time.
- Lethargy.
- Shortness of breath: most marked on exertion.
- Lightheadedness.
- Palpitations.

Causes of iron-deficiency anaemia	
Mechanism	Examples
reduced iron intake	poor diet malabsorption (gastrectomy, coeliac disease)
increased iron utilization	infancy, adolescence, pregnancy
abnormal iron loss	chronic bleeding from gastrointestinal tract, uterus, urinary tract

Fig. 25.1 Causes of iron-deficiency anaemia.

Causes of anaemia of chronic disease	
Mechanism	Examples
malignancy	breast, prostate, lung
inflammation	rheumatoid arthritis, temporal arteritis
chronic infection	tuberculosis, subacute bacterial endocarditis

Fig. 25.2 Causes of anaemia of chronic disease.

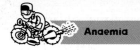

Causes of haemolytic anaemia		
	Mechanism	**Examples**
intrinsic	red blood cell membrane defects	hereditary spherocytosis hereditary elliptocytosis
	enzyme deficiencies	glucose-6-phosphate dehydrogenase deficiency pyruvate kinase deficiency
	abnormal haemoglobin	thalassaemia sickle cell disease
extrinsic	immune	ABO incompatibility (blood transfusion) haemolytic disease of the newborn autoimmune (warm): idiopathic, lymphoma, CLL, SLE, methyldopa autoimmune (cold): idiopathic, lymphoma, mycoplasma, Epstein–Barr virus drugs
	non-immune	mechanical heart valves burns malaria microangiopathic (DIC, TTP, pre-eclampsia) paroxysmal nocturnal haemoglobinuria hepatic or renal disease

Fig. 25.3 Causes of haemolytic anaemia. (CLL, chronic lymphocytic leukaemia; DIC, disseminated intravascular coagulation; SLE, systemic lupus erythematosus; TTP, thrombotic thrombocytopenic purpura.)

Causes of folate deficiency	
Mechanism	**Examples**
reduced intake	poor diet, e.g. old age, poverty, alcoholics
reduced absorption	coeliac disease, extensive Crohn's disease, tropical sprue, gastrectomy
increased utilization	physiological, e.g. pregnancy, lactation, prematurity increased cell turnover, e.g. malignancy, chronic inflammation, haemolysis, dialysis
drugs	trimethoprim, sulphasalazine, anticonvulsants, methotrexate

Fig. 25.4 Causes of folate deficiency.

Causes of vitamin B_{12} deficiency	
Mechanism	**Examples**
reduced intake	vegans
reduced absorption	stomach, e.g. gastrectomy, pernicious anaemia small intestine, e.g. Crohn's disease, ileal resection, ileal TB or UC
increased utilization	blind loop syndrome (bacterial overgrowth), fish tapeworm (*Diphyllobothrium latum*)
abnormal metabolism	transcobalamin II deficiency (autosomal recessive)
drugs	nitrous oxide, metformin

Fig. 25.5 Causes of vitamin B_{12} deficiency. (TB, tuberculosis; UC, ulcerative colitis)

Symptoms of complications

- Symptoms of cardiac failure (Chapters 1 and 2).
- Angina.
- Ischaemic claudication.
- Visual disturbance due to retinal haemorrhage: very rare—the anaemia must be severe.

Evidence to suggest underlying cause

- Specific symptoms: menorrhagia, change in bowel habit, dyspepsia, weight loss, headache.
- Pre-existing illness: rheumatoid arthritis, previous abdominal surgery, dialysis.
- Family history: haemolytic anaemia.
- Drug history: salicylates (iron deficiency), anticonvulsants (folate deficiency).
- Diet: vegans (vitamin B_{12} deficiency), alcoholics (folate deficiency).
- Pica (craving for specific and often bizarre foods): iron deficiency.
- Pregnancy: folate deficiency.

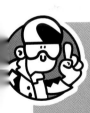

Dysphagia plus iron-deficiency anaemia: think of Plummer–Vinson or Paterson–Brown–Kelly syndrome (postcricoid oesophageal web).

EXAMINING THE ANAEMIC PATIENT

Signs of anaemia and its consequences

Fig. 25.6 summarizes the examination approach. The following signs of anaemia should be noted:

- Pallor: mucous membranes (mouth and conjunctivae), nails, skin creases.
- Hyperdynamic circulation: tachycardia, collapsing pulse, systolic flow murmur.
- Cardiac failure.
- Retinal haemorrhages.

Signs of underlying disease

A full general examination should always be performed, including breast examination and rectal examination in iron deficiency. Specific abnormalities include the following:

- Glossitis: megaloblastic anaemia, iron deficiency.
- Angular stomatitis: koilonychia, iron deficiency.
- Jaundice: haemolysis, megaloblastic anaemia (mild).
- Splenomegaly: haemolysis, megaloblastic anaemia (Chapter 21).
- Leg ulcers: sickle cell disease.
- Bone deformities: thalassaemia.
- Peripheral neuropathy, optic atrophy, subacute combined degeneration of the cord, dementia are all neurological sequelae of vitamin B_{12} deficiency.
- Blue line on the gums (Burton's line), peripheral motor neuropathy, encephalopathy are seen in lead poisoning.

Note the racial origin of the patient as thalassaemia is more common in people from South-East Asia and China, while sickle cell anaemia is more common among Africans.

INVESTIGATING THE ANAEMIC PATIENT

General investigations
Full blood count

- Haemoglobin: anaemia.
- Mean corpuscular volume: underlying pathologies.
- White cell count: if low, consider general bone marrow failure; if high, consider infection, inflammation or malignancy.
- Platelet count: if low, consider general bone marrow failure; if high, consider infection, inflammation or malignancy.

Erythrocyte sedimentation rate

The erythrocyte sedimentation rate will be raised in infection, inflammation, or malignancy.

Reticulocyte count

Reticulocytes are young erythrocytes that normally constitute only 0.5–2.0% of circulating RBCs. The reticulocyte count is increased if RBC production is increased and red cells are prematurely released into

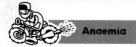
the circulation. This occurs following haemorrhage, in chronic haemolysis, or with vitamin B_{12}, folate, or iron replacement, when there has been a deficiency.

Blood film

The blood film can provide diagnostic information as shown in Fig. 25.7.

Bone marrow

- Not necessary when the diagnosis is obvious, e.g. iron deficiency.
- Bone marrow aspirate gives information regarding the development of different cell lines, the proportion

of these different cell lines, infiltration by abnormal cells (e.g. infiltration with metastatic carcinoma), and the presence of iron stores.

- Bone marrow trephine provides structural information regarding bone marrow architecture and infiltration.

Specific investigations

All patients with anaemia should have measurement of serum ferritin, vitamin B_{12}, and RBC folate, as more than one deficiency can occur at the same time. An algorithm is presented in Fig. 25.8 for the diagnosis of anaemia.

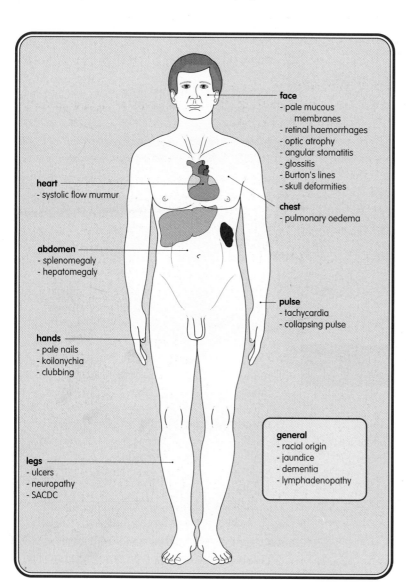

Fig. 25.6 Examining the anaemic patient. (SACDC, subacute combined degeneration of the cord.)

face
- pale mucous membranes
- retinal haemorrhages
- optic atrophy
- angular stomatitis
- glossitis
- Burton's lines
- skull deformities

heart
- systolic flow murmur

chest
- pulmonary oedema

abdomen
- splenomegaly
- hepatomegaly

pulse
- tachycardia
- collapsing pulse

hands
- pale nails
- koilonychia
- clubbing

general
- racial origin
- jaundice
- dementia
- lymphadenopathy

legs
- ulcers
- neuropathy
- SACDC

Abnormalities on the blood film in anaemia	
Abnormality	**Changes on blood film**
iron deficiency	hypochromic, microcytic RBCs, target cells, pencil cells, poikilocytosis (variation in RBC shape), anisocytosis (variation in RBC size), often thrombocytosis
vitamin B_{12}/folate deficiency	oval-shaped macrocytosis, neutrophil nuclei hypersegmented (greater than six lobes), poikilocytosis; white blood cell and platelet count may be low
haemolysis	reticulocytosis, microspherocytes, erythroblasts many spherocytes in hereditary spherocytosis elliptocytes in hereditary elliptocytosis
thalassaemia	hypochromic, microcytic RBCs, basophilic stippling, target cells, reticulocytosis
sickle cell disease	sickle cells, target cells features of hyposplenism in adults (Howell–Jolly bodies, Pappenheimer bodies, target cells)
anaemia of chronic disease	normochromic, normocytic RBCs neutrophilia and thrombocytosis may be present
liver disease	macrocytic RBCs, target cells features of iron deficiency and folate deficiency may also be present

Fig. 25.7 Abnormalities on the blood film in anaemia. (RBCs, red blood cells)

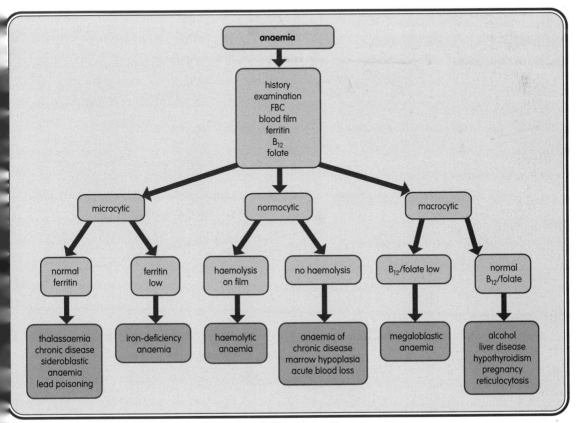

Fig. 25.8 Algorithm for the diagnosis of anaemia. (FBC, full blood count.)

Iron deficiency

- Serum ferritin: low in iron deficiency but raised in iron overload, haemochromatosis and anaemia of chronic disease (occasionally).
- Serum iron: low.
- Total iron-binding capacity: increased.
- Menorrhagia or pregnancy: no further investigations are necessary.
- If no menorrhagia or pregnancy: consider upper gastrointestinal endoscopy, rectal examination, and sigmoidoscopy with colonoscopy or barium enema.
- No obvious cause: consider mesenteric angiogram for angiodysplasia.

Vitamin B_{12} deficiency

- Serum vitamin B_{12}: low.
- Bilirubin: mildly raised—intramedullary destruction of abnormal RBCs.
- Lactate dehydrogenase (LDH): elevated—intramedullary destruction of abnormal RBCs.
- Gastric parietal antibodies: positive in 90% of patients with pernicious anaemia.
- Intrinsic factor antibodies: positive in approximately 50% of patients with pernicious anaemia.
- Schilling test: the patient is given a loading dose of 1000 mg vitamin B_{12} intramuscularly, followed by a small oral dose of radioactive vitamin B_{12}, and excretion is then measured in the urine; vitamin B_{12} malabsorption is corrected by giving intrinsic factor with labelled vitamin in pernicious anaemia, but persists despite the use of intrinsic factor in intestinal disease.
- Endoscopy or barium meal and follow through: may be necessary in underlying intestinal disease.

Folate deficiency

- RBC folate: more reliable than serum folate.
- Bilirubin: mildly raised—intramedullary destruction of abnormal RBCs.

- LDH: elevated—intramedullary destruction of abnormal RBCs.
- Tests for intestinal malabsorption: including jejunal biopsy, may be necessary when the diagnosis is not clear.

Haemolysis

- Serum bilirubin: raised and unconjugated.
- Serum haptoglobins: reduced or absent.
- Faecal stercobilinogen: raised.
- Urinary urobilinogen: raised.
- Reticulocyte count: raised.
- Haemoglobin electrophoresis: abnormal in thalassaemia and sickle cell disease.
- Coombs' test: positive in autoimmune haemolytic anaemias.
- Osmotic fragility: increased if spherocytes are present.
- Enzyme assays: available in specialist centres only for glucose-6-phosphate dehydrogenase and pyruvate kinase deficiencies.
- Ham's test: positive in paroxysmal nocturnal haemoglobinuria.

Anaemia of chronic disease

- Ferritin: high (ferritin is an acute phase protein).
- Serum iron: low.
- Total iron-binding capacity: low.
- Serum vitamin B_{12}: normal.
- RBC folate: normal.

Other investigations should be directed by the clinical scenario. Consider erythrocyte sedimentation rate, C-reactive protein, autoantibody screen, sepsis screen, and search for occult malignancy.

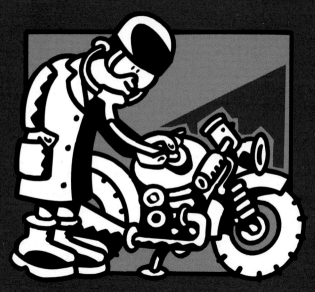

HISTORY, EXAMINATION, AND COMMON INVESTIGATIONS

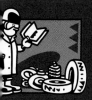

26. Taking a History

GENERAL PRINCIPLES—THE BEDSIDE MANNER

From the first meeting, a patient decides whether or not they think the doctor is trustworthy, based on the doctor's general manner and attitude. Mutual trust is the foundation of the good doctor–patient relationship.

There is no easy recipe for developing a good bedside manner but courtesy, patience, and letting the patient express their ideas, concerns, and expectations are essential ingredients.

Whenever you meet a patient, introduce yourself politely and do not forget relatives or friends who might also be present. Try to put the patient at ease, as visiting the doctor is very stressful for most people, particularly if they think that they have a serious illness. If you cannot speak the same language, try to get an interpreter. If a patient cannot hear you, do not assume they have dementia, but speak louder! Remember that the history is still the most useful tool the clinician has.

The aims of the history are as follows:

- To establish rapport with the patient.
- To obtain an accurate, sequential account of the patient's symptoms and create a differential diagnosis.
- To ask specific questions to focus on the most likely diagnoses.
- To determine risk factors for these possible diagnoses.
- To assess whether complications have occurred on the basis of associated symptoms.
- To put this problem or problems into the context of the patient's life.

We have outlined a standard approach to obtaining the history. However, the important thing is that you develop an approach with which you are comfortable and then practise it again and again. In this way you will not miss things out and you will be able to concentrate more on what the patient is telling you rather than what comes next.

Watch the patient closely, as facial expression and body posture can sometimes tell you more than the words themselves. If you are looking up, they will also feel that you are genuinely listening to what they are saying. It is important to strike a good balance between recording the history accurately and maintaining eye contact.

As a general principle, start the consultation by asking very open-ended questions, such as 'How are you?' or 'What symptoms have made you come to the clinic today?'. This gives the patient the opportunity to say what they want. Then ask more specific questions to clarify important aspects.

THE HISTORY

At the start of every history you should always:

- Document the date, time, and place of consultation. (Remember that the clerking is a legal document.)
- Record the age, sex, and occupation of the patient.
- Document who referred the patient and if they were seen as an emergency.

PRESENTING COMPLAINT

This should be a single sentence that concisely summarizes the main symptom(s) and the length of time they have been present, e.g. a 2-hour history of crushing retrosternal chest pain, or a 6-month history of alternating constipation and diarrhoea with a 4-month history of weight loss of 2 stone.

Resist the temptation to write the entire history in this section, particularly when there are multiple symptoms.

HISTORY OF PRESENTING COMPLAINT

Ask when the patient first had this symptom and what has happened since then. Make sure that you establish the following details.

Onset and offset

Find out whether or not the symptom came on suddenly or gradually, and discover what the patient was doing at the time. For example, chest pain on walking up a hill is likely to be angina, syncope on tilting the head upwards is likely to due to be vertebrobasilar insufficiency, etc.

As for the offset, did the complaint resolve gradually or quickly?

Duration

Find out whether the complaint is still present. If not, then how long did it last?

Relieving/exacerbating factors

These are particularly important in describing pain.

Associated symptoms

Did the patient notice anything else at the time? For example, sweating, clamminess, and vomiting, in association with cardiac chest pain, is usually seen in myocardial infarction rather than angina alone.

Pattern

Was the symptom a solitary event or a recurrent problem? Did it come on suddenly, and is it gradually settling? Is it getting progressively worse?

Note that the patient may often use medical terms to explain what has happened to them, so take time to ask what he or she actually means, e.g. when the term 'vertigo' is used it might actually mean true vertigo, lightheadedness, or unsteadiness of gait, which have very different underlying aetiologies.

It is often useful to list the risk factors for the likely diagnosis at the end of this section.

PREVIOUS MEDICAL HISTORY

Ask the patient if they have had any previous operations or medical problems. It is prudent to probe a little about each illness and how the diagnosis was made. Record the history in chronological order and, where possible, record the year, hospital and consultant involved (where appropriate) for each episode. Many patients may forget past illnesses, particularly if anxious, and it is worth asking them specifically about diabetes, hypertension, angina or heart disease, rheumatic fever, tuberculosis, epilepsy, asthma, jaundice, stroke, or transient ischaemic attacks.

SYSTEMS REVIEW

Patients occasionally focus on one minor symptom while omitting to tell you of another more significant symptom. In fact, this can be a deliberate act, asking the doctor to deal with a simple problem e.g. sore throat, while deciding whether to ask for help with the real worry such as impotence or chest pain. Performing a quick systems review will prevent you from missing other important diseases. The symptoms to ask about in each system are outlined below.

General symptoms
Fatigue

This is a non-specific symptom which can accompany many organic as well as psychiatric diseases. Look particularly for evidence of anaemia or hypothyroidism.

Appetite

Anorexia is a feature of many diseases, again organic and psychiatric; increased appetite despite weight loss is seen in hyperthyroidism.

Weight changes
Weight loss

Weight loss can be deliberate (dieting) or due to chronic disease. The causes are discussed in detail in Chapter 9.

Weight gain

Weight gain is seen in pregnancy, hypothyroidism, Cushing's syndrome, polycystic ovarian disease and 'comfort eating' due to anxiety or depression.

Sweats

Drenching sweats occurring at night are seen in lymphoma, chronic leukaemia, and tuberculosis. Sweats at any time of the day are a feature of the menopause.

Pruritus (itching)

Pruritus can be due to local skin disease or systemic disease as shown in Fig. 26.1.

Sleep pattern

If there is difficulty in sleeping, ask if the problem is in going to sleep or in waking early. Difficulty in getting off to sleep is often due to worry or anxiety, whereas early morning wakening is a feature of depression.

Cardiovascular symptoms
Chest pain
Establish the site, radiation, character, exacerbating and relieving factors, and severity discussed in detail in Chapter 1.

Dyspnoea
Exertional dyspnoea can be due to poor left ventricular function, pulmonary oedema, arrhythmia, or valvular disease.

Orthopnoea is breathlessness on lying flat (pulmonary venous congestion). Note that this symptom can be present in chronic obstructive airways disease, as diaphragmatic respiration is less efficient when the patient is lying flat.

Paroxysmal nocturnal dyspnoea is waking during the night due to severe breathlessness (pulmonary oedema).

Sudden onset of breathlessness, irrespective of body position or exercise, is often due to arrhythmia. See Chapter 2 for more information.

Syncope
Syncope is the transient loss of consciousness and motor tone, which may be due to arrhythmia, valvular heart disease, postural hypotension, or vertebrobasilar insufficiency (Chapter 18).

Palpitations
Ask the patient to tap out the rhythm (Chapter 3). Is the beat fast or slow, regular or irregular?

Causes of pruritus	
Cause	**Examples**
skin disease	scabies, eczema, lichen planus, urticaria, dry skin (elderly, hypothyroidism)
systemic disease	hepatic (biliary obstruction, pregnancy) malignancy (particularly lymphoma) haematological (polycythaemia, iron deficiency) chronic renal failure drugs (sensitivity, opiates) endocrine (diabetes mellitus, hyper/hypothyroidism, carcinoid syndrome) parasitic (trichinosis) neurological (multiple sclerosis) psychogenic

Fig. 26.1 Causes of pruritus.

Ankle swelling
This can be due to right ventricular failure, drugs (e.g. Ca^{2+} channel blockers), or it can be gravitational.

Calf swelling
This can be due to:
- Deep vein thrombosis: recent travel, immobility or surgery, pregnancy, combined oral contraceptive pill, family history, malignancy.
- Ruptured Baker's cyst: in elderly, secondary to osteoarthritis of the knee.
- Muscle trauma.
- Cellulitis.
- Tumour: sarcoma (rare).

Claudication
Intermittent claudication due to peripheral vascular disease causes calf, thigh, or buttock pain on exercise. The amount of exercise required to cause pain tends to be consistent although it often deteriorates slowly. It is relieved within a predictable period of time on rest.

Spinal claudication due to spinal stenosis also causes calf, thigh, or buttock pain on exertion, possibly by causing occlusion of the spinal arteries. However, the claudication distance tends to be variable. The pain can also be brought on by prolonged standing and is also often bilateral. The pain improves with rest (though improvement takes longer with ischaemic pain) or with lumbar spine flexion (less pain on climbing hills than going downhill).

Respiratory symptoms
Dyspnoea
See Chapter 2 for more information on dyspnoea.

Cough
Is the cough dry or productive? Is there diurnal variation (Chapter 5)?

Sputum
How much sputum is produced? There is often little sputum in bronchial carcinoma but copious amounts in bronchiectasis. Ask about its colour;
- Yellow: infection, acute asthma (due to eosinophils).
- Green: infection.
- Frothy: pulmonary oedema.
- Rusty: lobar pneumonia (pneumococcal).
- Blood: see Chapter 5.

- Taste: foul in bronchiectasis and abscess.
- Smell: foul in bronchiectasis.

Chest pain

Chest pain is usually pleuritic in chest disease (Chapter 1), and is often due to pneumonia, pneumothorax, and pulmonary embolus.

Wheeze

Patients with airways obstruction sometimes notice an audible expiratory wheeze.

Hoarse voice

This may be caused, for example, by recurrent laryngeal nerve palsy in bronchial carcinoma.

Gastrointestinal disease

Abdominal pain

Establish the site, radiation, character, exacerbating and relieving factors, and severity. This is discussed in detail in Chapter 11.

Dysphagia

Dysphagia means difficulty in swallowing. Ask about:

- Where do things get stuck? This may give a clue as to the site of the lesion.
- Is there difficulty with solids, fluids or both? Neuromuscular disorders tend to present with dysphagia for fluids at onset, whereas mechanical obstruction results in dysphagia for solids at onset.

The causes of dysphagia are outlined in Fig. 26.2.

Vomiting

What does the vomitus look like?

- Yellow–green: upper gastrointestinal (GI) contents plus bile.
- Brown (faeculent): lower small bowel contents.
- Bright-red blood: active upper GI bleeding (Chapter 7).
- Coffee grounds': 'old' upper GI bleeding.

Fig. 26.2 Causes of dysphagia.

Causes of dysphagia	
Disorder	**Examples**
oropharyngeal lesions	stomatitis, pharyngitis, quinsy, lymphoma
intrinsic oesophageal and gastric lesions	peptic stricture carcinoma of oesophagus or gastric fundus foreign body oesophageal web (Paterson–Brown–Kelly or Plummer–Vinson syndrome) infection (*Candida albicans*) pharyngeal pouch Schatzki's ring (oesophagogastric junction in hiatus hernia) leiomyoma of oesophageal muscle
extrinsic oesophageal compression	goitre with retrosternal extension intrathoracic tumours (lymphoma, bronchial carcinoma) enlarged left atrium
neuromuscular disorders	achalasia scleroderma diffuse oesophageal spasm diabetes mellitus myasthenia gravis myotonia dystrophica bulbar or pseudobulbar palsy diphtheria
psychological	globus hystericus

How 'violent' was the vomiting? Projectile vomiting indicates pyloric stenosis, most commonly seen in infants, but may arise as a consequence of duodenal ulceration in adults.

Indigestion

'Heartburn' or 'dyspepsia' is due to reflux of the gastric contents into the oesophagus.

Bowel habit

Has there been a change? Ask about diarrhoea and constipation, or the presence of one alternating with the other. For more on this, see Chapter 8.

Rectal bleeding

Is the bleeding with or without mucus? The causes of rectal bleeding are summarized in Fig. 26.3. Anal and rectal lesions result in fresh blood on the outside of the stool, on the paper on wiping, or in the pan. Higher lesions result in blood intermixed with the stool.

Tenesmus

Tenesmus is the painful desire to defecate when there is no stool in the rectum. This is due to a lesion in the lumen or wall of the rectum mimicking faeces.

Genitourinary symptoms

Dysuria

This is discomfort during or after micturition due to urinary tract infection or recent urethral instrumentation (catheter or cystoscope).

Urine

What does the urine look like?
- Cloudy: infection, precipitated urates or phosphates.
- Frothy: proteinuria.

- Orange: very concentrated urine, bilirubin, rifampicin.
- Red: haematuria, haemoglobinuria, myoglobinuria, rifampicin.
- Black: 'blackwater fever' due to *Plasmodium falciparum*.
- Dark on standing: porphyria.
- Green: drugs containing methylene blue (commercial analgesics).

See Chapter 13 for the causes of haematuria and proteinuria.

Frequency

Increased frequency of micturition can be due to:
- Bladder irritation: infection, stones, tumour.
- Outflow obstruction: prostatic hypertrophy, urethral stricture.
- Neurological: multiple sclerosis.

N.B. In polyuria there is an increased volume of urine as well as frequency of micturition.

Nocturia

This can be due to any of the causes of polyuria (see Chapter 12) and increased frequency.

Hesitancy

Hesitancy, followed by a poor stream with terminal dribbling, are features of prostatic enlargement.

Loin pain

This can be associated with renal disease (Chapter 11).

Incontinence

This can be either urge incontinence (e.g. detrusor instability) or stress incontinence (e.g. weak pelvic musculature following childbirth).

Menstruation

Determine the pattern of the normal cycle. Then ask about flow (heavy or light), intermenstrual bleeding, post coital bleeding, or dysmenorrhoea.

Discharge

Vaginal or penile discharge can indicate infection.

Causes of rectal bleeding

- haemorrhoids
- anal fissure
- carcinoma (anus, rectum, or colon)
- polyps
- diverticulitis (including Meckel's diverticulum) but not diverticulosis
- colitis (infective, ulcerative, Crohn's, ischaemic)
- angiodysplasia

Fig. 26.3 Causes of rectal bleeding.

Neurological symptoms

Headache
See Chapter 15.

Dizziness
This can also be unsteadiness (Chapters 18 and 22).

Limb weakness and sensory loss
These are covered in detail in Chapter 22.

Syncope
See Chapter 18.

Disturbed vision
Vision can be affected by lesions of the optic pathway or of the nerves controlling eye movements (3rd, 4th, 6th), or conjugate gaze.

Disturbed hearing
Ask about deafness, tinnitus, and vertigo (Chapter 24).

Disturbed smell
Anosmia can result from head injury, nasal polyps, following viral upper respiratory tract infections or frontal lobe tumours.

Altered speech
There are three types of disordered speech:
- Dysarthria: difficulty in articulating speech, but language content is completely normal.
- Dysphonia: difficulty in voice production.
- Dysphasia: difficulty in understanding or expressing language; caused by lesions affecting the dominant cerebral hemisphere (usually the left).

Fig. 26.4 shows the characteristic speech abnormalities that result from lesions at specific anatomical sites.

Metabolic and endocrine symptoms
Most symptoms will have been described in previous chapters. In particular, look for a history suggestive of hyper- or hypothyroidism (Fig. 26.5) and diabetes mellitus (Fig. 26.6).

Musculoskeletal symptoms
Weakness
This is covered in detail in Chapter 20.

Pain
Pain can arise in the muscles (Chapter 20), joints (Chapter 16), or bones (Fig. 26.7).

Stiffness
Stiffness, particularly after inactivity (e.g. early morning stiffness), is a feature of inflammation.

Joint swelling
This can be caused by infection, inflammation, blood (haemarthrosis), or crystal deposition.

Disability
How do the symptoms affect lifestyle? This is extremely important in patients with rheumatological diseases.

Skin symptoms
Rash
The distribution may be very helpful in determining the diagnosis (Chapter 17).

Pruritis
For the causes of pruritis, see Fig. 26.1.

Cause
Has there been any recent change in detergents, soap, shampoo, etc?

Haematological symptoms
These can be summarized as follows:
- Symptoms of anaemia: low haemoglobin (Chapter 25).
- Recurrent infections: low white cell count.
- Bleeding or bruising: low platelets (Chapter 23).

DRUG HISTORY

Record which drugs the patient is taking and at what dose. Ask if there have been any recent changes in medication. Has the patient had any adverse reactions (e.g. rash, facial swelling, or bronchospasm) to drugs or anaesthetics in the past? If so, record exactly what that reaction was as it may have not been a true allergy, e.g. thrush with broad-spectrum antibiotics.

Causes and features of abnormalities of speech		
Site of lesion	Causes	Features of speech
dysarthria mouth	ulcers, macroglossia	slurred
lower cranial nerve lesions (9th to 12th)	bulbar palsy (stroke, poliomyelitis, motor neuron disease, syringobulbia, malignancy)	nasal quality, slurred associated features such as dysphagia
upper cranial nerve lesions (9th to 12th)	pseudobulbar palsy (stroke, motor neuron disease, multiple sclerosis)	spastic speech, like 'Donald duck' associated features like dysphagia and emotional lability
cerebellum	multiple sclerosis, stroke, tumour, hereditary ataxias, alcohol, hypothyroidism	scanning ('staccato') speech flow is broken syllables explosive
extrapyramidal	parkinsonism	difficulty initiating speech monotonous and slightly slurred
toxic	acute alcohol intoxication	slurred
dysphonia neuromuscular junction	myasthenia gravis	weak, nasal speech deteriorates on repetition
vocal cord disease	tumour, viral laryngitis, tuberculosis, syphilis	weak volume, husky quality
vocal cord paralysis	recurrent laryngeal nerve palsy (mediastinal carcinoma, intrathoracic surgery or trauma, aortic aneurysm)	weak volume, husky quality
dysphasia Broca's area (inferior frontal gyrus)	infarction, bleeding, space-occupying lesion	expressive dysphasia comprehension intact difficulty in finding appropriate words and so speech non-fluent
Wernicke's area (superior temporal gyrus)	infarction, bleeding, space-occupying lesion	receptive dysphasia fluent speech but words are disorganized or unintelligible comprehension impaired
frontotemporoparietal lesion	infarction (left middle cerebral artery), bleeding, space-occupying lesion	global dysphasia marked receptive and expressive dysphasia
posterior part of superior temporal/inferior parietal lobe	infarction, bleeding, space-occupying lesion and raised intracranial pressure, dementia	nominal aphasia unable to name specific objects other aspects of speech preserved

g. 26.4 Causes and features of abnormalities of speech arising from lesions at pecific anatomical sites.

AMILY HISTORY

o any diseases 'run' in the patient's family? Record nesses in close relatives, including age of death where levant. Drawing a family tree can be helpful in some atients.

In some conditions, such as adult polycystic disease, the family history should be more detailed as family members may need to be screened and considered for genetic counselling.

Fig. 26.5 Differences in the history between hyperthyroidism and hypothyroidism.

Differences in the history between hyperthyroidism and hypothyroidism		
Symptom	Hyperthyroidism	Hypothyroidism
temperature intolerance	heat	cold
weight	decreased	increased
appetite	increased	decreased
bowel habit	diarrhoea	constipation
psychiatric	anxiety, irritability	poor memory, depression
menstruation	oligomenorrhoea	menorrhagia
others	palpitations, sweating, eye changes, pretibial myxoedema, acropachy	dry skin, brittle hair, arthralgia, myalgia

Symptoms of diabetes mellitus	
Mechanism	Symptoms
due to hyperglycaemia	polyuria polydipsia fatigue blurred vision recurrent infections, e.g. *Candida* weight loss (type I)
due to complications	peripheral neuropathy retinopathy vascular disease

Fig. 26.6 Symptoms of diabetes mellitus.

Causes of bone pain	
Cause	Example
tumour	primary tumour (benign or malignant), metastases
infection	osteomyelitis (*Staphylococcus, Haemophilus influenzae, Salmonella*, tuberculosis)
fracture	traumatic, pathological
metabolic	Paget's disease, osteomalacia

Fig. 26.7 Causes of bone pain.

SOCIAL HISTORY

The importance of this part of the history is to establish how the illness affects the patient's life and how they are coping at home. Ask about:
- Who is at home? If they have a partner, are they fit and well?
- Do they have dependent children? Who is looking after them at the moment?
- What is the home like? If the patient is elderly, is there a warden?
- If the patient is disabled, have appropriate modifications been made?
- Do they need help with daily tasks, such as washing, dressing, feeding, cleaning, or shopping?
- Is there a nearby relative who helps, or does the patient have meals-on-wheels, a home help, or a district nurse?
- In a diabetic patient with retinopathy, can they see to draw up their insulin and monitor BMs? If not, who does it for them?
- What is their occupation? Details of their past and present occupation can be important, e.g. industrial lung disease.
- Are they still able to work despite the current problem?
- Some diagnoses can be particularly important in relation to work, such as HGV drivers and epilepsy.
- Do they smoke? Smoking is a significant cause of many diseases.

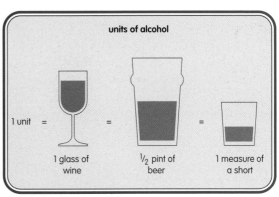

- Alcohol past and present. Record as units per week (Fig. 26.8).
- Do they use 'recreational' drugs? These have health, social, and financial implications.
- Have they recently been abroad? Thay may have been exposed to different infective agents.
- Do they have pets (particularly budgerigars, pigeons, and parrots)?
- Sexual history is not appropriate in every history but may be important, e.g. for hepatitis or HIV.

Fig. 26.8 Units of alcohol.

At the end of the history ask two questions:
- **'Is there anything else you are worried about or want to tell me?'** It is possible that the patient may now feel ready to tell you about their main concern.
- **'Is there anything that you are worried this might be?'** There is often visible relief when this question is asked and it enables you to address the patient's real feelings about his or her illness.

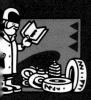

27. Examination of the Patient

INTRODUCTION

When it comes to examining patients, practice really does make perfect. Examiners will be able to tell whether you have examined many patients or not within the first 2 or 3 minutes of seeing you in action! Therefore, take every opportunity you have to rehearse your technique. The more you do it, the more comfortable you will be with the patient, you will use the right words to get the patient to do what you need and, as in history taking, you will stop worrying about what comes next and start thinking about which physical signs are absent or present.

FIRST THINGS FIRST

There are three essential things you must do whenever you see a patient:

- Introduce yourself, shake hands, and tell the patient what you are going to do, e.g. 'Hello Mr Bloggs, my name is Dr— and I would like to examine your chest'.
- Ask the patient to move into the position required for the system you are looking at, expose the area concerned, and then make sure that the patient is comfortable.
- From the moment you first see the patient, try to decide whether they look well or ill. There is plenty of time while an examiner introduces you to the patient, and while the patient undresses and gets on to the couch, for you to gain a lot of information. Can the patient walk? Can they undo buttons? Are they breathless? Are they in pain? Can they see? Are they deaf? Are there any handy clues around the bed (diabetic drinks, wheelchair, nebulizer, catheter)? Taking time to do this has several advantages: it will help you with the diagnosis, it helps to prioritize your approach as a practising clinician, and it will calm your nerves in clinical examinations.

You will probably find that all clinical teachers will show you a slightly different format for examination technique. The important thing is to develop an approach that you are comfortable with and then keep practising it until it becomes second nature.

In examinations you will almost always be asked to examine a particular system: 'Examine this gentleman's chest', 'What do you notice about this lady's face?' This chapter describes the technique for each system and how to interpret the clinical signs you will find. When, as a doctor, you see a patient you will need to be able to examine the whole patient and focus your attention on relevant areas.

GENERAL INSPECTION

It is medical etiquette that all clinical examinations are performed from the right hand side of the patient. The most important thing is to decide is how well or ill the patient is, as described above. Other specific abnormalities should then be looked for.

Cyanosis

This is a bluish discoloration which is seen when the concentration of reduced (deoxygenated) haemoglobin in the blood rises above 5g/dL. Central cyanosis is seen best in the tongue and lips. It is caused by underlying respiratory or cardiovascular disease. Peripheral cyanosis can be due to either central cyanosis or reduced peripheral circulation, as poorly perfused peripheral tissue will take up oxygen more readily. Reduced peripheral circulation is seen in shock, cold weather, and vascular abnormalities. Cyanosis is seen rarely in anaemia but occurs more readily in polycythaemia.

Jaundice

Jaundice is the yellow discoloration of the skin, sclera, and mucous membranes due to serum bilirubin concentrations greater than 30 µmol/L, which becomes more obvious at concentrations greater than 50 µmol/L. Jaundice can be due to increased bilirubin production, abnormal bilirubin metabolism in the liver, or reduced bilirubin excretion (Chapter 10).

Yellow skin (particularly palms and soles) with normal sclera can be due to carotenaemia (excessive consumption of carrots, or hypothyroidism).

Pallor

Generalized pallor can be racial, inherited (albinism), or due to anaemia, shock, myxoedema, or hypopituitarism. Localized pallor is seen in disruption of the arterial supply, as in Raynaud's phenomenon.

Hydration

Signs of dehydration include dry mucous membranes, tachycardia, postural hypotension, decreased skin turgor, and altered consciousness level if severe. If the patient is in hospital, hydration status should be monitored more accurately using weight, fluid balance charts, and central venous pressure (if very ill).

Overhydration can sometimes result from the overenthusiastic administration of intravenous fluids, particularly in the elderly. Clinical signs include raised jugulovenous pressure (JVP), pulmonary oedema, and peripheral oedema.

Temperature

Fever can accompany numerous infectious, inflammatory, and malignant diseases. If associated with an acute infection the patient often looks flushed, sweaty, and unwell. A swinging pyrexia may be a feature of lymphoma and is known as Pel–Ebstein fever. A fever that recurs every few days is seen in malaria. (For more on this, see Chapter 6.)

Hypothermia is a particular problem of the elderly, alcoholics, and patients with dementia. A patient becomes hypothermic when the core temperature falls below 35°C. The causes are summarized in Fig. 27.1.

Pigmentation

Generalized pigmentation is usually of racial origin but may also arise in haemochromatosis (greyish-bronze), occupational exposure (slate-grey appearance with argyria in silver workers), and with some drugs (slate-grey with amiodarone).

Localized pigmentation is seen in Addison's disease (brown lesions in the buccal mucosa, skin creases, and sites of pressure, e.g. beneath the bra strap), Peutz–Jeghers syndrome (brown lesions around the lips), and neurofibromatosis (*café-au-lait* patches).

Localized areas of depigmentation, particularly affecting the back of the hand and neck, are seen in vitiligo, an autoimmune disease of the skin affecting melanocytes. It may be associated with other autoimmune diseases.

Breast examination

Breast examination should be performed in women who have symptoms of breast disease or when an underlying malignancy is suspected. Do not forget that breast tissue extends into the axillae. It is not always appropriate to examine the breasts and male students (and doctors) should have a female chaperone when possible.

Lymphadenopathy

Examine all lymph node sites (Fig. 27.2). Always examine the cervical lymph nodes standing behind the patient. The causes for generalized and localized lymphadenopathy are discussed in Chapter 21. If lymphadenopathy is present, pay special attention to examination of the spleen and liver.

THE FACE AND BODY HABITUS

Examiners will often take you to a patient and simply ask 'What is the diagnosis in this patient?' or 'What do you notice about this gentleman's face?' Consider the diagnoses listed in Fig. 27.3.

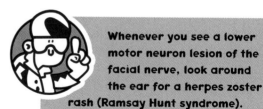

Whenever you see a lower motor neuron lesion of the facial nerve, look around the ear for a herpes zoster rash (Ramsay Hunt syndrome).

Causes of hypothermia	
Cause	**Examples**
exposure	at home in patients who are immobile on treks or after prolonged water immersion in the young
infection	septicaemia from any cause
endocrine	hypothyroidism, hypopituitarism
toxic	alcohol abuse, drug overdose
drugs	hypnotics, e.g. benzodiazepines
stroke	failure of thermoregulation

Fig. 27.1 Causes of hypothermia.

THE NECK

When asked to examine the neck, there will usually be a thyroid mass or lymphadenopathy. However, do not forget the salivary glands, branchial cyst, pharyngeal pouch, cervical rib, carotid body tumour, and cystic hygroma. Causes of lymphadenopathy are described in Chapter 21. Fig. 27.4 lists the causes of thyroid enlargement.

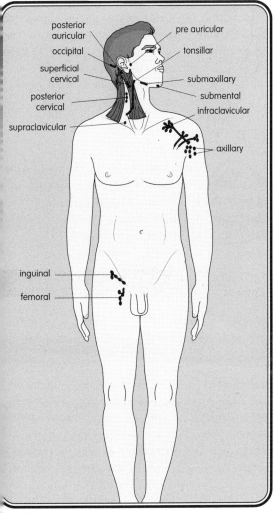

Fig. 27.2 Examination of lymph node sites.

Diseases causing typical abnormalities of the face and body habitus	
Disease	**Examples**
endocrine	hypothyroidism, hyperthyroidism, acromegaly, Cushing's syndrome
metabolic	Paget's disease
neuromuscular	Parkinson's disease, myotonia dystrophica, facial nerve palsy, Horner's syndrome
connective tissue	SLE, scleroderma, Marfan's syndrome
hereditary	Turner's syndrome, Klinefelter's syndrome, achondroplasia
cardiovascular	mitral facies
physiological	chloasma of pregnancy
haematological	thalassaemia
infection	congenital syphilis

Fig. 27.3 Diseases causing typical abnormalities of the face and body habitus. (SLE, systemic lupus erythematosus)

Fig. 27.4 Causes of thyroid gland enlargement.

Causes of thyroid gland enlargement	
Form of enlargement	**Causes**
diffuse enlargement (goitre)	• idiopathic • physiological—puberty, pregnancy • autoimmune—Hashimoto's and Graves' diseases • iodine deficiency—endemic, e.g. Derbyshire neck • thyroiditis—de Quervain's (viral), Riedel's (autoimmune) • drugs—carbimazole, lithium, sulphonylureas • genetic—dyshormonogenesis (Pendred's syndrome)
solitary nodule	• prominent nodule in multinodular goitre • adenoma • cyst • carcinoma (papillary, follicular, anaplastic, medullary) • lymphoma

Firstly, look very carefully at the neck, lifting the hair out of the way if necessary. Look for obvious masses, scars, skin changes, or deformity. If there is a mass in the region of the thyroid gland, ask the patient to take a sip of water into their mouth and then swallow—a goitre will move upwards on swallowing. Also ask the patient to open the mouth and then watch as they protrude the tongue forward—a thyroglossal cyst will move upwards. If a mass is present, determine the properties shown in Fig. 27.5. Percussion is useful to determine retrosternal extension of a goitre. Bruits may be audible in the thyroid gland (thyrotoxicosis) or carotid artery (atheroma). If you find a thyroid mass, you should go on to assess thyroid status as shown in Fig. 27.6.

If you find no abnormality in the neck examine the jugulovenous pressure, listen to the carotid artery for bruits, and re-examine for cervical rib.

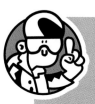

Always palpate the neck from behind the patient with the neck slightly flexed to relax the sternocleidomastoid muscles.

Features of any mass

- site
- shape
- size including upper, lower and lateral limits
- consistency
- tenderness
- fluctuance
- fixation to underlying or overlying structures
- transillumination (where appropriate)
- local lymph node involvement
- bruit

Fig. 27.5 Features to determine for any mass.

THE HANDS

The hands can provide a wealth of information for the alert clinician. When you are asked to examine the hands, consider the normal structures present and examine them in turn. Where appropriate, go on to examine the functional use of the hand, e.g. undoing a button or picking up a pen. This is particularly importan

Examination of thyroid status		
	Hyperthyroidism	**Hypothyroidism**
mood	irritability, anxiety	depression, slowness
weight	thinness	overweight
hands	fine tremor, palmar erythema, sweaty palms, acropachy	puffiness, anaemia, Tinel's sign (carpal tunnel syndrome)
pulse	tachycardia, atrial fibrillation	bradycardia
face	lid lag, lid retraction, exophthalmos, ophthalmoplegia, chemosis	loss of outer third of eyebrow, puffy eyes, 'toad-like' facies, xanthelasmata
skin	pretibial myxoedema (shins)	dry, thin hair
neuromuscular	proximal myopathy	delayed ankle jerks, cerebellar signs

Fig. 27.6 Examination of thyroid status.

n neurological abnormalities and destructive arthritides, e.g. rheumatoid arthritis (RA).

Hands
- Blue: peripheral cyanosis.
- Pallor: anaemia (skin creases) and Raynaud's phenomenon.
- Pigmentation: Addison's disease (skin creases).
- Depigmentation: vitiligo.
- Palmar erythema (Fig. 27.7).

Nails
- Koilonychia: spoon-shaped nails seen in iron deficiency.
- Leuconychia: white nails due to hypoalbuminaemia (Fig. 27.8).
- Clubbing: an increase in angle between nail-plate and fold to over 180°. The causes are shown in Fig. 27.9.
- Splinter haemorrhages: terminal lesions usually due to trauma, proximal lesions found in subacute bacterial endocarditis (SBE), and vasculitis.
- Quincke's sign: capillary pulsation in the nail-bed due to aortic regurgitation.
- Beau's lines: horizontal grooves in the nails caused by temporary arrest of nail growth due to acute severe illness.
- Onycholysis: separation of the nail from the nail-bed due to psoriasis, trauma, fungal infections, and hyperthyroidism.
- Yellow nails: yellow nail syndrome with lymphatic hypoplasia (peripheral oedema and pleural effusions).
- Half-and-half nails where the proximal nail is white and the distal nail is brown or red due to chronic renal failure.

Tendons
- Xanthomata: hypercholesterolaemia.
- Dupuytren's contractures (thickening of the palmar fascia): associated with alcoholic liver disease, epileptics treated with phenytoin, vibrating tools, and familial and idiopathic causes.

Joints
- Destructive arthropathy: RA, psoriasis, gout.
- Heberden's nodes: osteophytes of the distal interphalangeal joints.
- Bouchard's nodes: osteophytes of the proximal interphalangeal joints.

Causes of palmar erythema	
Causes	**Examples**
physiological	pregnancy puberty familial
pathological	chronic liver disease rheumatoid arthritis thyrotoxicosis oral contraceptive pill polycythaemia

Fig. 27.7 Causes of palmar erythema.

Causes of hypoalbuminaemia	
Causes	**Examples**
reduced intake	malnutrition
reduced synthesis	liver disease
increased utilization	chronic illness
increased loss	nephrotic syndrome (kidneys) protein-losing enteropathy (gut) severe burns (skin)

Fig. 27.8 Causes of hypoalbuminaemia.

Causes of clubbing	
Causes	**Examples**
respiratory	tumour: bronchial carcinoma, mesothelioma chronic suppuration: abscess, bronchiectasis, empyema fibrosis: from any cause vascular: arteriovenous malformation
cardiovascular	congenital cyanotic heart disease subacute bacterial endocarditis atrial myxoma
gastrointestinal	inflammatory bowel disease lymphoma cirrhosis
endocrine	thyrotoxicosis (acropachy)
familial	autosomal dominant

Fig. 27.9 Causes of clubbing.

Muscles
- Localized wasting: ulnar or median nerve lesions.
- Generalized wasting: T_1 lesion (brachial plexus, root) or RA.
- Myotonia: failure to relax after voluntary contraction seen in myotonia dystrophica.

Other signs
- Sclerodactyly (tightening of the skin causing tapering of the fingers): look also for **C**alcinosis, **R**aynaud's phenomenon, (o)**E**sophageal dysmotility (ask the patient if they have difficulty on swallowing), and **T**elangiectasia—hence CREST syndrome (where the **S** stands for sclerodactyly).
- Spade hands: acromegaly.
- Asterixis: a coarse flapping tremor seen when the hand is oustretched with the wrist extended and fingers apart. It is caused by metabolic encephalopathy, e.g. liver failure, carbon dioxide retention, uraemia.

When examining the hands always look at the elbows for a psoriatic rash, rheumatoid nodules, or gouty tophi.

THE CARDIOVASCULAR SYSTEM

General inspection
- Does the patient look well or ill?
- Are they lying flat?
- Are they cachectic (cardiac cachexia)?
- Do they have Marfan's syndrome (aortic regurgitation, mitral regurgitation) or Down's syndrome (atrial septal defect)?

Position
Help the patient to adopt a comfortable position at 45° with the chest exposed. In women cover the chest until ready to examine the praecordium.

Hands
- Clubbing: SBE and congenital cyanotic heart disease.
- Cyanosis: peripheral vasoconstriction, pulmonary oedema, and right-to-left shunt.
- Splinter haemorrhages: SBE.
- Janeway's lesions: non-tender macules in the palms due to SBE.
- Osler's nodes: painful nodules on the pulps of the fingers due to SBE.
- Quincke's sign: aortic regurgitation.
- Xanthomata: hypercholesterolaemia—vascular disease.

Radial pulse
- Rate: normally between 60 and 100 beats per minute (see Chapter 3).
- Rhythm: regular or irregular (Chapter 3).
- Radioradial delay: dissecting thoracic aortic aneurysm
- Radiofemoral delay: coarctation of the aorta.
- Character: best determined by palpation of a larger artery, e.g. brachial or carotid arteries.

Blood pressure
- Level: hypertension is a risk factor for vascular disease
- Lying and standing: postural hypotension.
- Right and left: left may be lower than right in aortic dissection.
- Wide pulse pressure: in the elderly and aortic regurgitation.
- Narrow pulse pressure: aortic stenosis.
- Pulsus paradoxus: exaggerated fall in pulse pressure during inspiration resulting in a faint or absent pulse in inspiration; caused by severe asthma or cardiac tamponade.

Brachial and carotid artery
- Character: collapsing (Fig. 27.10), slow-rising (aortic stenosis), bisferiens (mixed aortic valve disease), alternans (severe left ventricular failure), and jerky (hypertrophic obstructive cardiomyopathy).
- Corrigan's sign: prominent carotid pulsation due to aortic regurgitation.

When assessing JVP, the patient should be at 45° with their head rested on a pillow (this relaxes the sternocleidomastoid muscles). Pulsation should be up to 3cm above the sternal angle (8cm above right atrium). Differences between JVP and carotid pulsation in normal subjects are shown in Fig. 27.11. JVP acts as manometer for right atrial pressure and is raised when

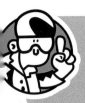

When looking at the JVP, concentrate on the a and v waves. These are the easiest and most reliable to detect.

Causes of a collapsing pulse	
Causes	Examples
physiological	elderly pregnancy exercise
pathological	aortic regurgitation patent ductus arteriosus fever thyrotoxicosis anaemia arteriovenous shunts

Fig. 27.10 Causes of a collapsing pulse.

ight atrial pressure is raised (Fig. 27.12). Abnormalities n the waveform result from specific underlying pathologies (Fig. 27.13).

Face

- Central cyanosis: pulmonary oedema and right-to-left shunt.
- Anaemia: possible high output cardiac failure.
- Malar flush: pulmonary hypertension due to mitral valve disease.
- Jaundice: haemolysis due to mechanical valves.
- Xanthelasmata: hypercholesterolaemia (vascular disease).
- Teeth: source in bacterial endocarditis.
- Mouth: high-arched palate in Marfan's syndrome.
- De Musset's sign: head nodding due to aortic regurgitation.
- Roth's spots in the retina: bacterial endocarditis.

Praecordium

ook for scars and deformities, including:
- Sternotomy scar: arterial bypass grafts and valve replacements.

- Mitral valvotomy scar under the left breast: always look for it as it indicates a previously closed mitral valvotomy.
- Skeletal deformities—can cause an ejection systolic flow murmur.

Apex beat

The apex beat should be at the mid-clavicular line in the fifth left intercostal space.
- Lateral displacement: left or severe right ventricular dilatation.
- Impalpable: obesity, pleural effusion, pericardial effusion, chronic obstructive airways disease, and dextrocardia (palpable on the right!).
- Tapping: mitral stenosis (palpable first heart sound).

Differences between JVP and carotid pulsation		
Feature	Carotid pulsation	JVP
palpable	yes	no
number of visible peaks	one	two
occlusion by gentle pressure	no	yes (fills from above)
sitting upright	no change	height falls
lying flat	no change	height rises
gentle pressure on liver	no change	height rises (hepatojugular reflex)
deep inspiration	no change	height falls

Fig. 27.11 Differences between jugulovenous pulsation (JVP) and carotid pulsation.

Causes of a raised JVP
• right ventricular failure
• volume overload (overenthusiastic intravenous fluids)
• superior vena caval obstruction (JVP is non-pulsatile)
• tricuspid valve disease (stenosis and regurgitation)
• pericardial effusion
• constrictive pericarditis

If you cannot see the JVP, look for pulsation of the ear lobe, as it may be this high!

Fig. 27.12 Causes of a raised jugulovenous pressure (JVP).

- Heaving: 'pressure overload' in aortic stenosis, or hypertension.
- Thrusting: 'volume overload' in aortic regurgitation, pulmonary regurgitation (ventricle usually markedly displaced); diffuse: left ventricular dilatation, double impulse: left ventricular aneurysm (uncommon).

Palpation

Parasternal heave is caused by the enlargement or hypertrophy of the left atrium or right ventricle.

A thrill is a palpable murmur and indicates significant valve disease; it can be systolic or diastolic. Palpate in all valve areas (Fig. 27.14).

Auscultation

- Listen in all four areas with the bell and diaphragm (Fig. 27.14).
- Roll the patient to the left hand side to listen with the bell at the axilla for mitral stenosis.
- Sit the patient forward to listen with the diaphragm

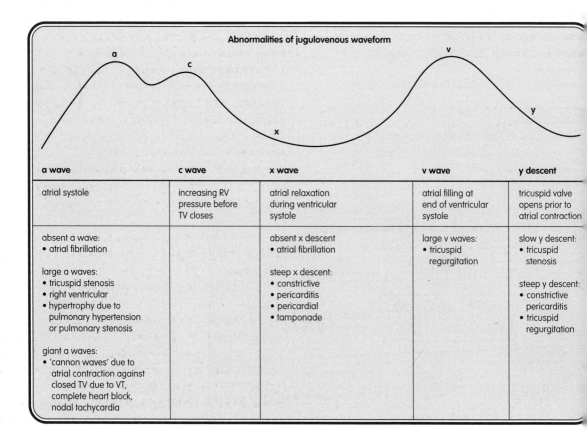

Abnormalities of jugulovenous waveform

a wave	c wave	x wave	v wave	y descent
atrial systole	increasing RV pressure before TV closes	atrial relaxation during ventricular systole	atrial filling at end of ventricular systole	tricuspid valve opens prior to atrial contraction
absent a wave: • atrial fibrillation large a waves: • tricuspid stenosis • right ventricular • hypertrophy due to pulmonary hypertension or pulmonary stenosis giant a waves: • 'cannon waves' due to atrial contraction against closed TV due to VT, complete heart block, nodal tachycardia		absent x descent: • atrial fibrillation steep x descent: • constrictive • pericarditis • pericardial • tamponade	large v waves: • tricuspid regurgitation	slow y descent: • tricuspid stenosis steep y descent: • constrictive pericarditis • tricuspid regurgitation

Fig. 27.13 Abnormalities of jugulovenous waveform. (VT, ventricular tachycardia; TV, tricuspid valve.)

at the left sternal edge in expiration for aortic regurgitation.

- Listen to the first and second sounds, then for third and fourth sounds.
- Are there any murmurs? (See Chapter 4.)
- Listen for additional sounds including opening snap, ejection click, pericardial knock or rub, and mechanical valves.
- Time any abnormalities against the carotid pulsation.
- Listen to the carotid arteries for bruits (atheroma) or radiation of aortic stenotic murmur.

Evidence of cardiac failure

- Examine lung bases for pulmonary oedema and pleural effusions indicating left ventricular failure.
- Sacral oedema occurs in right ventricular failure.
- Hepatomegaly occurs in right ventricular failure; it will be pulsatile if there is tricuspid regurgitation.
- Pitting oedema occurs in right ventricular failure and is almost always bilateral.

Peripheral pulses

Pulses in the legs may be diminished in peripheral vascular disease. Systolic and diastolic

There are four main features of Horner's syndrome. Remember that everything 'gets smaller'.

murmurs may be heard in the femoral arteries due to aortic regurgitation (pistol shots and Duroziez's sign).

THE RESPIRATORY SYSTEM

General inspection

- Does the patient look well or ill? Is the patient alert?
- Cachexia: underlying malignancy.
- Sputum pot: examine (see p. 135).
- Nebulizer: bronchospasm.
- Distress: breathless at rest and moving around in the bed.
- Voice: hoarse in bronchial carcinoma (recurrent laryngeal nerve palsy).
- Lymphadenopathy: supraclavicular, cervical, and axillary.
- Respiratory rate: normally around 14–18 breaths per minute.

Position

Help the patient to adopt a comfortable position at 45° with the chest exposed. In women cover the chest until you are ready to examine it.

Hands

- Clubbing: malignancy, fibrosis, and chronic suppuration.
- Cyanosis: peripheral vasoconstriction and respiratory failure.
- Wasting of small muscles: infiltration of T_1 by bronchial neoplasm.
- Nicotine-stained fingers: increased likelihood of malignancy and obstructive airways disease.
- Asterixis: carbon dioxide retention.
- Hypertrophic pulmonary osteoarthropathy: swelling and pain, particularly in wrists or ankles, due to bronchial carcinoma (particularly squamous cell).

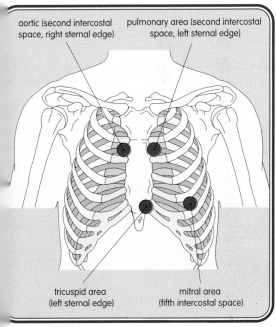

aortic (second intercostal space, right sternal edge)

pulmonary area (second intercostal space, left sternal edge)

tricuspid area (left sternal edge)

mitral area (fifth intercostal space)

Fig. 27.14 Positions of auscultation of the cardiac valves.

Pulse

- Tachycardia: severe respiratory disease, e.g. acute asthma or pneumonia.
- Bounding: carbon dioxide retention.
- Atrial fibrillation: malignancy and pneumonia.

Blood pressure

Pulsus paradoxus is seen in severe acute asthma.

JVP

- Right ventricular failure: chronic respiratory disease with pulmonary hypertension.
- Superior vena caval obstruction: bronchial carcinoma.
- Large a waves: cor pulmonale.

Face

- Central cyanosis: respiratory failure.
- Anaemia: chronic respiratory disease, particularly malignancy.
- Horner's syndrome: bronchial malignancy (Fig. 27.15).
- Fine tremor: β-agonists.
- Plethoric facies: polycythaemia.

Trachea

Warn the patient before you palpate the trachea! Note the following:

- Tracheal deviation (Fig. 27.16).
- Feel for tracheal tug in acute respiratory distress.
- The distance from the cricoid cartilage to the suprasternal notch should be three to four finger breadths—this distance reduces in hyperinflation.
- Check the position of the apex beat to confirm mediastinal shift.

Inspection

Perform inspection, palpation, percussion, and auscultation on the front of the chest first. Then sit the patient forward, palpate for lymphadenopathy, and then repeat the examination on the back of the chest. Typical patterns of respiratory abnormalities are shown in Fig. 27.17.

On inspecting the chest assess the following:

- Respiration: use of accessory muscles (respiratory distress).
- Recession: intercostal and subcostal (respiratory distress).
- Scars: including previous surgery and chest drains.
- Deformity: in particular Harrison's sulci (indrawn costal margins) and pectus carinatum due to severe childhood asthma; barrel chest is seen in long-standing airways obstruction due to hyperinflation.
- Radiotherapy: markings or skin changes indicate previous treatment for underlying malignancy.

Expansion

- Ask the patient to take a deep breath in and out and watch closely.
- Place your hand firmly on the chest laterally with fingers apart and thumbs lifted off the chest wall touching each other.
- The lungs should expand by at least 5 cm on deep inspiration.
- Any significant pulmonary disease will reduce expansion.
- In unilateral disease, the affected side will move less than the other.
- Note any chest wall tenderness, which is usually caused by musculoskeletal abnormalities.

Vocal fremitus

Ask the patient to say '99' and palpate with the ulnar border of the hand. Increased vocal fremitus indicates consolidation (sometimes fibrosis and above pleural effusion); decreased indicates pleural effusion or collapse.

Features of Horner's syndrome
Ipsilateral • partial ptosis • enophthalmos • pupillary constriction • reduced sweating

Fig. 27.15 Features of Horner's syndrome. These result from interruption of the sympathetic innervation of the eye.

Causes of tracheal deviation	
Towards lesion	**Away from lesion**
collapse	tension pneumothorax
apical fibrosis	massive pleural effusion
pneumonectomy	large mass (e.g. thyroid)

Fig. 27.16 Causes of tracheal deviation.

Findings on clinical examination of common respiratory diseases						
Pathology	General signs	Tracheal deviation	Palpation	Percussion note	Breath sounds	Causes
pneumothorax	tachycardia and hypotension in tension pnueumothorax	away from affected side if tension	reduced expansion, reduced TVF	normal or hyper resonant	reduced or absent	spontaneous (particularly tall healthy males and Marfan's syndrome), trauma, airways obstruction, cystic fibrosis, pulmonary abscess
consolidation	pyrexia, tachycardia	none	reduced expansion, increased TVF	dull	bronchial breathing, inspiratory crepitations	pneumococcus, *Haemophilus influenzae, Staphylococcus aureus, Klebsiella, Pseudomonas, Mycoplasma, Legionella, Influenza type A, Aspergillus*
pleural effusion		away from affected side if large	reduced expansion, reduced TVF	stony dull	absent	transudate (<30g/L protein): cardiac failure, liver failure, nephrotic syndrome, Meigs' syndrome, myxoedema exudate (>30g/L protein): malignancy, pneumonia, pulmonary embolus, rheumatoid arthritis, SLE, subphrenic abscess, pancreatitis, trauma, Dressler's syndrome
collapse		towards affected side	reduced expansion, reduced TVF	dull	reduced or absent	foreign body or mucus plugs (asthma, aspergillosis) within the bronchial lumen, bronchial carcinoma arising from the bronchus itself, extrinsic compression by enlarged lymph nodes (malignancy, tuberculosis)
fibrosis	clubbing	towards affected side if apical disease	reduced expansion, increased TVF	normal or dull	fine inspiratory crepitations	cryptogenic fibrosing alveolitis, sarcoidosis, drugs (amiodarone, bleomycin), radiation, inhalation of dusts (asbestos, coal), extrinsic allergic alveolitis, ankylosing spondylitis, rheumatoid arthritis, systemic sclerosis, tuberculosis
bronchiectasis	clubbing, purulent sputum	normal	normal or reduced expansion, normal or increased TVF	normal or dull	coarse inspiratory crepitations, occasional polyphonic wheeze	congenital (cystic fibrosis, Kartagener's syndrome, hypogammoglobulinaemia), idiopathic, bronchial obstruction (foreign body, carcinoma, lymphadenopathy), infection (childhood measles or whooping cough, tuberculosis, aspergillosis, postpneumonia)
bronchospasm	hyperexpanded chest, tremor, Harrison's sulci, pectus excavatum	normal	reduced expansion, normal TVF	normal, hyper resonant over bullae, reduced liver dullness	polyphonic wheeze, crepitations in chronic obstructive airways disease	asthma, chronic bronchitis, emphysema (cardiac failure—'cardiac asthma')

27.17 Findings on clinical examination of common respiratory diseases. (TVF, tactile vocal fremitus.)

Percussion

Compare one side with the other and remember the axillae. The following signs are important:

- Hyperresonant: pneumothorax.
- Dull: solid organ (liver or heart), consolidation, collapse, pleural thickening, peripheral tumours, and fibrosis.
- Stony dull: pleural effusion.

Auscultation

- Vesicular breath sounds: these are normal.
- Bronchial breathing: consolidation (sometimes fibrosis and above pleural effusion).
- Wheeze: airways obstruction (polyphonic or generalized), bronchial carcinoma (monophonic or localized), and cardiac failure.
- Fine crepitations: pulmonary fibrosis.
- Medium crepitations: cardiac failure.
- Coarse crepitations: infection.
- Absent breath sounds: pleural effusion.
- Pleural rub: pleural irritation due to pneumonia or pulmonary embolus.
- Click: during systole this is occasionally heard in pneumothorax (Hamman's sign).
- Whispering pectoriloquy: consolidation (sometimes fibrosis and above pleural effusion).

Other signs

- The liver may be palpable liver if it is pushed down by hyperexpanded lungs (ptosis), enlarged due to right ventricular failure, or if there are metastases from a bronchial carcinoma.
- Pitting oedema indicates right ventricular failure.
- Peak flow should be assessed if available.

The upper border of the liver is normally at the sixth rib in the right midclavicular line. If the percussion note remains resonant below this, the lungs are hyperinflated.

THE ABDOMEN

General inspection

- Appearance: does the patient look well or ill?
- Pain.
- Patient's position: think of peritonism if very still, appendicitis (psoas irritation) if right knee flexed, and renal colic if rolling around in agony.
- Cachexia: chronic disease, particularly malignancy
- Drowsy: encephalopathy (hepatic or uraemia).
- Hydration (see p. 144).

Position

Ask the patient if they are comfortable lying flat. If so, help the patient to do this with the head on one pillow and arms relaxed by the sides. Expose from below the breasts (in women) or the nipples (in men) down to the symphysis pubis.

Hands

- Clubbing: cirrhosis, inflammatory bowel disease and gastrointestinal lymphoma.
- Leuconychia: liver failure, nephrotic syndrome, protein-losing enteropathy.
- Koilonychia: chronic iron deficiency, consider occult neoplasm particularly in the stomach and caecum.
- Palmar erythema: cirrhosis.
- Asterixis: hepatic encephalopathy and uraemia.
- Dupuytren's contracture: alcoholic liver disease.
- Half-and-half nails: renal failure.
- Bullae (blisters): porphyria cutanea tarda due to alcoholic liver disease.

Arms

- Scratch marks: obstructive jaundice (particularly primary biliary cirrhosis) and lymphoma.
- Muscle wasting: proximal myopathy due to alcohol, steroid excess, or underlying malignancy (paraneoplastic).
- Bruising: hepatic impairment.

Always look at the patient's face when palpating the abdomen—it will often tell you a lot!

Face
- Jaundice: prehepatic, hepatic, or posthepatic (Chapter 10).
- Anaemia: from any cause (Chapter 25).
- Xanthelasmata: hypercholesterolaemia (primary biliary cirrhosis or nephrotic syndrome).
- Kayser–Fleischer rings: Wilson's disease (best seen by slit-lamp examination).

Mouth
- Hydration.
- Glossitis: iron deficiency and megaloblastic anaemia.
- Pigmentation: Addison's disease and Peutz–Jeghers syndrome.
- Telangiectasia: hereditary haemorrhagic telangiectasia (Osler–Weber–Rendu syndrome).
- Crohn's disease: lip swelling and mucosal ulceration.
- Gingival hypertrophy (Fig. 27.18).

Neck
Look for left supraclavicular lymphadenopathy—caused by metastasis from underlying gastrointestinal carcinoma (Virchow's node or Troisier's sign).

Trunk
Spider naevi arise in the distribution of the superior vena cava—five or more suggest underlying chronic liver disease, pregnancy, or hyperthyroidism.

Gynaecomastia and sexual hair loss indicates chronic liver disease.

Inspection
Ask the patient to breathe in and then out—watch carefully for the following:
- Scars: previous surgery or trauma.
- Distension (Fig. 27.19).
- Obvious mass: including movement with respiration.
- Bruising: Cullen's (paraumbilical) and Grey Turner's (flanks) signs in acute pancreatitis.
- Dilated veins: inferior vena cava (venous flow is upwards).
- Caput Medusae: portal hypertension (venous flow is away from the umbilicus).
- Pulsation: abdominal aortic aneurysm.
- Striae: pregnancy or Cushing's syndrome.
- Node: umbilical nodule (Sister Mary Joseph's nodule) is a metastasis from intra-abdominal malignancy.
- Peristalsis: if visible this indicates an obstruction, though it may be normal in a thin or elderly patient.

Palpation
Before you touch the patient, ask if they are tender anywhere and start palpation away from that area. Feel gently in each of the four quadrants, noting tenderness or masses. Then feel more deeply in each quadrant to determine the characteristics of any mass found (Fig. 27.5).

If a mass is present, consider what structures normally lie at that site and what disease processes might affect that structure (Chapter 11). Next, palpate for hepatomegaly and splenomegaly starting in the right iliac fossa. Examine for renal masses by bimanual palpation. If hepatomegaly or splenomegaly are

Causes of gingival hypertrophy	
Cause	**Examples**
acute myeloid leukaemia	monocytic, myelomonocytic
drugs	cyclosporin, phenytoin, nifedipine
infection	gingivitis
scurvy	see p. 117
physiological	pregnancy

Fig. 27.18 Causes of gingival hypertrophy.

Causes of generalized abdominal swelling	
Cause	**Aetiology**
fluid	ascites
faeces	constipation
fetus	pregnancy
flatus	bowel obstruction
fat	obesity
fibroids	and any other tumour or organomegaly

Fig. 27.19 Causes of generalized abdominal swelling.

present, comment on consistency and size in centimetres (not finger breadths) beneath the costal margin (the causes of hepatomegaly are shown in Fig. 27.20); the causes of splenomegaly are discussed in detail in Chapter 21.

Do not forget the distinguishing features of the spleen and kidney (see Fig. 21.2); the causes of a renal mass are summarized in Fig. 27.21.

Finally, palpate for abdominal aortic aneurysm and examine the groins for lymphadenopathy and hernias.

Percussion

Always percuss from resonance to dullness. Use percussion to determine the size of the liver and spleen starting at the chest, moving inferiorly. Percuss over any masses to determine their consistency. Always assess for ascites by looking for a fluid thrill and shifting dullness. Fig. 27.22 summarizes the causes of ascites.

Auscultation

- Bowel sounds may be normal, increased, or decreased: increased in bowel obstruction (high-pitched and

tinkling) and absent in the ileus (functional motor paralysis of the bowel) due to any cause (Fig. 27.23).
- Arterial bruits: may be heard over stenosed vessels such as renal arteries.
- Venous hum in the epigastrium: portal hypertension.
- Friction rubs: may rarely be heard over the liver (infarction, tumour, or gonococcal perihepatitis) or spleen (infarction).
- Succussion splash: pyloric stenosis.

Other signs

- Look at the legs for pitting oedema (Fig. 27.24).
- In the clinical examinations, if you say that you would also like to examine the genitalia and perform

Causes of unilateral and bilateral palpable kidneys	
Type	**Cause**
unilateral	tumour (hypernephroma, nephroblastoma) hydronephrosis, pyonephrosis hypertrophy of single functioning kidney, perinephric abscess or haematoma, polycystic disease (only one kidney palpable)
bilateral	polycystic kidneys (autosomal dominant in adults, autosomal recessive in children) amyloidosis bilateral hydronephrosis

Fig. 27.21 Causes of unilateral and bilateral palpable kidneys.

Causes of hepatomegaly	
Cause	**Examples**
cirrhosis	any cause, particularly primary biliary cirrhosis and haemochromatosis
tumour	benign, malignant, primary (hepatocellular carcinoma), and metastases
venous congestion	right ventricular failure, Budd–Chiari syndrome, tricuspid stenosis
infection	viral hepatitis, abscess, syphilis, Weil's disease, hydatid disease
cysts	polycystic disease
haematological	lymphoproliferative disease, myeloproliferative disease
metabolic	storage diseases, amyloidosis
inflammatory	sarcoidosis

Fig. 27.20 Causes of hepatomegaly. Remember the 'Cs' for common causes: **c**irrhosis, **c**arcinoma, and **c**ardiac failure. Note that the liver may appear large in the absence of true hepatomegaly when it is pushed down by a hyperinflated lung (as in acute asthma or chronic obstructive airways disease) and when a Riedel's lobe is present (normal anatomical variation of the right hepatic lobe).

Causes of ascites	
Type	**Cause**
transudate (protein <25 g/L)	cardiac failure liver failure nephrotic syndrome Meigs' syndrome myxoedema constrictive pericarditis (rare)
exudate (protein >25 g/L)	intra-abdominal malignancy cirrhosis with portal hypertension infection (tuberculosis, perforation, spontaneous) pancreatitis Budd–Chiari syndrome lymphatic obstruction (chylous)

Fig. 27.22 Causes of ascites.

a rectal examination, you will usually be taken to the next case. When seeing patients as a practising clinician, always consider whether these examinations are appropriate. In some circumstances, they are essential, such as rectal bleeding, iron deficiency, or change in bowel habit.

- If there is hepatosplenomegaly, go on to examine all lymph node sites, bearing in mind lymphoproliferative disorders, sarcoidosis, and viruses such as Epstein–Barr virus.

Causes of ileus

- following intra-abdominal surgery where the gut has been handled
- peritonitis
- pancreatitis
- hypokalaemia
- uraemia
- diabetic ketoacidosis
- intra-abdominal haemorrhage
- retroperitoneal haematoma
- retroperitoneal trauma, e.g. surgery for aortic aneurysm
- anticholinergic drugs

Fig. 27.23 Causes of ileus.

Causes of lower limb oedema

Cause	Examples

pitting	unilateral:
	  deep venous thrombosis
	  unilateral compression of veins (nodes, tumour)
	
	bilateral:
	  right ventricular failure
	  tricuspid stenosis
	  constrictive pericarditis
	  hepatic failure
	  nephrotic syndrome
	  protein-losing enteropathy
	  inferior vena cava obstruction (thrombosis, nodes, tumour)
	  immobility
	  kwashiorkor

lymphatic (non-pitting)	obstruction by nodes, tumour or infection (filariasis) congenital hypoplasia (Milroy's disease) myxoedema

Fig. 27.24 Causes of lower limb oedema.

THE NERVOUS SYSTEM

All medical short case examinations will involve at least one neurology case—this usually fills medical students and membership candidates with fear and dread!

Although it is true that neuroanatomy is complicated and many different diseases can affect each part, the end result is a limited repertoire of patterns of signs. The best approach is to identify which signs are present using a well-rehearsed technique and consider where the lesion is likely to be. You can then think of which diseases affect that part of the nervous system and look for additional evidence to support the diagnosis.

Chapter 22 has discussed in detail the clinical signs and common diseases associated with different parts of the nervous system. This section covers a practical approach to the examination technique itself. It is particularly important to practice this routine over and over again as it is the most difficult to perform competently and will be all the more impressive if you can do it well!

General inspection

- Appearance: does the patient look well or ill?
- Level of consciousness: is the patient conscious or unconscious?
- Age: a young patient is more likely to have multiple sclerosis or an inherited disease; an elderly patient is more likely to have had a stroke.
- General clues: is there a wheelchair (the problem also affects the legs) or diabetic drinks (peripheral neuropathy or stroke)?
- Posture: how is the patient sitting? Is the patient leaning towards one side (hemiparesis)? Is there a tremor at rest (parkinsonism)?
- Speech: when the patient speaks does the speech sound normal? (See Fig. 26.4.)

Cranial nerves

Features and examinations of the cranial nerves include the following.

1st cranial nerve (olfactory)

- Sensory only.
- This is not routinely tested, but ask the patient if they have noticed anything abnormal about their sense of smell.
- Sense of smell can be tested using bottles containing

essences, though this test is rarely performed. (N.B. Ammonia should not be used as it also stimulates the trigeminal nerve.)

- Anosmia can result from head injury (fracture of the cribriform plate), upper respiratory tract infection, tumour (olfactory groove meningioma or glioma), or Kallmann's syndrome (anosmia with hypogonadotrophic hypogonadism).

2nd cranial nerve (optic)

- Sensory only.
- Visual acuity: ask the patient to read some print or Snellen's chart (with spectacles if normally worn). Test each eye separately. Any lesion from the cornea, lens, retina, optic nerve, optic chiasm, optic radiation, or occipital cortex can result in reduced acuity.
- Visual fields: test each eye individually. Make sure your eyes are on the same level as the patient's. Move your fingers from beyond your visual field inwards and ask the patient to tell you when they can see them. Check each quadrant. Use a red hat pin to determine the blind spot. Typical field defects are shown in Fig. 27.25. Vision can be formally assessed using perimetry.
- Fundoscopy: common abnormalities on fundoscopy are papilloedema (Fig. 27.26), optic atrophy (Fig. 27.27), diabetic retinopathy (Fig. 27.28), hypertensive retinopathy, and retinitis pigmentosa. Retinitis pigmentosa is associated with Refsum's disease, hereditary ataxias, abetalipoproteinaemias,

Laurence–Moon–Biedl syndrome, and mitochondrial cytopathies.

3rd, 4th, and 6th cranial nerves

- Control the eye's movements.
- Ask the patient to follow your finger with their eyes and tell you if they 'see double'.
- Look for nystagmus (see p. 123) and failure of eye movements.
- Assess conjugate gaze by asking the patient to look at your hand and then to a finger on your other hand and then from one to the other as quickly as possible. If there is an internuclear ophthalmoplegia (a lesion in the medial longitudinal fasciculus) there will be slow movement in the adducting eye and nystagmus in the abducting eye. Internuclear ophthalmoplegia is usually caused by multiple sclerosis but may occasionally result from vascular lesions.
- Diplopia in all directions of gaze may result from myasthenia gravis or disease in the surrounding tissue of eye, such as Graves' disease, tumour, or orbital cellulitis.

3rd cranial nerve (oculomotor)

- Motor supply to levator palpebrae superioris, all orbital muscles except the superior oblique and lateral rectus muscles, and parasympathetic tone to pupillary reflex.
- Controls pupillary reflexes, in addition to the 2nd cranial nerve. Test the reaction to light and accommodation.

Visual field defects		
Defect	**Site of lesion**	**Causes**
tunnel vision	retina	glaucoma, retinitis pigmentosa, laser therapy for diabetic retinopathy
enlarged blind spot	optic nerve	papilloedema (due to any cause)
central scotoma	macular, optic nerve	optic atrophy, optic neuritis, retinal disease affecting macula
monocular visual loss	eye, optic nerve	optic nerve infarction, optic neuritis, optic atrophy, extensive retinal disease
bitemporal hemianopia	optic chiasm	pituitary tumour, craniopharyngioma, sella meningioma
quadrantic hemianopia	temporal lobe (superior) parietal lobe (inferior)	stroke, tumour
homonymous hemianopia	occipital cortex, optic tract	stroke, tumour

Fig. 27.25 Visual field defects.

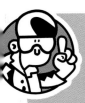

> **Patients with a fourth cranial nerve palsy have difficulty with vision when walking downstairs or reading a book.**

- There is diplopia on abduction of the affected eye with two images side by side.
- 6th cranial nerve lesions are caused by mononeuritis multiplex, demyelination, tumour, infarction, thiamine deficiency (Wernicke's encephalopathy), raised intracranial pressure (false localizing sign), and neurosyphilis.

- Lesion of this nerve results in ptosis and a dilated pupil with no reaction to light or accommodation. The eye looks 'down and out' at rest and is unable to look upwards or inwards.
- Causes of 3rd cranial nerve lesions are infarction, posterior communicating artery aneurysm, mononeuritis multiplex (see p. 109), demyelination, tumour, and neurosyphilis.

4th cranial nerve (trochlear)
- Motor supply to the superior oblique muscle.
- Patient may have the head tilted away from the lesion.
- Diplopia on looking down and away from the lesion with one image at an angle to the other.
- 4th cranial nerve lesions are usually associated with 3rd cranial nerve lesions and have a similar aetiology.

6th cranial nerve (abducens)
- Motor supply to the lateral rectus.

Causes of papilloedema	
Cause	**Examples**
raised intracranial pressure	tumour, abscess, hydrocephalus, haematoma, benign intracranial hypertension, cerebral oedema (trauma)
venous occlusion	central retinal vein thrombosis, cavernous sinus thrombosis
malignant hypertension	grade IV hypertensive retinopathy
acute optic neuritis	multiple sclerosis, sarcoidosis
metabolic	hypercapnia, hypoparathyroidism
haematological (rare)	severe anaemia, acute leukaemia

Fig. 27.26 Causes of papilloedema.

Causes of optic atrophy	
Cause	**Examples**
pressure on optic nerve	tumour, glaucoma, aneurysm, Paget's disease
demyelination	multiple sclerosis
vascular	central retinal artery occlusion
metabolic	diabetes mellitus, vitamin B_{12} deficiency
toxins	methyl alcohol, tobacco, lead, quinine
trauma	including surgery
consecutive	due to extensive retinal disease such as choroidoretinitis
hereditary prolonged papilloedema	Friedreich's ataxia, Leber's optic atrophy

Fig. 27.27 Causes of optic atrophy.

Stages of diabetic retinopathy	
Stage	**Features**
background	dot haemorrhages (microaneurysms), blot haemorrhages, hard exudates
preproliferative	all of the above, plus soft exudates (cotton wool spots), flame haemorrhages, venous beading and loops
proliferative	all of the above, plus new vessel formation on retina or iris (rubeosis iridis), retinal detachment, preretinal or vitreous haemorrhage, glaucoma (with rubeosis iridis)
maculopathy	hard exudates at maculae (sometimes form rings)

Fig. 27.28 Stages of diabetic retinopathy. Note that cataracts are also more common in diabetes, and that retinopathy may have been treated by laser photocoagulation (burns around the periphery of the retina, destroying ischaemic tissue and thus reducing the drive for new vessel formation).

5th cranial nerve (trigeminal)
- Sensation to the face (ophthalmic, maxillary, and mandibular branches).
- Motor supply to the muscles of mastication (temporalis, masseter, and pterygoid muscles).
- Test sensation in the distribution of each division comparing one side with the other.
- Remember the corneal reflex, which requires intact motor function of the 3rd cranial nerve for blinking.
- Ask the patient to clench the teeth.
- Ask them to hold the mouth open while you try to push it shut.
- Test jaw jerk, which is increased in pseudobulbar palsy, and reduced or absent in bulbar palsy.
- The causes of 5th cranial nerve lesions are shown in Fig. 27.29.

7th cranial nerve (facial)
- Sensation of taste from the floor of the mouth, the soft palate, and anterior two-thirds of the tongue.
- Motor supply to the muscles of facial expression and the stapedius muscle.
- Parasympathetic supply to the salivary and lacrimal glands.
- Ask the patient to wrinkle the forehead, screw the eyes tightly shut, show the teeth, and blow the cheeks out.
- In lower motor neuron lesions all the muscles are affected.
- In upper motor neuron lesions the upper half of the face and emotional expressions are spared, e.g. normal eye closure and wrinkling of the forehead.
- Taste is not usually examined formally but ask if the patient has noticed any recent change.
- Fig. 27.30 summarizes the causes of facial nerve palsies.

8th cranial nerve (vestibulocochlear)
- Sensory to the utricle, saccule, and semicircular canals (vestibular), and to the organ of Corti (cochlea).

Causes of a trigeminal nerve lesion	
Cause	**Examples**
brainstem	tumour, infarction, demyelination, syringobulbia
cerebellopontine angle	acoustic neuroma, meningioma
petrous temporal bone	trauma, tumour, middle ear disease, herpes zoster
cavernous sinus	tumour, thrombosis, aneurysm of internal carotid artery
peripheral	meningeal tuberculosis, syphilis, lymphoma, carcinoma, sarcoid

Fig. 27.29 Causes of a trigeminal nerve lesion.

Causes of facial nerve palsies	
Cause	**Examples**
upper motor neuron central	stroke, tumour
lower motor neuron pons	stroke, tumour, demyelination, motor neuron disease
cerebellopontine angle	acoustic neuroma, meningioma
petrous temporal bone	Bell's palsy, herpes zoster
middle ear disease	infection, tumour
peripheral	trauma, parotid disease, mononeuritis multiplex, sarcoid

Fig. 27.30 Causes of facial nerve palsies.

- Ask if the patient has noticed any difficulty with hearing.
- Rub your fingers in front of each of the patient's ears and ask if he or she can hear it.
- Rinne's test: place a vibrating tuning fork on the mastoid process and then at the external auditory meatus—the test is positive if the sound is louder when the fork is held at the external auditory meatus (i.e. air conduction) than when placed on the mastoid process (i.e. bone conduction). This is normal. An abnormal test (Rinne negative) indicates conductive deafness.
- Weber's test: place a vibrating tuning fork at the centre of the forehead; the sound will be heard towards the normal ear in sensorineural deafness or towards the affected ear in conductive deafness.
- The causes of vestibular disease are shown in Fig. 24.1.
- The causes of conductive and sensorineural deafness are described in Fig. 27.31.

9th and 10th cranial nerves

- Look at palatal movement (ask the patient to say 'Aah').
- No palatal elevation on the affected side, with the uvula pulled towards the normal side.
- Check the gag reflex (9th, sensory; 10th, motor).
- Fig. 27.32 summarizes diseases affecting these nerves.

9th cranial nerve (glossopharyngeal)

- Sensory to pharynx and carotid sinus and taste to the posterior third of the tongue.
- Motor supply to the stylopharyngeus muscle.
- Parasympathetic to the parotid gland.

10th cranial nerve (vagus)

- Sensory to the larynx.
- Motor supply to the cricothyroid and the muscles of the pharynx and larynx.
- Parasympathetic to the bronchi, heart, and gastrointestinal tract.

11th cranial nerve (accessory)

- Cranial root provides the motor supply to some muscles of the soft palate and larynx.
- Spinal root provides the motor supply to the trapezius and sternocleidomastoid muscles.
- Ask the patient to shrug the shoulders and test against resistance.
- Ask the patient to turn his or her head to each side and test against resistance.

Causes of deafness	
Cause	Examples
conductive	wax, foreign body, otitis externa, injury to tympanic membrane, otitis media, otosclerosis, middle ear tumour (e.g. cholesteatoma)
sensorineural	presbycusis (due to old age), noise induced, drugs (aminoglycosides, aspirin overdose), infection (meningitis, syphilis, measles), congenital (maternal rubella, cytomegalovirus, toxoplasmosis), Ménière's disease, acoustic neuroma, trauma, Paget's disease

Fig. 27.31 Causes of deafness. (CMV, cytomegalovirus.)

Causes of glossopharyngeal, vagus and accessory nerve palsies	
Cause	Examples
central (brainstem)	tumour, infarction, syringobulbia, motor neuron disease
peripheral	tumour or aneurysm near the jugular foramen, trauma of skull base, Guillain–Barré syndrome, poliomyelitis

Fig. 27.32 Causes of glossopharyngeal, vagus, and accessory nerve palsies.

12th cranial nerve (hypoglossal)
- Provides the motor supply to the styloglossus, hyoglossus, and all intrinsic muscles of the tongue.
- Ask the patient to open the mouth. Look for wasting and fasciculation, indicating a lower motor neuron lesion of the tongue.
- Then ask the patient to protrude the tongue. If there is a unilateral lesion the tongue will deviate towards the side of the lesion.
- Upper motor neuron lesions are due to stroke, tumour, or motor neurone disease.
- Lower motor neuron lesions are due to diseases in the posterior fossa, skull base, and the neck, including tumour, motor neuron disease, syringobulbia, trauma, and poliomyelitis.

The upper limbs
Inspection
- Wasting: lower motor neuron lesion, muscle disease, and disuse.
- Fasciculation: lower motor neuron lesion.
- Scars: particularly from surgery.
- Deformity: may cause mononeuropathy by entrapment, and contractures may be the result of neurological disease.
- Tremor (Fig. 27.33).

Pronator drift
- Ask the patient to hold his or her arms outstretched before them with the palms facing upwards.
- Marked weakness due to any cause will become immediately apparent.

- Ask the patient to keep their arms still and close their eyes.
- If there is an upper motor neuron lesion (affecting the parietal lobe), the arm will drift downwards and the palms will turn downwards.

Tone
Reduced tone is a feature of a lower motor neuron lesion or cerebellar lesion. Tone may be increased throughout a movement, when it is called 'lead pipe' rigidity (as in parkinsonism) or more pronounced at the beginning of a movement, so-called 'clasp knife' rigidity (as with an upper motor neuron lesion).

Power
All muscle groups should be tested and scored (Fig. 27.34). You will need to learn the root value for each movement (Fig. 27.35). Remember to compare muscle power of one side to the other for each group.

When assessing coordination
Ask the patient to alternately touch their nose and your finger. In cerebellar disease there will be an intention tremor and past pointing, i.e. the patient overshoots the examining clinician's finger consistently towards the side of the lesion. Ask the patient to tap one palm with alternating sides of the other hand as quickly as possible (demonstrate to the patient what you would

Do not confuse the asterixis of metabolic encephalopathy with a tremor.

Fig. 27.33 Causes of tremor.

Causes of tremor		
Type	**Features**	**Causes**
resting	seen when patients relaxed with hands at rest	parkinsonism
postural	seen when hands held outstretched	benign essential tremor anxiety thyrotoxicosis β_2-agonists
intention	seen when patients try to touch examiner's finger with their own finger	cerebellar disease

like them to do). In cerebellar disease this will be slow, poorly coordinated, and the action of the moving hand has a high amplitude—this is dysdiadochokinesis.

Reflexes

Practice as often as you can. Learn the root value of each reflex—these are clinically useful as well as helpful in examinations! (Fig. 27.36). Reflexes can be reduced normal or increased. They will be reduced or absent in lower motor neuron lesions, sensory neuropathy, and severe muscle disease (disruption of reflex arc), and will be exaggerated in upper motor neuron lesions.

Grading muscle power	
Grade	**Features**
0	no movement at all
1	flicker of movement only
2	movement only when gravity excluded
3	movement against gravity only
4	movement against gravity and some additional resistance
5	normal power

Fig. 27.34 Grading muscle power.

Fig. 27.35 Roots for each muscle group movement.

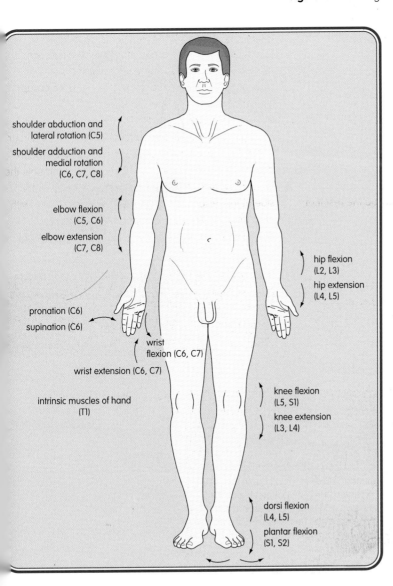

shoulder abduction and lateral rotation (C5)
shoulder adduction and medial rotation (C6, C7, C8)
elbow flexion (C5, C6)
elbow extension (C7, C8)
pronation (C6)
supination (C6)
wrist flexion (C6, C7)
wrist extension (C6, C7)
intrinsic muscles of hand (T1)
hip flexion (L2, L3)
hip extension (L4, L5)
knee flexion (L5, S1)
knee extension (L3, L4)
dorsi flexion (L4, L5)
plantar flexion (S1, S2)

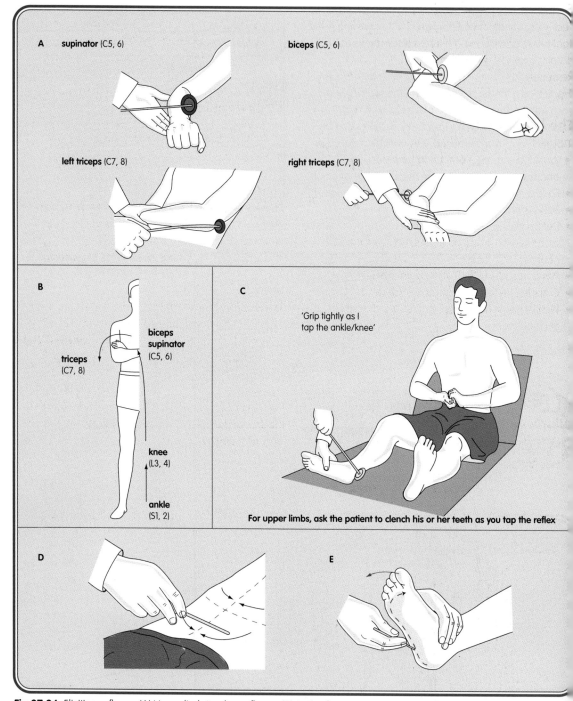

Fig 27.36 Eliciting reflexes. (A) Upper limb tendon reflexes. (B) A simple way to remember root values of reflexes. (C) Testing ankle jerk with reinforcement. (D) Abdominal reflexes: test in four quadrants shown. (E) The normal response is a downgoing hallux. In an upper motor neuron lesion, the hallux dorsiflexes and other toes fan out (the Babinski response).

Sensation

Test each dermatome (Fig. 27.37) for the sensation of light touch, pinprick, and temperature. Then, starting distally, check vibration and joint position sense. Remember the different pathways these senses take (Fig. 27.38).

The lower limbs

Inspection

- Wasting: lower motor neuron lesion, muscle disease, and disuse.
- Fasciculation: lower motor neuron lesion.
- Scars: particularly from surgery.
- Deformity: may cause mononeuropathy by entrapment, and contractures may be the result of neurological disease.
- Pes cavus: Charcot–Marie–Tooth disease.
- Catheter: neurogenic urinary incontinence.
- Walking aids: wheelchair and stick indicating degree of disability.

S2,3,4 feels your bottom on the floor!

Gait

- Ask the patient to walk for 2–3 metres, turn and walk back, then walk heel to toe (cerebellar ataxia), and finally stand on toes and on heels (any muscle weakness will now manifest itself).
- Make sure you walk with the patient so you can catch them if they fall.
- An immense amount of information can be gained by careful study of these aspects of gait (Fig. 22.2).

Tone

Reduced tone is a feature of a lower motor neuron lesion or cerebellar lesion. Tone may be increased in an upper motor neuron lesion or parkinsonism. Test for clonus, signifying an upper motor neuron lesion.

Power

All muscle groups should be tested and scored (Fig. 27.34). Learn the roots for each movement (Fig. 27.35). Remember to compare muscle power of one side to the other for each group.

Coordination

Ask the patient to gently run the heel of one leg down the shin of the other. In cerebellar disease this will be slow and clumsy

Fig. 27.37 Dermatome testing.

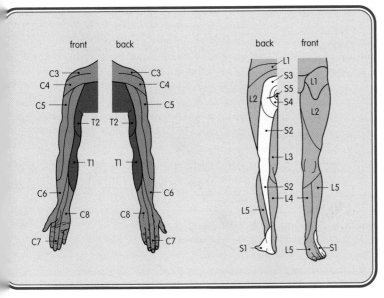

Reflexes

Learn the root value of each reflex (Fig. 27.36). Reflexes will be reduced or absent in lower motor neuron lesions, sensory neuropathy, and severe muscle disease, and will be exaggerated in upper motor neuron lesions. Check plantar response, which is normally downgoing but will be upgoing in upper motor neuron lesions.

Sensation

Test each dermatome (Fig. 27.37) for sensation of light touch, pinprick, and temperature. Then, starting distally check vibration and joint position sense. Check specifically for peripheral neurology—'stocking' distribution.

The sensory pathways are shown in Fig. 27.38.

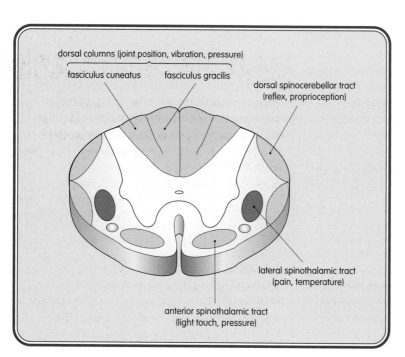

Fig. 27.38 (A) Anatomy of sensory pathways within the spinal cord.

Sensory pathways			
Sensation	**Tested using**	**Pathway**	**Level of decussation**
pain	neurotip	lateral spinothalamic tract	at level of sensory root within one spinal segment
temperature	tuning fork for cold	lateral spinothalamic tract	at level of sensory root within one spinal segment
light touch	cotton wool	anterior spinothalamic tract	at level of sensory root within several spinal segments
vibration	tuning fork	posterior columns (fasciculus gracilis and fasciculus cuneatus)	medulla oblongata
joint position sense	move fixed joints	posterior columns (fasciculus gracilis and fasciculus cuneatus)	medulla oblongata
two-point discrimination	orange stick	posterior columns (fasciculus gracilis and fasciculus cuneatus)	medulla oblongata

Fig. 27.38 (B) Tests for different sensory modalities.

THE JOINTS

Examination

Diseases affecting the musculoskeletal system and how to distinguish between different disease processes on clinical examination have been discussed in detail in Chapter 16. However, remember the following broad components to the examination of joints.

General
- Does the patient look well or ill?
- Anaemia: chronic disease, blood loss (peptic ulcer due to non-steroidal use), bone marrow suppression (immunosuppressive therapy), haemolysis (autoimmune associated with systemic lupus erythematosus), and hypersplenism (Felty's syndrome in RA).
- Face: scleroderma, systemic lupus erythematosus, cushingoid facies (long-term steroid therapy).
- Stooped: ankylosing spondylitis and osteoporosis.

Look
- Deformity.
- Scars: previous surgery.
- Erythema: acute inflammation or infection.
- Swelling: osteophytes, synovial hypertrophy, and acute inflammation.
- Muscle wasting: disuse, nerve entrapment, mononeuritis multiplex, or long-term steroid therapy.

Feel
- Increased temperature: acute inflammation or infection.
- Tenderness.
- Effusions.
- Crepitus on movement.

Move
- Active and passive movement.
- Is pain associated with movement?
- Is the joint stable? Are there intact ligaments and supporting musculature?

What is the underlying cause?
- Psoriatic rash.
- Subcutaneous rheumatoid nodules: particularly at the elbow.

- Gouty tophi: on the pinna and elbow.
- Look for evidence of long-term steroid treatment (Fig. 27.39).

Disability

It is very important to get an impression of how limiting the joint problem is. For example, in a patient with RA, ask the patient to undo some buttons or write their name with a pen.

THE SKIN

The clinical approach to skin rashes has been discussed in detail in Chapter 17. When asked to look at a rash, you will be awarded marks for giving a good description, even if you are unable to make a diagnosis. Remember to describe the following:
- Distribution: this can be diagnostic in itself.
- Shape.
- Size.
- Colour.
- Consistency.
- Temperature.
- Tenderness.
- Margins.
- Relation to the surface: raised, flat, or ulcerated.
- Fixation to underlying structures.

Fig. 27.40 summarizes skin disorders associated with underlying systemic disease.

Problems of long-term steroid therapy

- Cushing's syndrome (thin skin with easy bruising, moon-like facies, central obesity)
- proximal myopathy
- osteoporosis
- psychosis
- oedema (sodium retention)
- hypertension
- diabetes mellitus
- avascular necrosis of femoral head
- peptic ulceration

Fig. 27.39 Problems of long-term steroid therapy.

Skin disorders associated with underlying systemic disease	
Disease	**Skin manifestation**
diabetes mellitus	necrobiosis lipoidica diabeticorum, granuloma annulare, acanthosis nigricans
sarcoidosis	lupus pernio, scar infiltration, erythema nodosum
malignancy	dermatomyositis, acanthosis nigricans, necrolytic migratory erythema (glucagonoma), erythema gyratum repens (usually bronchial carcinoma), thrombophlebitis migrans (pancreatic carcinoma)
liver disease	spider naevi, palmar erythema, leukonychia, porphyria cutanea tarda
renal disease	uraemic frost (rare), pale yellow pigmentation, half-and-half nails
hyperlipidaemia	xanthelasmata, tendon xanthomata, eruptive xanthomata
neurofibromatosis	*café-au-lait* patches, axillary freckling, neurofibromas, plexiform neuromas

Fig. 27.40 Skin disorders associated with underlying systemic disease.

28. The Clerking

INTRODUCTION

The doctor's 'clerking' is a written summary of the patient's history and examination. It is a legal document and should be precise, complete, and legible. Avoid using abbreviations—although the meaning may be obvious to you, they may be interpreted very differently in a different speciality or hospital.

At the end of the clerking, the salient points should be emphasized in a summary statement. You should then, always, compile a 'problem list'. This is often forgotten by students and junior doctors alike, but is invaluable in planning appropriate investigations and management. In some patients it will not be appropriate, or even possible, to take a full history and perform a full clinical examination, e.g. in an emergency situation. We have outlined a clinical example.

As a student it is good practice to be very thorough as it helps you to learn the relevant questions and to avoid missing anything important. However, with practice, you will learn to tailor carefully the clinical approach to each patient based on their individual, and often very different, needs.

MEDICAL SAMPLE CLERKING

CHECKLIST	EXAMPLE
Date:	1st January 2000
Time:	0720
Place:	A & E
Age:	47
Sex:	male
Occupation:	HGV driver
Referred by:	'999' call

PC (presenting complaint)

4 hour crushing retrosternal chest pain

HPC (history of presenting complaint)

Onset: 4 hours crushing retrosternal chest pain, radiating to neck and both arms, gradual onset over 5–10 mins.

Duration: persistent since onset.

Relieving/exacerbating factors:

GTN provided no relief although normally relieves pain in mins, no other relieving/exacerbating factors.

Associated symptoms:

nausea, vomiting (x 2), sweating, dizzy.

Relevant previous history:

1986 myocardial infarction, full recovery
1997 exertional chest tightness and dyspnoea initially controlled on atenolol
1/12 symptoms worse, exercise tolerance 200 yards on flat, limited by chest pain, no rest pain, no orthopnoea or PND

169

Risk factors

Hypertension	—no.
Smoking	—20 cigarettes per day from 16 years.
FH	—father died of 'heart attack' at 52 years.
Diabetes	—no.
Cholesterol	—never checked.
Ischaemic heart disease	—angina, previous MI.

PMH (past medical history)

1963: appendectomy.
1972: duodenal ulcer (no symptoms since).
1989: gout (quiescent on treatment).
NO diabetes, hypertension, rheumatic heart disease, tuberculosis, epilepsy, asthma, jaundice, cerebrovascular disease.

-S/E (systems enquiry)

General
Fatigue lately, appetite unchanged, weight stable, no sweats or pruritus, sleeping well.

CVS
As above.

RS
Dyspnoea on exertion, particularly uphill, but not limiting. No cough/sputum/wheeze

GIT
No current indigestion. No symptoms like previous duodenal ulcer. No vomiting/dysphagia/abdominal pain.

GUS
No change in bowel habit/rectal bleeding. No urinary symptoms.

NS
No headache/syncope. No dizziness/limb weakness/sensory loss. No disturbed vision/hearing/smell/speech.

MS
No painful gout for 5 years. No joint pain/stiffness/swelling. No disability.

Skin
No rash/pruritus/bruising.

Drug history
Atenolol 100 mg once daily.
Allopurinol 300 mg nocte.
GTN as required.
Not taking aspirin.
Allergies: Penicillin: skin rash.

FH (family history)
Father died of 'heart attack' age 52.
Mother died of old age at 76.

SH (social history)
Lives with wife who is fit and well.
Own house.
Completely independent.
Smoking 20 cigs/day for many years.
Alcohol: 24 units per week.
Sexual history: not appropriate.
Overseas travel: not appropriate.
Pets: not appropriate.
Occupation: heavy goods vehicle driver.

O/E (on examination)
General:
unwell, sweaty, clammy, no cyanosis/jaundice.
Temperature: 37.5 °C.
Cigarette-stained fingers.
No arcus/xanthomas/xanthelasma

CVS
Pulse 104 bpm regular, normal character.
BP 110/70 mmHg (right), 112/74 mmHg (left).
JVP normal.
No praecordial scars/chest deformities.
Apex beat displaced to anterior axillary line 6th intercostal space.
No parasternal heave/thrills.
Auscultation: Heart sounds normal, but soft pansystolic murmur at apex radiating to axilla,

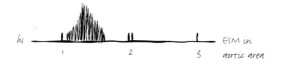

and ejection systolic murmur in aortic area with no
radiation.

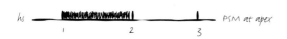

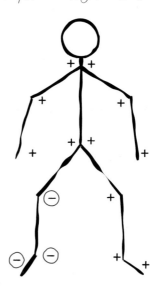

peripheral pulses: absent right popliteal to dorsalis pedis.
No sacral or ankle oedema.

RS
Trachea central.
Respiratory rate 15/min, no respiratory distress.
Expansion symmetrical and normal.
Vocal fremitus normal.
Percussion note normal.
Breath sounds vesicular throughout, no added sounds.

Abdomen
No scars/veins/distension.
Palpation: soft, but tender LIF (left iliac fossa).
Percussion note normal.
Auscultation bowel sounds normal.
Genitalia not examined.
Rectal examination: not performed.

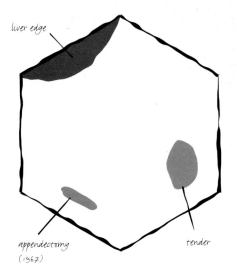

liver edge

appendectomy (1967)

tender

NS
Higher function normal.
Cranial nerves:
    I: normal.
    II: PERRLA (pupils equal in reaction to light and accomodation)/normal fundi and visual fields.
    III,IV,VI: no diplopia/nystagmus.
    V, VII, VIII, IX, X, XI, XII: normal.
Upper and lower limbs: power, tone, coordination, sensation all normal.

Reflexes

	Right	Left
Biceps	++	++
Supinator	++	++
Triceps	++	++
Knee	++	++
Ankle	+	+
Plantar	↓	↓

Joints and skin
Normal.

SUMMARY
47 year old male smoker, with a family history and previous history of ischaemic heart disease, presents with a 4 month history of increasing exertional chest pain and a 4 hour history of persistent, severe pain at rest which is unrelieved by GTN and associated with nausea, vomiting and sweating. On examination he has a resting taccycardia and evidence of left ventricular dilatation with a displaced apex beat and possible secondary mitral regurgitation. The most likely diagnosis is acute myocardial infarction.

PROBLEM LIST
Chest pain? myocardial infarction
Known ischaemic heart disease (myocardial infarction, post-infarct angina)
Clinical left ventricular enlargement with secondary mitral regurgitation
Previous duodenal ulcer but quiescent for years-no contraindications to thrombolysis
Gout (can be precipitated by the diuretics prescribed for cardiac failure)

29. Common Investigations

INTRODUCTION

By the time it comes to organizing investigations, the good clinician will already have a fairly clear idea of what he or she is likely to find. The investigation plan should be well structured, starting with simple non-invasive tests designed to answer specific questions. Remember two important rules:

- Do not request a test if you do not know why you are doing it. There is nothing worse than getting an abnormal result and wondering whether it is important or not!
- If a test is worth requesting, always make sure you see the result—it may be the clue you need.

If you are given an investigation to comment on in any examination, always describe what the investigation is, the patient's name, and the date it was performed. This is a good habit to get into, as the name will usually tell you what sex the patient is and possibly their ethnic background, which may be useful. As a practising clinician, it is also important as patients' results occasionally find their way into the wrong set of notes.

THE CARDIOVASCULAR SYSTEM

Cardiac enzymes

The enzymes released by necrotic myocardium following myocardial infarction (MI) include creatinine kinase (CK), aspartate aminotransferase (AST), and lactate dehydrogenase (LDH). Each enzyme is released and reaches a peak level at different times and can help to determine when the infarct occurred (see p. 7). Unfortunately these enzymes are also present in other tissues and are not specific (Fig. 29.1). Isoenzymes of CK (CK-MB) and LDH (LDH₁) can be measured and are more indicative of acute MI.

Electrocardiogram

The 12-lead electrocardiogram (ECG) is an assessment of the electrical activity of the heart. Twelve electrodes are attached to the patient, as shown in Fig. 29.2, giving 12 different 'views' of the heart (Fig. 29.3). Diagnostic information is obtained by considering the different components of the ECG.

Tissues containing 'cardiac enzymes' and the differential diagnosis of raised levels			
Enzyme	Creatinine kinase	Aspartate aminotransferase	Lactate dehydrogenase
tissues found in	cardiac muscle skeletal muscle smooth muscle brain	cardiac muscle skeletal muscle liver kidney red blood cells	cardiac muscle skeletal muscle liver kidney brain red blood cells
raised levels in	myocardial infarction muscle trauma postintramuscular injection muscular dystrophy hypothyroidism following surgery severe head injury	myocardial infarction hepatitis cirrhosis malignant hepatic infiltration muscle disease following surgery severe haemolytic anaemia	myocardial infarction megaloblastic anaemia lymphoma acute leukaemia malignancy muscle disease pulmonary embolus hepatitis renal infarction

Fig. 29.1 Tissues containing 'cardiac enzymes' and the differential diagnosis of raised levels.

Rate

Divide 300 by the number of large squares between two QRS complexes to give the number of beats per minute (each large square represents 0.2 seconds). Normal rate is 60–100 beats per minute. Causes of sinus tachycardia and bradycardia are shown in Fig. 29.4.

Rhythm

Are the QRS complexes regular? Is each QRS preceded by a p wave (Chapter 3)?

In tachycardia

In sinus tachycardia a P wave preceeds each QRS complex and the rhythm is regular. If there are no P waves and the rhythm is irregular, consider atrial fibrillation, atrial flutter with variable block, and frequent ectopic beats.

If no p waves are present and the rhythm is regular, consider atrial tachycardia, atrial flutter with 2:1 block, and ventricular tachycardia.

In bradycardia

If P waves are small or absent, check for hyperkalaemia. In sinus bradycardia P waves are present and the rhythm is regular.

In first-degree heart block, P waves are present with a regular rhythm, but the PR interval is prolonged.

In second-degree heart block two or more P waves are present between each QRS (2:1 or 3:1 heart block). In

Mobitz I (second-degree heart block) the PR interval gradually lengthens until one P wave is not conducted. In Mobitz II, the PR interval is constant with dropped beats.

In third-degree heart block, P waves are present but are completely independent of QRS complexes, creating an irregular rhythm (see Chapter 30—cardiovascular disease).

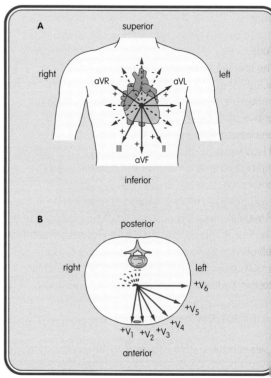

Fig. 29.3 The 12 different views of the heart given by a 12-lead electrocardiogram. (A) Superior perspective. (B) Posterior perspective.

Causes of sinus tachycardia and sinus bradycardia	
Sinus tachycardia	**Sinus bradycardia**
anxiety	physical fitness
exercise	sinoatrial node disease
anaemia	hypothermia
shock	hypothyroidism
fever	cholestatic jaundice
pregnancy	raised intracranial pressure
thyrotoxicosis	postmyocardial infarction
pulmonary embolus	drugs, e.g. β-blockers
cardiac failure	
drugs, e.g. β-agonists	

Fig. 29.2 The position of the anterior electrodes for a 12-lead electrocardiogram.

Fig. 29.4 Causes of sinus tachycardia and sinus bradycardia

Check whether the complexes are regular by marking five QRS complexes on a piece of paper. Move it along by one complex and your marks should coincide exactly.

Axis

The axis is the average direction of spread of electrical activity through the ventricles. The normal axis lies between -30° and +90° (Fig. 29.5). Look at leads I, II, and III. If the axis in normal, all three will have a predominantly upwards or positive deflection (i.e. R>S). If lead I is negative (with the others positive), there is right axis deviation. If lead II is negative (with I positive and III negative), there is left axis deviation.

P wave

The P wave represents electrical activity of the right and left atria.

It is tall in P pulmonale (i.e. >2.5 mm), which is caused by hypertrophy of the right atrium, as in

tricuspid stenosis or pulmonary hypertension. The P wave is bifid (like an 'm') in P mitrale, which is caused by hypertrophy of the left atrium as in mitral stenosis.

PR interval

The PR interval represents the time for electrical activity to pass from the sinoatrial node to the atrioventricular (AV) node—it should be 0.12–0.2 seconds (3–5 small squares).

It is prolonged in heart block (see above) and shortened in Wolff–Parkinson–White and Lown–Ganong–Levine syndrome due to accessory pathways connecting the atria and ventricles. In Wolff-Parkinson-White syndrome there is also a slurred upstroke of the R wave, which is called a delta wave.

QRS complex

The QRS complex represents ventricular depolarization; it should last less than 0.12 seconds (3 small squares).

It is broad if depolarization has spread through an abnormal route, either due to disruption of the pathway, as in bundle branch block, or because it has started somewhere other than the AV node, as in ventricular ectopic beats or ventricular tachycardia.

Q waves result from depolarization of the septum and should be less than 0.04 seconds (1 small square) and less than 2 small squares deep. Abnormally wide and deep Q waves are permanent features of MI.

The height of the R wave in V_5 and V_6 should be less than 25 mm. The R wave may be abnormally tall in left ventricular hypertrophy (Fig. 29.6); the QRS complexes may be abnormally small in pericardial effusion.

ST segment

The ST segment should not be greater than 1 mm above or below the isoelectric line. (Causes of ST elevation are shown on p. 7.) ST depression is an indication of myocardial ischaemia.

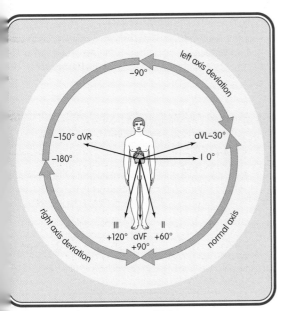

Fig. 29.5 Axis determination on ECG.

Features of left ventricular hypertrophy
• S wave in V_1 and R wave in V_5 or $V_6 \geq 35$ mm • R wave in $V_{5-6} > 27$ mm • S wave in $V_{1-3} > 30$ mm • ST depression in I, aVL, V_{4-6} • T wave inversion in I, aVl, V_{4-6} • left axis deviation

Fig. 29.6 Features of left ventricular hypertrophy.

T wave

The T wave represents ventricular repolarization and should be less than 10 mm in height. Peaked T waves are seen in acute MI and hyperkalaemia. Small, flattened T waves may be seen in hypokalaemia. Inverted T waves are a feature of myocardial ischaemia, infarction, and digitalis effect (reverse tick sign).

QT interval

The QT interval is the time from ventricular depolarization (start of QRS) to complete ventricular repolarization (end of T wave). It should be less than 0.44 seconds (which is 2 large squares). The QT interval varies inversely with heart rate (e.g. shortens in tachycardia). It can be corrected for rate by calculating $QT/_{R-R}$.

The QT interval is increased in hypocalcaemia, hypomagnesaemia, drugs (amiodarone, β-blockers, tricyclics), or severe myocardial disease.

U wave

The U wave is often a normal variant but is more prominent in hypokalaemia.

Exercise electrocardiogram

The resting ECG is taken. The patient then performs exercise until symptoms develop or the protocol is complete. Regular pulse, blood pressure, and ECGs are recorded. Evidence of myocardial ischaemia (ST depression and T wave inversion) and rate induced arrhythmias are looked for.

The test is useful for the following:
- Assessment of severity of ischaemic heart disease.
- Prognosis following MI.
- Exercise-induced palpitations.
- Diagnosis of atypical chest pain—is it angina or not?

24-Hour electrocardiogram

The 24-hour ECG records cardiac rhythm over a 24-hour period while the patient continues with their normal daily activities. It will detect transient arrhythmias and is useful in the investigation of episodic syncope, palpitations, dizziness, and dyspnoea.

Chest X-ray

Chest X-ray (CXR) can give much information regarding both the underlying diagnosis, as well as subsequent complications. This information is summarized in Fig. 29.7. Further related details are shown for mitral valve disease in Fig. 29.8, and for pulmonary oedema in Fig. 29.9.

Echocardiography

Echocardiography is an ultrasound technique that can be performed via a transthoracic or transoesophageal approach. It gives structural information of the heart.

Underlying diagnoses and complications in the cardiovascular system detectable on chest X-ray		
Region	Diagnosis	X-ray findings
pericardium	tuberculosis or constrictive pericarditis	calcification
myocardium	effusion left ventricular dilatation right ventricular dilatation left atrium left ventricular aneurysm	globular cardiomegaly cardiomegaly with left ventricle displaced inferolaterally cardiomegaly with apex beat elevated double right heart border; splaying of carina calcified mural thrombus
endocardium	rheumatic heart disease	calcification
valves	valve replacement mitral valve disease atheroma	sternal wires; metallic valves; surgical clips Fig. 29.8 calcification
aorta	coarctation dissection	rib notching widened mediastinum
lungs	pulmonary oedema	Fig. 29.9

Fig. 29.7 Underlying diagnoses and complications in the cardiovascular system detectable on chest X-ray.

Chest X-ray features of mitral stenosis
• calcified mitral valve • dilated left atrium (makes the left heart border look straight) • splayed carina with elevation of left main bronchus • prominent pulmonary arteries indicating pulmonary hypertension • pulmonary oedema may be present

Fig. 29.8 Chest X-ray features of mitral stenosis.

Chest X-ray features of pulmonary oedema
• upper lobe veins dilatation • Kerley B lines • bat's wing shadowing (perihilar oedema) • fluid in the horizontal fissure • pleural effusion (usually bilateral but can be unilateral)

Fig. 29.9 Chest X-ray features of pulmonary oedema.

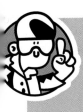

To make a definite diagnosis of left ventricular hypertrophy, voltage criteria in addition to repolarization abnormalities must be present.

Colour doppler can be used to look at blood flow and pressure gradients across valves. It is useful in the diagnosis of the following:
- Pericardium: effusion.
- Myocardium: left ventricular hypertrophy, left ventricular dysfunction, cardiomyopathies.
- Endocardium: atrial myxoma, vegetations, thrombus.
- Valves: stenosis and regurgitation with estimation of pressure across valves.
- Congenital heart disease: including atrial and ventricular septal defects.
- Aorta: aneurysm.

Thallium perfusion scan

Thallium perfusion scan monitors cardiac uptake of radioactive thallium. Areas with a poor coronary blood supply are identified as 'cold spots'. This test can be used in patients unable to use a treadmill, such as those with osteoarthritis affecting the lower limbs.

Cardiac catheterization

The right side of the heart is catheterized via the femoral vein (usually the right). The left side of the heart and coronary arteries are catheterised via the femoral artery. It provides the following information:
- Pressure in different chambers of the heart and the great vessels.
- Pressure gradient across the valves.

- Anatomy of the coronary arteries: following injection of radiopaque dye.
- Assessment of blood flow: valvular regurgitation or across septal defects.
- Oxygen concentrations: in different heart chambers in assessment of shunts.

Therapeutic measures include:
- Angioplasty (Fig. 29.10).
- Valvotomy.
- Arterial stent insertion.

THE RESPIRATORY SYSTEM

Chest X-ray

You should develop your own routine for looking at a CXR so as not to miss important features, particularly when there is a glaring abnormality that immediately demands attention. This should include the trachea, mediastinum (nodes, vessels), cardiac outline, diaphragms (including the costo- and cardiophrenic angles), lung fields themselves, bones, and soft tissues. The radiological findings for common respiratory diseases are outlined in Fig. 29.11.

If you cannot see any abnormality, look specifically at the apices for a small pneumothorax or cervical rib, behind the heart for a hiatus hernia (air–fluid level), at the soft tissues for unilateral mastectomy, and below the diaphragms for free gas.

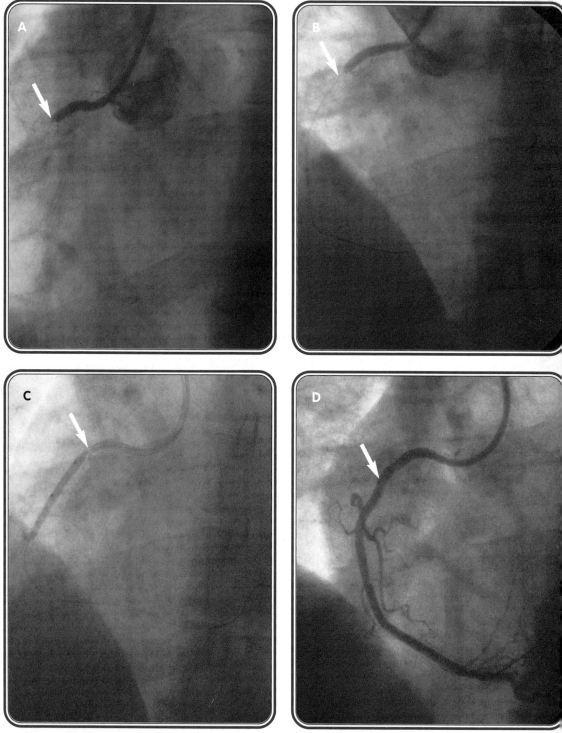

Fig. 29.10 Percutaneous transluminal coronary angioplasty (PTCA) of the right coronary artery. (A) The right coronary artery is occluded proximally. (B) A guide wire is introduced into the artery. (C) A balloon is inflated over the site of the obstruction, and a stent is deployed. (D) The whole artery is patent at the end of the procedure.

Always look at a chest X-ray in a systematic way as outlined in this section. Never comment on heart size unless the film is a posterior–anterior (PA) projection.

Spirometry

Measurements of airflow rates and forced vital capacity are obtained using a spirometer. The patient breathes in to maximum inspiration and then exhales into the spirometer as quickly and for as long as possible. The volume expelled is plotted against time.

The FEV$_1$ (forced expiratory volume in 1 second) is the volume exhaled in the first second of the test. The FVC (forced vital capacity) is the total volume exhaled. Both

measurements are related to age, sex, and height, and nomograms are used to provide predicted or 'normal' parameters. The FEV$_1$ is expressed as a percentage of the FVC and is 70–80% in normal subjects.

Where there is obstruction to airflow, as in bronchospasm due to chronic bronchitis, the FEV$_1$ is very much reduced. Although the total lung volume is increased, the FVC will also be slightly reduced due to air trapping as the small airways collapse. However, the reduction in FEV$_1$ is much greater than that for FVC and the FEV$_1$/FVC ratio is reduced (Fig. 29.12).

A repeat test should be performed after the administration of bronchodilators to determine if there is a reversible element present.

Restrictive defects due to pulmonary fibrosis are characterized by reduced lung volumes and reduced FVC. The FEV$_1$ will be normal or slightly reduced. The FEV$_1$/FVC ratio is therefore normal or increased (Fig. 29.12).

Radiological findings associated with common respiratory diseases	
Abnormality	**Radiological findings**
airways obstruction (asthma, emphysema, chronic bronchitis)	lungs hyperexpanded with flat hemidiaphragms allowing visualization of anterior aspects of sixth ribs; apical bullae may be seen in emphysema; look specifically for pneumothorax which may complicate bronchospasm or for evidence of infection which may have caused it
pneumonia	hazy opacification, often limited to one lobe or segment but may be diffuse; bronchi remain patent and may form air bronchograms; sometimes associated with collapse or pleural effusion
pulmonary embolus	often no abnormality; elevated hemidiaphragm, local oligaemia, wedge atelectasis, and pleural effusions may be seen
tumour	localized opacification; look for small rounded opacifications or hilar lymphadenopathy suggesting metastases
pleural effusion	dense opacity in the lower zone with edges curved upwards (meniscus); hemidiaphragm and heart border not visible; mediastinum may shift if effusion massive; look for causes of effusion such as tumour; need at least 500 ml of fluid before detectable on chest X-ray
fibrosis	diffuse 'ground glass', nodular or reticular may progress to honeycomb lung if severe; mediastinum may shift towards disease due to loss of lung volume
pneumothorax	increased translucency due to absence of vascular shadowing and visible visceral pleura; mediastinum will shift only if pneumothorax massive or under tension; look for underlying pathology such as airways obstruction
tuberculosis	apical mass with hilar lymphadenopathy with or without pleural effusion; may become calcified; apical fibrosis and miliary mottling indicate postprimary disease
bronchiectasis	may be normal; thickened bronchi may be visible as tramline or ring shadows; look for dextrocardia (Kartagener's syndrome)
pulmonary oedema	see Fig. 29.9

Fig. 29.11 Radiological findings associated with common respiratory diseases.

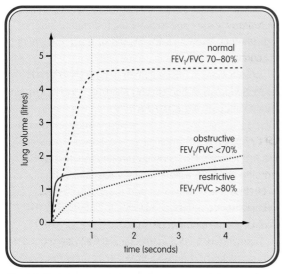

Fig. 29.12 Spirometry in normal patients, and those with obstructive and restrictive pulmonary defects.

When looking at blood gas results, remember these three handy tips:
- If the pCO_2 is high the problem is poor ventilation.
- If the pCO_2 is high, look at the HCO_3^-. If there is chronic carbon dioxide retention, it will be high due to renal compensation. Giving oxygen to these patients can be disastrous as they rely on hypoxic drive to maintain respiration.
- Administration of oxygen to hypoxic patients will improve or correct the pO_2 in all causes except right-to-left shunt.

Transfer factor

Transfer factor (TCLO) is a measurement of the diffusing capacity of a low concentration of carbon monoxide. The diffusion is across the alveolar–capillary membrane (i.e. movement from the alveolus to the blood) and is dependent on three conditions:
- An adequate blood supply to the areas of lung ventilated, i.e. ventilation–perfusion (V/Q) matching.
- Efficient diffusion across the alveolar–capillary membrane.
- Adequate amounts of normal haemoglobin.

TLCO should be corrected for the haemoglobin concentration. If it remains abnormal, it indicates that the pathology present has disrupted diffusion.

TLCO will be low when any of the three above steps are affected, as in emphysema, pulmonary fibrosis (from any cause), and *Pneumocystis carinii* pneumonia in patients with acquired immuno-deficiency syndrome. It will be raised in polycythaemia, left-to-right shunts, and pulmonary haemorrhage.

Arterial blood gases

The partial pressures of oxygen and carbon dioxide in the blood are dependent on the following factors:
- Neuromuscular control of ventilation.
- Patent airways for ventilation.

- Diffusion across the alveolar–capillary membrane.
- Pulmonary capillary blood flow matching the areas of ventilation.

Oxygen is carried in the blood in an easily reversible combination with haemoglobin. Carotid and aortic body chemoreceptors detect low partial pressures of oxygen pO_2.

Carbon dioxide is carried in the blood mainly as bicarbonate (reaction catalysed by carbonic anhydrase principally in the red blood cells [RBCs]) but is also bound to protein or dissolved. It therefore has a profound effect on the acid–base balance. Increased levels are detected by central chemoreceptors (increasing hydrogen ions) and peripheral chemoreceptors (increasing partial pressure of carbon dioxide [pCO_2] and falling pH).

Arterial blood is sampled from a peripheral artery (usually the radial artery). The pO_2, pCO_2, pH, bicarbonate (HCO_3^-), and oxygen saturations can be measured. The pO_2 will be low if atmospheric oxygen is low (e.g. at high altitude), if ventilation is poor (see below), if diffusion is reduced (interstitial lung disease), there is a V/Q mismatch (pulmonary embolus [PE]), or there is a right-to-left shunt (ventricular septal defect with Eisenmenger's phenomenon).

The pCO_2 will be high if ventilation is inadequate. This may be due to reduced central drive (sedative drugs, cerebral trauma), neuromuscular disease (Guillain–Barré syndrome, myasthenia gravis), thoracic wall abnormalities (kyphoscoliosis, ankylosing spondylitis) or airways obstruction (chronic bronchitis).

The pCO_2 will be low in hyperventilation due to anxiety or panic.

Respiratory failure

Respiratory failure is defined by a pO_2 of less than 8 kPa and can be subdivided according to the pCO_2.

In type I respiratory failure there is a low pO_2 with normal pCO_2. This can be caused by lung disease (pneumonia, pulmonary fibrosis, pulmonary oedema), V/Q mismatch (PE), or right-to-left shunts.

If the pO_2 is very low, ventilation will increase and the pCO_2 may also be low.

In type II respiratory failure there is a low pO_2 with high pCO_2. This results from inadequate ventilation (see above).

Ventilation–perfusion scan

Technetium-99m-(^{99m}Tc)-labelled albumin is injected intravenously and detected in the lungs by a gamma camera—this is the perfusion scan. Areas not perfused are identified as 'cold spots'.

Pulmonary ventilation is demonstrated by the inhalation of xenon-133 (^{133}Xe), which is also detected by a gamma camera.

In PE, an area of well-ventilated lung is deprived of its blood supply. This will create a discrepancy ('mismatch') in the V/Q scans which is diagnostic of PE. Where a V/Q scan is not possible, a pulmonary angiogram should be considered. In other pulmonary diseases, such as pneumonia, both ventilation and perfusion are reduced. This results in a non-specific 'matched' defect.

V/Q scans are reported in most centres as showing high, intermediate, or low probability of PE. When the probability is intermediate or low, careful clinical re-evaluation and further investigations are usually required.

Computed tomography scan

Most lung pathology can be detected by a standard CXR. However, computed tomography (CT) scanning provides more detailed information regarding the mediastinum and pleura and is particularly valuable in two scenarios:

- Demonstration and staging of bronchogenic carcinoma.
- Demonstration of pulmonary disease not detectable by CXR, e.g. industrial lung disease, lymphangitis carcinomatosis, sarcoidosis.

Bronchoscopy

Fibre-optic bronchoscopy is performed under local anaesthetic and allows direct visualization of the bronchial tree. It is important in the diagnosis and sometimes treatment of pulmonary disease.

Central tumours can be visualized and biopsied. Transbronchial biopsy of the lung will provide diagnostic tissue in interstitial lung disease.

Bronchoalveolar lavage is important in the diagnosis of some infections (tuberculosis, *P. carinii*), peripheral tumours, and some unusual diseases (e.g. histiocytosis X).

Laser therapy can obliterate small endobronchial tumours and palliate large symptomatic tumours that have not responded to other therapeutic modalities.

Lung biopsy

Biopsy may be necessary in the diagnosis of tumours, interstitial lung disease, and infections when other techniques have failed to provide adequate information. The tissue can be obtained by transthoracic needle biopsy under ultrasound or CT guidance, mediastinoscopy, mediastinotomy, thoracoscopy, and open biopsy at thoracotomy.

THE GASTROINTESTINAL SYSTEM

Serum amylase

Amylase breaks down starch to glycogen and maltose. It is found at highest concentrations in saliva and pancreatic juice and is excreted in the urine. It is used as an indicator of acute pancreatitis where levels may be very high (i.e. greater than five times normal upper limit). However, serum amylase may also be elevated in the conditions listed in Fig. 29.13.

Plain abdominal X-ray

Plain X-rays are of limited use in gastrointestinal (GI) disease. Fig. 29.14 shows radiological changes that may be found in specific diseases.

Ultrasound scan, CT scan, and magnetic resonance imaging

These are useful in defining intra-abdominal anatomical abnormalities and pathologies such as fluid (ascites, abscess), tumour and stones (biliary, urinary tract). Ultrasound is cheaper, more accessible and, is often used as the first-line investigation. CT and magnetic resonance imaging (MRI) are particularly helpful in examining the deeper structures that are not always adequately visualized on ultrasound, which include the pancreas and retroperitoneum.

Barium swallow

The progress of swallowed barium is recorded. This procedure is used in the investigation of dysphagia. It should be performed prior to endoscopy in these patients to demonstrate oesophageal anatomy and prevent perforation by the endoscope. It will demonstrate anatomical lesions in the oesophagus including strictures, carcinoma, web, or pharyngeal pouch, and motility abnormalities such as achalasia.

Barium meal

Barium is taken with effervescent tablets producing a double-contrast image of the stomach and proximal duodenum. This will demonstrate anatomical abnormalities including ulcers and polyps. However, most patients with gastric pathology will need a histological diagnosis and endoscopy with the option of biopsy is the investigation of choice.

Small bowel contrast studies

Barium can be introduced into the small bowel in two ways—in a small bowel follow-through, barium is swallowed and its journey to the terminal ileum is recorded; and in a small bowel enema, barium is delivered to the distal duodenum via a nasojejunal tube. It is useful in the diagnosis of small bowel polyposis, Crohn's disease, and malignancies, such as lymphoma.

Causes of a raised serum amylase

- acute pancreatitis
- perforated peptic ulcer
- ruptured ectopic pregnancy
- acute cholecystitis
- diabetic ketoacidosis
- severe glomerular disease
- myocardial infarction
- mumps
- salivary calculi

Fig. 29.13 Causes of a raised serum amylase.

Radiological abdominal abnormalities associated with gastrointestinal diseases	
Diagnosis	**Radiological abnormality**
intestinal obstruction	proximal bowel distension; absent bowel gas distally; air–fluid levels on the erect film
perforation of a viscus	subdiaphragmatic free gas on the erect film
sigmoid volvulus	grossly distended loop of sigmoid colon often extending from the pelvis to the xiphisternum (looks like a coffee bean)
acute pancreatitis	'sentinel loop' of dilated adynamic small bowel; 'ground glass' appearance if ascites present
chronic pancreatitis	pancreatic calcification
calculi	90% of urinary tract stones and 10% of gallstones are radiopaque
abdominal aortic aneurysm	calcified aneurysmal abdominal aorta

Fig. 29.14 Radiological abdominal abnormalities associated with gastrointestinal diseases.

Barium enema

A double-contrast picture of the colon and terminal ileum is produced by introducing barium and air into the rectum. The rectum is poorly visualized and should be examined by sigmoidoscopy. Typical abnormalities will be seen in polyps, malignancy, ulcerative colitis, and Crohn's disease.

Endoscopy

Various 'scopes' are now available, enabling direct visualization of the whole GI tract with the exception of the third part of the duodenum to the terminal ileum (Fig. 29.15).

As well as visualizing pathology, biopsies can be taken for histological diagnosis. Contrast can also be injected into the pancreatic and biliary tree (endoscopic retrograde cholangiopancreatogram [ERCP]).

Endoscopy is also important in treatment for the following reasons:

- Strictures can be dilated.
- Stents and prosthetic tubes can be placed through malignant lesions causing obstruction (oesophagus, urinary tract, ampulla of Vater).
- Varices can be injected with sclerosing agents.
- Polyps can be removed.
- Bleeding lesions can be cauterized.

THE URINARY SYSTEM

Urine

Urine should be collected by taking a midstream specimen which minimizes contamination by skin commensals.

The urine should have a dipstick test which gives an indication of urinary pH, specific gravity, protein, glucose, ketones, and blood. Causes of proteinuria and haematuria are discussed in detail in Chapter 13. Glycosuria is usually due to high plasma glucose concentration (diabetes mellitus) though it may rarely be due to renal glycosuria, an autosomal dominant condition characterized by a reduction in tubular glucose reabsorption.

Heavy ketonuria is a feature of diabetic ketoacidosis, though ketones will become present in the urine on testing for several hours.

Microscopy is performed to determine the number of RBCs and white blood cells (WBCs), and the presence of bacteria or casts. A urinary tract abnormality is likely to be present if there is more than 2 RBC or 5 WBCs per high-powered field, RBC or WBC casts, or a large number of bacteria ($>1 \times 10^5$/mL). The urine can be cultured to confirm a urinary tract infection and to determine sensitivities to available antibiotics. If tuberculosis is suspected, three early morning specimens should be examined.

Urea and creatinine

Urea is produced by the liver from amino acids, while creatinine is a product of tissue breakdown; both are excreted by the kidneys. Levels of both in the plasma are dependent on a balance between production and excretion.

In renal failure, urea and creatinine will be raised proportionally. In an upper GI bleed, urea will be raised but creatinine remains normal (high protein intake—blood absorbed by the small intestine). The urea:creatinine ratio is also raised in dehydration and tetracycline administration. A low ratio occurs in chronic liver disease, low-protein diet, and haemodialysis. Creatinine may also be low in those with reduced muscle bulk.

Plain X-ray

A plain X-ray ('KUB' film) is most useful in the diagnosis of renal stones, of which 90% are radiopaque. It also demonstrates renal size, shape, and position.

Renal ultrasound

Renal ultrasound is good at detecting renal size, cysts, stones, tumours, and urinary outflow obstruction (hydronephrosis), but gives little

'Scopes' used to examine the gastrointestinal tract	
'Scope'	**Bowel visualized**
oesophagogastroscope	oesophagus, stomach, first two parts of duodenum
colonoscope	rectum, entire colon, terminal ileum
flexible sigmoidoscope	rectum, descending colon
rigid sigmoidoscope	rectum, lower sigmoid colon
proctoscope	anus, lower rectum

Fig. 29.15 'Scopes' used to examine the gastrointestinal tract.

information regarding the pelvicalyceal system and is a poor predictor of renal artery stenosis. It provides no information about renal function.

Intravenous urography

Renally excreted contrast is injected intravenously and a series of X-rays are taken at specific time intervals. Information regarding anatomy and excretion are gained by following the movement of contrast from the renal parenchyma, through the pelvicalyceal system, to the ureters and bladder. It detects renal scarring due to chronic parenchymal disease, pelvicalyceal pathology, the location of calculi and is a good predictive indicator of renal artery stenosis.

CT scan

CT scan provides detailed anatomical information. It is important in staging malignancy and the examination of regions poorly visualized by other techniques, such as the retroperitoneal and perinephric areas.

Radioisotope studies

Renal scintigraphy can provide information about gross renal anatomy, obstruction, the relative contribution of each kidney to overall renal function, and features suggestive of renal artery stenosis. Its accuracy is increased by the coadministration of Captopril—the 'Captopril renogram'.

Renal angiography

Contrast is injected directly into the renal arteries via a catheter introduced into the femoral artery. This is the gold standard test for the diagnosis of renovascular disease.

Cystoscopy

Cystoscopy allows the direct visualization of the bladder mucosa. It is useful in the diagnosis and sometimes treatment of bladder carcinoma.

A slightly elevated creatinine may indicate significant renal impairment.

Renal biopsy

Renal biopsy is performed transcutaneously under ultrasound guidance. It is particularly useful in the assessment of rapidly deteriorating renal function, nephrotic syndrome, and assessment of transplanted kidneys. It may be complicated by significant haematuria, pain, and, in the long term, arteriovenous malformation. Biopsy material should be evaluated by light microscopy, electron microscopy, and immunofluorescence.

THE NERVOUS SYSTEM

Tests useful in the diagnosis of neurological disease have been described in Chapter 22.

METABOLIC AND ENDOCRINE DISORDERS

Diabetes mellitus

Diabetes mellitus (DM) is characterized by chronic hyperglycaemia. It can be primary, as in type 1 (IDDM—insulin-dependent DM) and type 2 (NIDDM—non-insulin dependent DM), or secondary to pancreatic disease (chronic pancreatitis, haemochromatosis, cystic fibrosis), endocrine disease (Cushing's syndrome, acromegaly), pregnancy, or drugs (steroids, thiazide diuretics).

Diagnosis

Diagnostic criteria for diabetes mellitus include:
- Fasting blood glucose >6.7 mmol/L (7.8 mmol/L in plasma).
- On two separate occasions, random blood glucose >10 mmol/L (11.1 mmol/L in plasma).
- Oral glucose tolerance test >10 mmol/L 2 hours after ingestion of 75 g oral glucose (11.1 mmol/L in plasma).

Monitoring response to diet or treatment

Glycated haeomoglobin (HBA1c) gives a measurement of overall glycaemic control over the previous 2–3 months. Fructosamine gives a measurement of overall glycaemic control over the previous 1–3 weeks.

Hypothalamus–pituitary–adrenal axis

Fig. 29.16 summarizes the normal control of cortisol. Excess circulating cortisol causes the clinical picture of Cushing's syndrome. It may result from increased release of adrenocorticotrophic hormone (ACTH) from an anterior pituitary adenoma (Cushing's disease), ectopic ACTH from a bronchogenic carcinoma or carcinoid tumour, excess cortisol production by an adrenal adenoma or carcinoma, or by the oral administration of corticosteroids. Pseudo-Cushing's syndrome may arise in alcohol abuse and endogenous depression.

Reduced circulating cortisol results from reduced pituitary ACTH production (tumour, infarction, prolonged corticosteroid therapy), or reduced adrenal cortisol production (autoimmune Addison's disease, tuberculosis, metastases, amyloidosis, Waterhouse–Friderichsen syndrome).

Tests useful for determining the site of the lesion in cortisol excess and deficiency are given in Fig. 29.17.

Plasma cortisol

Plasma cortisol will vary throughout the day in normal individuals and should be measured at 9am and 11pm. Normal circadian rhythm will be lost and levels raised in Cushing's syndrome. Very low or absent cortisol levels at a time of suspected addisonian crisis confirms hypoproduction of cortisol.

Tests for cortisol excess

Urinary cortisol
24-hour estimation of urinary free cortisol is a better predictor of Cushing's syndrome than plasma cortisol.

Plasma ACTH
This is very high in ectopic ACTH production, moderately raised in Cushing's syndrome (pituitary adenoma), and very low in adrenal adenoma or carcinoma.

Overnight dexamethasone suppression test
Here, 2 mg oral dexamethasone is taken at 11pm; plasma cortisol is measured at 9am the next morning. In normal patients, ACTH and cortisol production will be suppressed by negative feedback, and plasma levels of cortisol will be <190 nmol/L.

In all cases of Cushing's syndrome suppression will not occur. In patients with Cushing's disease the feedback mechanism is less sensitive than normal as ACTH levels are chronically elevated. Ectopic ACTH production has no feedback mechanism; ACTH is always suppressed in those with an adrenal cause.

High-dose dexamethasone suppression test
Plasma cortisol is measured; 2 mg oral dexamethasone is taken every 6 hours for 2 days. After 48 hours from the first dose, plasma cortisol is remeasured. In normal individuals the plasma cortisol should be suppressed to at least half its initial value. This dose of dexamethasone should overcome the less sensitive feedback mechanism in Cushing's disease but will not cause suppression in ectopic ACTH production and adrenal hyperfunction.

Tests for cortisol deficiency

Short Synacthen stimulation test
Plasma cortisol is measured (>170 nmol/L normally) and 0.25 mg Synacthen (which has the same biological action as ACTH) is given intramuscularly or intravenously. Plasma cortisol is remeasured after 60 minutes. In normal patients, cortisol will rise by a minimum of 190 nmol/L to at least 580 nmol/L. The response will be poor in any case of cortisol hypoproduction.

Long Synacthen stimulation test
Here, 1 mg Synacthen is given by intramuscular injection daily for 3 days. Adrenal glands suppressed by the

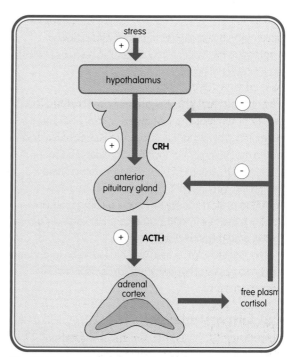

Fig. 29.16 Hypothalamus–pituitary–adrenal axis. (ACTH, adrenocorticotrophic hormone; CRH, corticotrophin-releasing hormone.)

Investigations in abnormalities of the hypothalamus–pituitary–adrenal axis					
	Cushing's disease	**Ectopic ACTH production**	**Adrenal hyperproduction of cortisol**	**Pituitary hypoproduction of ACTH**	**Adrenal hypoproduction of cortisol**
causes	pituitary adenoma	bronchial carcinoma, carcinoid tumour	adenoma, carcinoma	tumour, infarction, corticosteroids	Addison's disease, amyloid, TB, metastases, Waterhouse–Friderichsen syndrome
plasma cortisol	high	high	high	low	low
plasma ACTH	high	very high	very low	low	high
urinary free cortisol	high	high	high	low	low
overnight dexamethasone suppression test	no suppression	no suppression	no suppression	not applicable	not applicable
high-dose dexamethasone suppression test	suppression	no suppression	no suppression	not applicable	not applicable
short Synacthen test	not applicable	not applicable	not applicable	no stimulation	no stimulation
long Synacthen test	not applicable	not applicable	not applicable	stimulation	no stimulation

Fig. 29.17 Investigations in abnormalities of the hypothalamus–pituitary–adrenal axis. (ACTH, adrenocorticotrophic hormone.)

prolonged admistration of corticosteroids show a response to this level of stimulation. No response will be seen in adrenal hypofunction.

The hypothalamus–pituitary–thyroid axis

Fig. 29.18 summarizes the normal control of thyroid hormones. Thyroid status can now be easily assessed by the measurement of thyroid-stimulating hormone (TSH), total thyoxine (T_4) and total tri-iodothyronine (T_3) (Fig. 29.19). Around 99% of circulating T_4 and T_3 is bound to protein (mostly thyroxine-binding globulin—TBG). It is the free T_4 and T_3 that is physiologically active and can be measured separately.

The TRH stimulation test, which used to be important in the diagnosis of hyperthyroidism, is now almost never necessary.

Calcium metabolism

Calcium homoeostasis is dependent on the normal availability of calcium and vitamin D and normal functioning of the parathyroid glands, kidneys, and gut (Fig. 29.20).

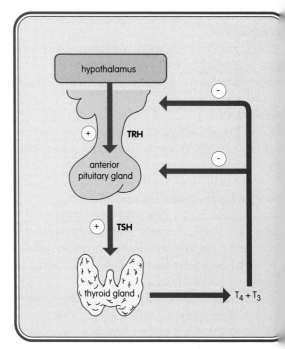

Fig. 29.18 Hypothalamus–pituitary–thyroid axis. (TRH, thyrotropin-releasing hormone; TSH, thyroid-stimulating hormone.)

Biochemical abnormalities in thyroid disease				
	Primary thyrotoxicosis	**Secondary thyrotoxicosis**	**Primary hypothyroidism**	**Secondary hypothyroidism**	**Sick euthyroid syndrome**
causes	thyroiditis, toxic adenoma, multinodular goitre, carcinoma, amiodarone	pituitary adenoma	thyroiditis, iodine deficiency, dyshormonogenesis, antithyroid drugs, postirradiation/^{131}I therapy	hypopituitarism, isolated TSH deficiency	acute severe illness
TSH	low	high	high	low	normal or low
total or free T$_4$ and T$_3$	T$_3$ high (first) then T$_4$ high	T$_3$ high (first) then T$_4$ high	T$_4$ low (first) then T$_3$ low	T$_4$ low (first) then T$_3$ low	T$_4$ and T$_3$ low

Fig. 29.19 Biochemical abnormalities in thyroid disease. (T$_3$, tri-iodothyronine; T$_4$, thyroxine; TSH, thyroid-stimulating hormone.)

Fig. 29.20 Calcium homeostasis. (PTH, parathyroid hormone.)

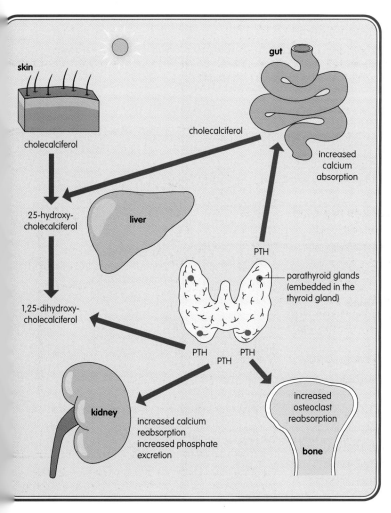

Plasma calcium

Total plasma calcium is measured and should be adjusted for albumin concentration (half is protein bound but it is the unbound that is physiologically active). The most accurate measurement is in the fasted patient with a sample taken without a cuff. Causes of hypercalcaemia and hypocalcaemia are shown in Figs 29.21 and 29.22.

Phosphate

Phosphate levels are dependent on a balance between release from bone by osteoclastic activity, and renal tubular reabsorption. Parathyroid hormone (PTH) increases phosphate release from bone but reduces renal reabsorption, with the overall effect of lowering phosphate concentrations.

Hyperphosphataemia occurs in renal disease and hypoparathyroidism.

Hypophosphataemia occurs as a result of hyperparathyroidism, reduced intake due to dietary deficiency or long-term parenteral feeding, and increased phosphate loss as in renal tubular acidosis.

Causes of hypercalcaemia	
Mechanism	**Example**
increased calcium intake	milk–alkali syndrome
increased vitamin D intake	self-administered, iatrogenic
increased activity of vitamin D	sarcoidosis, lymphoma, Addison's disease
increased production of PTH	primary hyperparathyroidism (adenoma, hyperplasia, carcinoma), tertiary hyperparathyroidism (hyperplasia)
production of PTH-related peptide	squamous carcinoma, renal cell carcinoma
increased osteoclastic activity	osteolytic metastases, multiple myeloma
increased bone turnover	hyperthyroidism
increased renal tubular calcium reabsorption	familial hypocalciuric hypercalcaemia (autosomal dominant)

Fig. 29.21 Causes of hypercalcaemia. (PTH, parathyroid hormone.)

Causes of hypocalcaemia	
Mechanism	**Example**
reduced calcium intake	dietary deficiency, malabsorption
reduced vitamin D intake/production	dietary deficiency, malabsorption, reduced sunlight exposure
reduced activation of vitamin D	renal disease, liver disease
increased inactivation of vitamin D	enzyme induction by anticonvulsants
reduced production of PTH	surgical removal of parathyroid glands, autoimmune, congenital (DiGeorge syndrome)
resistance to PTH	pseudohypoparathyroidism
hypoalbuminaemia	shock

Fig. 29.22 Causes of hypocalcaemia. (PTH, parathyroid hormone.)

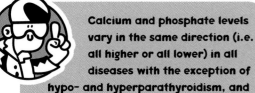

Calcium and phosphate levels vary in the same direction (i.e. all higher or all lower) in all diseases with the exception of hypo- and hyperparathyroidism, and renal failure.

Urinary calcium

Hypercalciuria will occur whenever there is hypercalcaemia if glomerular function is normal or if the renal tubules 'leak' calcium (idiopathic hypercalciuria).

Alkaline phosphatase

Alkaline phosphatase is found in osteoblasts, liver, and the placenta. Isoenzymes can be measured to determine the origin of high levels. Alkaline phosphatase concentrations will be increased in bone disease if there is an increase in the number or activity of osteoblasts, as Paget's disease, osteomalacia, metastases, healing fractures, and hyperparathyroidism.

Parathyroid hormone

PTH concentrations can be measured by radioimmunoassay. They are elevated in

hyperparathyroidism and pseudohypoparathyroidism, and low or undetectable in primary hypoparathyroidism.

The overall pattern of abnormalities in these investigations are typical, as shown in Fig. 29.23.

MUSCULOSKELETAL AND SKIN DISEASE

Muscle disease is investigated by measuring muscle enzymes, electromyography, and muscle biopsy, as described in Chapter 22. The investigation of joint and connective tissue diseases is described in Chapter 16, and characteristic findings on investigation of skin pathology are discussed in Chapter 17.

HAEMATOLOGICAL DISORDERS

Full blood count
Haemoglobin

Normal values for haemoglobin are 13.5–17.5 g/dL in men and 11.5–15.5 g/dL in women. Anaemia is present when the haemoglobin level falls below these values. The causes and investigation of anaemia are described in Chapter 25.

In polycythaemia, haemoglobin levels are above the normal range. It may be true where the total RBC volume

Pattern of biochemical abnormalities in bone disease				
Disease	Calcium	Phosphate	Alkaline phosphatase	PTH
osteoporosis	N	N	N	N
osteomalacia	↓	↓	↑	N or ↑
Paget's disease	N	N	↑↑	N
metastases	↑	↑	↑	PTH-rp may be ↑
renal failure	↓	↑	N or ↑	N or ↑
primary hyperparathyroidism	↑	↓	N (slightly ↑)	↑
primary hypoparathyroisism	↓	↑	N	↓
pseudo-hypoparathyroidism	↓	↑	N	↑

Fig. 29.23 Pattern of biochemical abnormalities in bone disease. (N, normal; PTH-rp, parathyroid hormone resorption.)

is increased, or relative where the total RBC volume is normal but the plasma volume is decreased (Fig. 29.24).

Mean corpuscular volume

Normal values for mean corpuscular volume are 80–95 fL. The causes of a raised and low mean corpuscular volume are described in Chapter 25.

Reticulocytes

Reticulocytes normally comprise 0.5–20% of the RBCs; they are immature RBCs that still contain ribosomal RNA. They are demonstrated by supravital staining with methylene blue. They are present in the peripheral blood for up to 2 days after leaving the bone marrow before they become mature RBCs. The number of reticulocytes present in the peripheral blood will increase when the bone marrow is producing large numbers of RBCs. This is seen 2–3 days after acute blood loss and in haemolysis.

Total white cell count

The normal range for total white cell count is 4.0–11.0 x 10⁹/L. The total count comprises neutrophils, lymphocytes, monocytes, eosinophils, and basophils (Fig. 29.25).

Platelet count

The normal range for platelet count is 150–400 x 10⁹/L. The causes of thrombocytopaenia are discussed in Chapter 23, and the causes of thrombocytosis are shown in Fig. 29.26.

Erythrocyte sedimentation rate

The erythrocyte sedimentation rate (ESR) is a measure of the rate of RBC sedimentation over 1 hour. The normal

A 'reactive' blood picture consists of a normochromic normocytic anaemia, neutrophilia, thrombocytosis and raised erythrocyte sedimentation rate. It suggests underlying inflammation, infection or malignancy.

range varies between laboratories, increases with age, and is higher in women. It is a non-specific indicator of inflammation, infection, and malignancy.

Bone marrow examination

Aspirate and trephine are usually taken from the poster iliac crest under local anaesthesia (aspirate may also be obtained from the sternum). A smear of bone marrow cells is made from the aspirate, allowing a detailed examination of the proportion and differentiation of different cell lines in the bone marrow. Infiltration by oth cells (carcinoma) and iron reserves can also be assesse Cytogenetic analysis of the aspirate may give diagnostic and prognostic information. The trephine consists of a core of bone containing marrow cells, is important in determining marrow cellularity and infiltration.

Coagulation assessment

Coagulation is assessed by measurement of the prothrombin time, activated partial thromboplastin tim thrombin time, and bleeding time (Chapter 23).

Causes of polycythaemia		
Primary polycythaemia (myeloproliferative disorder)	**Secondary polycythaemia (↑ erythropoietin production)**	**Relative (↓ plasma volume)**
polycythaemia rubra vera	chronic hypoxia: pulmonary disease, cyanotic heart disease, high altitudes, obesity (pickwickian syndrome), methaemoglobinaemia inappropriate erythropoietin: renal disease, cerebellar haemangioblastoma, hepatocellular carcinoma, uterine myomata, phaeochromocytoma	stress polycythaemia dehydration plasma loss (burns)

Fig. 29.24 Causes of polycythaemia.

Causes of abnormalities of the white cell count			
White cell	**Normal value ($\times 10^9$/L)**	**Increased**	**Decreased**
neutrophils	2.5–7.5	bacterial infections, uraemia, inflammation, malignancy, steroids, acute haemorrhage, myeloproliferative disorders	bone marrow failure, hypersplenism, infections (HIV, typhoid), racial, drugs (phenytoin, tolbutamide), connective tissue disease (SLE, rheumatoid arthritis)
lymphocytes	1.5–3.5	infections (viral, TB, brucellosis), CLL, ALL, non-Hodgkin's lymphoma, thyrotoxicosis	bone marrow failure, HIV, drugs (cytotoxics)
monocytes	0.2–0.8	infection (TB, brucellosis), inflammation (UC, Crohn's disease), connective tissue disease (SLE, rheumatoid arthritis), AML, malignancy	bone marrow failure
eosinophils	0.04–0.44	allergy (urticaria, drugs), parasite infection (filariasis, amoebiasis), skin disease (psoriasis, dermatitis herpetiformis), polyarteritis nodosa, Hodgkin's disease, pulmonary eosinophilia, eosinophilic leukaemia	bone marrow failure
basophils	0.01–0.1	infection (varicella), hypothyroidism, myeloproliferative disorders	bone marrow failure

Fig. 29.25 Causes of abnormalities of the white cell count. (ALL, acute lymphoblastic leukaemia; AML, acute myeloid leukaemia; CLL, chronic lymphocytic leukaemia; HIV, human immunodeficiency virus; SLE, systemic lupus erythematosus; TB, tuberculosis; UC, ulcerative colitis.)

Computed tomography scan

Deep intra-abdominal and mediastinal lymphadenopathy are well demonstrated on CT scans and often missed on other imaging techniques such as ultrasound. CT scans are useful in the staging of haematological malignancies such as lymphoma.

Causes of thrombocytosis	
primary	essential thrombocythaemia
secondary	inflammation malignancy chronic infection postsplenectomy haemorrhage surgery or trauma

Fig. 29.26 Causes of thrombocytosis.

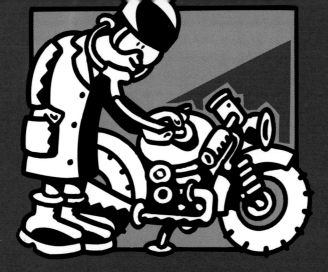

DISEASES AND DISORDERS

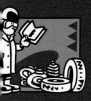

30. The Cardiovascular System

ISCHAEMIC HEART DISEASE

Ischaemic heart disease (IHD) is the result of an imbalance between myocardial oxygen supply and demand. The term covers a group of clinical syndromes that includes angina pectoris, acute myocardial infarction (MI), and sudden death. The commonest underlying pathology is atherosclerosis of the coronary arteries. More rarely, IHD can result from coronary artery spasm, embolis, coronary ostial stenosis, aortic stenosis, hypertrophic obstructive cardiomyopathy, arrhythmias causing decreased coronary perfusion pressures, and anaemia.

Ischaemia may also occur with normal coronary arteries, and is then termed syndrome X. It is thought to be due to abnormalities of small coronary vessels resulting in a reduction of coronary flow reserve.

The incidence of IHD shows large geographical variations, ranging from a mortality rate below 100 in 100 000 in Japan to 600 in 100 000 in Finland and Northern Ireland. The incidence appears to be declining in Western Europe although there has been a noticeable increase in IHD mortality rates in several Eastern European countries. In England and Wales, 1 in men aged 40–44 years have some evidence of IHD; at 55–59 years, this rises to 1 in 3, showing the increase in prevalence with age.

Risk factors for ischaemic heart disease

A number of predictors have been found to be associated with an increased likelihood of developing IHD, and are called risk factors (Fig. 30.1).

The complete list of possible risk factors for IHD is extremely long and includes environmental factors as well as personal characteristics. Not all these factors will ultimately be shown to be truly causal. For example, obesity may act as a risk factor because it is associated with raised serum cholesterol, hypertension, and decreased glucose tolerance.

Age

Mortality from IHD rises steeply with increasing age. This may be due to the accumulative effects of raised serum total cholesterol, hypertension, cigarette smoking, and other factors over time.

Sex

The rate in young men is about six times higher than in women of the same age, though this difference diminishes with increasing age. Premenopausal women are thought to be protected by their hormonal status, and this protection diminishes progressively during and after the menopause.

Family history

The effect of family history appears to be independent of other major risk factors if first-degree relatives below the age of 50 years are affected. Although high levels of serum total cholesterol may cluster in families, only a very small proportion of these are associated with genetically conditioned 'familial hypercholesterolaemia'.

Cigarette smoking

The risk of developing coronary artery disease is directly proportional to the number of cigarettes smoked. The rate of IHD in current smokers is about three times that of those who have never smoked. Giving up smoking leads to an initial rapid decrease in the risk of developing IHD followed by a more gradual decline in risk, so that the risk of IHD is almost the same as a non-smoker after about 10 years.

Major risk factors for coronary artery disease	
Type	**Risk factors**
fixed	age male sex positive family history race
modifiable	cigarette smoking hyperlipidaemia hypertension diabetes mellitus left ventricular hypertrophy

Fig. 30.1 Major risk factors for coronary artery disease.

Blood lipids

The risk of IHD increases as serum total cholesterol and low density lipoprotein (LDL) cholesterol increases. High density lipoprotein (HDL) cholesterol is be 'protective' for IHD, and the risk of IHD decreases as HDL increases. Triglycerides are also positively related to IHD risk, although when the relationship of IHD to other blood lipids is taken into account, the independent contribution of triglycerides to IHD is very small.

Hypertension

Both systolic and diastolic hypertension are associated with the risk of developing IHD, as well as hypertensive heart disease, stroke, and renal failure. Treatment of hypertension with drugs reduces the incidence of cardiac events by about 16% overall, with a greater benefit obtained in the elderly.

Diabetes mellitus

In countries where IHD is prevalent, diabetes mellitus (DM) is associated with an approximately two-fold increase in the risk of a major IHD event. The role of asymptomatic hyperglycaemia is uncertain.

Race

The prevalence of IHD in British Asians is high compared with their family members remaining in the Indian subcontinent. The explanation is only partly accounted for by a low HDL cholesterol and a higher prevalence of DM and glucose intolerance.

Overweight

Overweight individuals have twice the risk of a major IHD event. This is probably mediated through increased blood pressure levels, total cholesterol, insulin resistance, and with decreased HDL and physical activity.

Psychosocial factors

Although stress and other strong emotional responses can precipitate major IHD events in individuals with severe atherosclerosis, it remains to be shown whether stress plays a role in the pathogenesis of coronary artery disease in the absence of other standard risk factors.

Combining risk factors is a more accurate way of predicting those at risk from IHD than relying on any one individual risk factor. Many models and scoring systems have been devised incorporating the different risk factors so that those at high risk may be targeted for preventative treatment. This should be accompanied by population-based measures to reduce the risk of IHD.

Pathology

Atherosclerosis is a slowly progressive focal proliferation of connective tissue within the intima, which begins early in life. It is linked to high lipid levels, although the principal constituent of atherosclerotic plaques is collagen synthethised by smooth muscle cells.

The initial process consists of endothelial dysfunction in association with a high circulating cholesterol, inflammation, shear forces, and chemical irritants from tobacco smoke. Macrophages enter the arterial wall between endothelial cells. The accumulation of lipid-laden macrophages in the subendothelial zone leads to the formation of fatty streaks. Toxic products released from the macrophages lead to the adhesion of platelets and results in smooth muscle cell proliferation and thrombus formation. This then becomes organized, leading to the development of an atherosclerotic plaque surrounded by a fibrotic cap. Progressive enlargement of these lesions leads to segmental narrowing of the lumen, which, when sufficient to be flow limiting on exercise, causes stable exertion-associated angina. Atherosclerotic plaques are liable to rupture resulting in sudden thrombosis, which is responsible for the acute manifestations of IHD. Factors associated with plaque disruption and consequent thrombosis include a large lipid core, a high monocyte density, and low smooth muscle cell density.

The onset or worsening of angina is due predominantly to intraplaque thrombosis leading to rapid plaque growth. Extension of thrombus into the lumen results in unstable angina or non-Q wave MI.

Investigations

Electrocardiogram

A normal electrocardiogram (ECG) does not exclude a diagnosis of angina. During attacks, there may be ST segment depression or symmetrical T wave inversion. wave inversion in leads V_{1-3} often indicates a critical left anterior descending coronary artery (LAD) stenosis. The ECG may show signs of an old MI or left ventricular hypertrophy.

Exercise electrocardiogram

The exercise ECG is a useful indicator of exercise performance and is an independent indicator of prognosis. It is contraindicated in unstable angina, recent (within 7 days) MI, severe aortic stenosis, severe pulmonary hypertension, and significant rhythm disturbances. Relative contraindications include infirmity and ataxia.

The test is usually regarded as positive if there is more than 1 mm of J point depression, the junction of the ST segment and the T wave. If the pretest probability of angina is high, the number of false positives is low. Causes of false positive tests include hyperventilation, digoxin and other antiarrhythmic agents, hypokalaemia, hypertension, valvular heart disease, left ventricular hypertrophy, and pre-excitation syndromes. The test should be terminated if there is a fall in blood pressure, ventricular tachycardia, or if the patient becomes pale, indicating peripheral circulatory collapse. Relative contraindications for termination include ST segment depression of more than 4 mm, incoordination, or paroxysmal rhythm disturbances other than ventricular tachycardias (VTs).

Echocardiography

This can be used to assess ventricular function and localize areas of ventricular wall involvement. In patients with angina but no evidence of infarction, the echocardiogram may be normal. With diffuse ischaemic changes, left ventricular function may be globally impaired. Exercise or pharmacological stress echocardiography may be used to detect areas of 'hibernating' myocardium. These are areas that show reduced function on exercise, due to decreased blood flow secondary to decreased coronary flow reserve, but which show improved function at rest.

Nuclear imaging

This technique may be used to assess myocardial structure and function. A radioactive isotope, e.g. thallium, is injected during exercise and an image is taken soon after. The isotope is taken up by healthy myocardium whereas areas of infarction show up as 'cold spots'.

Repeat images are taken at rest to obtain a redistribution image. The disappearance of the cold spot implies ischaemia provoked by exertion and reversed by rest; a fixed cold spot indicates infarction. It is a useful technique when the exercise test is equivocal or contraindicated, or to indicate the clinical significance of angiographically equivocal stenoses.

Coronary angiography and cardiac catheterization

This is a technique for radiographically visualizing the coronary arteries, and measuring intracardiac pressures, blood oxygen saturation in different cardiac chambers, and cardiac output. The test is usually used to determine the exact coronary anatomy and is used to decide on further management, i.e. medical therapy, coronary angioplasty, or coronary artery bypass surgery. It is usually reserved for patients with:
- Angina resistant to medical treatment.
- Strongly positive exercise tests indicating a poor prognosis.
- Unstable angina.
- Persisting angina after MI.

More rarely, coronary angiography is used as a diagnostic test when other non-invasive tests have not been helpful and symptoms persist.

The mortality from the procedure is about 1 in 1000. Complications include:
- Haemorrhage at the site of arterial puncture.
- Emboli into arteries resulting in MI.
- Stroke.
- Arrhythmias.
- Coronary artery dissection.
- Infection.

Treatment
General measures

It is important to explain the condition to the patient, emphasizing that the prognosis is generally good and that treatment can alleviate symptoms. The diagnosis can lead to severe emotional upset, and patients should be encouraged to return for discussion. Non-coronary causes for angina, e.g. valvular heart disease, calcific aortic stenosis, intermittent tachycardias, hyperthyroidism, or anaemia, should be sought and treated appropriately.

Risk factors should be evaluated and steps taken to correct them. All patients should be advised to stop smoking and should lose weight if overweight. Dietary control of hyperlipidaemia should be considered if total cholesterol is above 4.8 mmol/L.

Factors precipitating angina, e.g. cold weather or emotion, should be avoided, although exercise within the patient's limits should be encouraged to promote the formation of a collateral cardiac circulation.

Drugs

All patients should be prescribed aspirin 75–300 mg daily as this lowers the incidence of subsequent MI and death. If cholesterol is more than 4.8 mmol/L after diet, patients will also benefit from HMG-CoA reductase inhibitors (statins) to lower cholesterol. During an acute attack the patient should be advised to stop any precipitating factors such as exercise and to take sublingual glyceryl trinitrate (GTN); the acute attack usually subsides within 5 minutes. Patients may also be advised to take sublingual GTN prophylactically before exertion.

When angina occurs frequently, regular prophylactic therapy should be advised. This consists of ß-adrenoreceptor blockers, nitrates, calcium antagonists, and potassium channel openers.

ß-Blockers

These act by reducing sympathetic tone, depressing myocardial contractility (negatively inotropic), and reducing the heart rate (negatively chronotropic). In addition to these effects (which reduce the oxygen demand), ß-blockers may also increase the perfusion of the ischaemic area because the decrease in heart rate increases the duration of diastole and hence the time available for coronary blood flow.

Typical ß-blockers include atenolol 50–100 mg daily or metoprolol 25–50 mg t.d.s. if a shorter half-life is required. Contraindications include asthma, peripheral vascular disease with skin ulceration, and second and third degree heart block.

Nitrates

Nitrates cause peripheral vasodilatation, especially in the veins. This reduces venous return and the ventricular volume is decreased. Reduction in the distension of the heart wall decreases oxygen demand resulting in relief of pain. Sublingual GTN acts for about 30 minutes. Nitrates work by conversion to nitric oxide, a free radical, which activates guanylate cyclase. This results in an increase in intracellular cyclic GMP in the

smooth muscle; by stimulating calcium binding processes the free calcium available to trigger muscle contraction is reduced.

Longer-acting nitrates are more stable and can be effective for several hours. Isosorbide dinitrate (ISDN) is rapidly metabolized by the liver to the mononitrate, which is the main active metabolite. Isosorbide mononitrate (ISMN) may avoid the variable absorption and unpredictable first-pass metabolism of the dinitrate.

Typical doses include ISMN 10–60 mg b.d. or slow-release ISMN 60–120 mg o.d. Adverse effects are normally due to arterial dilatation and include headaches, flushing, hypotension, and rarely fainting.

Calcium channel blockers

Calcium antagonists have direct actions on the heart but they relieve angina mainly by causing peripheral arteriolar dilatation and afterload reduction. They are especially useful if there is some degree of coronary artery spasm. The dihydropyridines such as nifedipine can cause reflex tachycardia and should not generally be used without a ß-blocker. Typical doses are slow-release nifedipine 10–40 mg b.d. Diltiazem has slight negative inotropic and chronotropic effects, and the patient should be closely monitored if on concomitant ß-blockers for the development of heart block. Verapamil is the drug of choice if ß-blockers are contraindicated, e.g. in patients with asthma, or for patients who have supra-ventricular tachycardias in addition to angina. They are contraindicated in heart block and heart failure. Constipation is a frequent side effect.

Side effects with the dihydropyridines include headache, flushing, dizziness, and gravitational oedema.

Potassium channel activators

This is a new class of drug with arterial and venous vasodilating properties. It may be useful in patients refractory to treatment with other antianginal agents. The only licensed drug in this group at present is nicorandil 10–30 mg b.d.

Side effects include headache, flushing, nausea, vomiting, and dizziness.

Unstable angina

Angina which occurs with increasing frequency and severity, even at rest, is termed unstable. Patients should be admitted to hospital to facilitate rapid adjustments to drug therapy. Antianginal therapy should be added and titrated to control symptoms, and the patient should be on bed rest. Aspirin reduces the incidence of death and MI.

Intravenous ISDN is useful for patients who do not settle on oral treatment, and intravenous heparin or high-dose, low molecular weight heparin may reduce the incidence of occlusive coronary thrombosis and MI. If the patient still does not settle, it may be appropriate to proceed to coronary angiography with a view to urgent angioplasty or coronary artery bypass surgery.

Coronary angioplasty

Angioplasty is a similar technique to diagnostic angiography except that a fine wire is passed through the obstructing lesion, followed by a small catheter with a non-elastic balloon near its tip. The balloon is inflated to a pressure of several atmospheres to dilate the lesion and hence relieve the obstruction. If there are no complications the patient is mobilized the next day and allowed home. The technique is used on selected patients, ideally with a discrete stenosis of a major vessel, including lesions of bypass grafts. One exception is stenosis of the left main stem as occlusion during attempted angioplasty is likely to be catastrophic.

The procedure may be carried out in multiple vessels, and repeat procedures can be undertaken. Complications occur in about 5% of cases, usually resulting from acute occlusion at the lesion within a few hours following the procedure. This may be due to spasm, thrombosis, or dissection of the artery. About 2% of patients will require urgent coronary artery bypass surgery and/or will sustain a MI. The mortality is less than 1%.

About one-third of lesions will restenose within the first 6 months. This can be dealt with by repeat angioplasty, although a substantial proportion will eventually require coronary artery bypass surgery. Some lesions are now amenable to coronary artery 'stenting', which involves the insertion of a metal tube mounted on the balloon and inflated over the stenosis.

Surgical management

Surgery should be considered in patients whose symptoms persist despite optimal medical management. The commonest operation involves harvesting the saphenous vein from the leg, and bypassing the coronary obstruction by suturing the vein between the aorta and the coronary artery distal to the obstruction. The internal mammary artery may also be used as a conduit and has a lower occlusion rate than vein grafts. The overall mortality with surgery is about 2%, and certain factors confer a reduced risk or mortality compared to medical treatment (Fig. 30.2).

The main determinants of risk are increasing age, the degree of ventricular damage, the extent and diffuseness of coronary artery disease, and gender, with females at higher risk. Seventy per cent of patients obtain total relief, and 20% have improved symptoms, although pain returns to 50% in 5 years.

All patients should be given aspirin 75–300 mg daily, and treated with an HMG-CoA reductase inhibitor if total cholesterol is greater than 4.8 mmol/L.

Prognosis

The mortality of patients with some evidence of IHD in the general population is less than 1% per year. In those with definite angina who are treated with aspirin, the risk of a major coronary heart disease event is about 3% per year. Mortality increases with multivessel disease and with left ventricular dysfunction. It is highest in those with left main stem stenosis, where the mortality is over 10% per year. In unstable angina the annual mortality is up to 40% per year.

Poor prognostic factors include pain lasting for more than 48 hours, heart failure, an enlarged heart, persistent ST/T changes in the ECG, and a long past history of IHD.

Patient factors associated with reduction in mortality with surgery

- left main stem stenosis
- triple vessel coronary artery disease
- two vessel disease with proximal LAD disease
- benefit is greater in those with left ventricular impairment

Fig. 30.2 Factors associated with reduction in mortality with coronary artery bypass surgery compared to medical management of patients with coronary artery disease. (LAD, left anterior descending coronary artery.)

MYOCARDIAL INFARCTION

Myocardial infarction (MI) affects 5 in 1000 of the general population per year in the UK and is the most common cause of mortality in the Western world. Ninety per cent of transmural MIs are caused by an occlusive intracoronary thrombus overlying an ulcerated or fissured stenotic plaque. Underlying most cases there is a dynamic interaction between severe coronary atherosclerosis, an acute atheromatous plaque change, superimposed thrombosis, platelet activation, and vasospasm. The microscopic changes of acute MI follow a predictable sequence (Fig. 30.3).

The overall fatality from acute MI in community studies is 50% in the first month. About half these deaths occur within the first 2 hours, while in-patient mortality is about 20%. After the first 6 months the annual mortality, with appropriate prophylactic treatment, is about 2%.

Adverse risk factors in patients admitted to hospital with acute MI are:

- Older age.
- Previous medical history (diabetes, previous MI).
- Indicators of a large infarct size, including the site of infarction (anterior versus inferior).
- Low initial blood pressure.
- The presence of pulmonary congestion.
- The extent of ischaemia as expressed by ST elevation with or without depression on the ECG.

Diagnosis

The diagnosis of acute MI is based on two or three out of: the history (see p. 3), ECG changes, and enzyme changes.

Cardiac enzymes

Cardiac enzymes are intracellular enzymes which leak out of infarcted myocardium into the bloodstream (Fig. 30.4):

- Creatinine kinase (CK) peaks within 24 hours. It is a cardiac enzyme that is also produced by skeletal muscle and brain. In cases of doubt, the myocardial bound isoenzyme fraction of CK—i.e. CKMB—can be requested which is specific for heart muscle damage. The site of the infarct is related to the serum level of enzyme.
- Aspartate aminotransferase (AST) peaks at 24–48 hours. It is also released by damaged red blood cells (RBCs), kidney, liver and lungs.
- Lactate dehydrogenase (LDH) peaks at 3–4 days. The predominant isoenzyme released with cardiac necrosis is ∝-hydroxybutarate dehydrogenase (HBD). LDH is also released from the liver, skeletal muscle, and RBCs.
- Troponin 'T' is a regulatory protein with high specificity for cardiac injury. It is released within 2 hours of myocardial infarction. It is not yet widely available as a diagnostic tool.

Electrocardiogram

The earliest ECG changes or 'hyperacute' changes consist of tall, pointed, upright T waves, followed by elevation of the ST segment. This is shortly followed by T wave

Elevation of cardiac enzymes after a myocardial infarction is CPK, then AST, then LDH. Remember this as C AST Le.

Changes induced by acute myocardial infarction		
Time after onset of symptoms	Macroscopic changes	Microscopic changes
up to 18 hours	none	none
24–48 hours	pale oedematous muscle	oedema, acute inflammatory cell infiltration, necrosis of myocytes
3–4 days	yellow rubbery centre with haemorrhagic border	obvious necrosis and inflammation, early granulation tissue
3–6 weeks	silvery scar becoming rough and white	dense fibrosis

Fig. 30.3 Changes induced by acute myocardial infarction.

nversion, the R wave voltage decreases, and Q waves develop. After weeks or months the T wave may become upright again but the Q waves remain (Fig. 30.5).

The site of the infarction may also be deduced from the affected leads on the ECG.

- Inferior MI involves leads II, III, and aVF.
- Anterior MI: affects the precordial leads.
- Anteroseptal MI: affects leads V_{1-3}.
- Lateral MI: affects leads I and aVF.
- Posterior MI; there is a tall R wave in leads V_1 and V_2 with ST segment depression and upright T waves.

There may also be 'reciprocal' ECG changes with ST segment depression in leads opposite to the site of infarction. The absence of Q waves in a proven infarct denotes a subendocardial or 'non-Q wave' infarct, and is represented by T wave inversion in any lead.

Other investigations to help with management include:

- A full blood count (FBC) to exclude anaemia.
- Urea and electrolytes (U&Es) to exclude electrolyte abnormalities.
- A chest X-ray (CXR) to exclude aortic dissection, to look for signs of heart failure, and to assess changes in cardiac size.

Management

Emergency care

The main aims are to prevent or treat cardiac arrest, and to relieve pain—the patient should ideally be managed on a coronary care unit and an intravenous

cannula should be inserted for emergency medicines. Intravenous opiates, such as diamorphine 2.5–10 mg i.v., are given for pain relief. This relieves pain not only for humane reasons but alleviates sympathetic activation associated with the pain which causes vasoconstriction and increases the work of the heart.

Side effects include nausea and vomiting, hypotension with bradycardia, and respiratory depression. Antiemetics should be administered concurrently with opiats, e.g. metoclopramide 10 mg i.v., cyclizine 50 mg i.v., or prochlorperazine 12.5 mg i.v. If respiratory depression occurs, intravenous naloxone, which is a specific opioid antagonist, should be given. High-dose oxygen should be given via a face-mask or nasal cannula, especially to those who are breathless or who have any features of heart failure or shock.

Anxiety is a natural response to the pain and to the circumstances surrounding a heart attack. Reassurance of patients and those closely associated with them is therefore of great importance.

Early care
The aims are to initiate reperfusion therapy, limit infarct size, prevent infarct extension, and to treat life-threatening arrhythmias.

Thrombolytic treatment
Within 12 hours of the onset of pain, treatment with thrombolysis should be given for patients with ST elevation or bundle branch block. This prevents 30 deaths in 1000 patients treated within 6 hours, or 20 deaths if treated between 7 and 12 hours. The benefit from aspirin is additive so that 50 lives are saved in 1000 patients treated.

The largest benefit is seen for those at highest risk, e.g:

- The elderly.
- Those with presenting systolic blood pressure of below 100 mmHg.
- Those with anterior infarction.

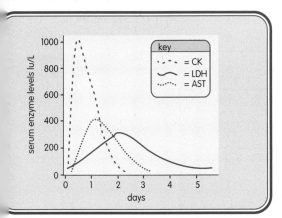

g. 30.4 The pattern of serum enzymes after acute myocardial infarction. (AST, aspartate aminotransferase; , creatinine kinase; LDH, lactate dehydrogenase.)

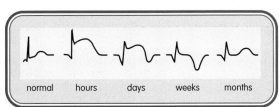

Fig. 30.5 Progressive ECG changes in myocardial infarction.

- Those treated soonest after the onset of thrombolysis.

Contraindications to thrombolytic therapy are given in Fig. 30.6.

Streptokinase is the most frequently used fibrinolytic agent but it increases the patient's antistreptokinase antibody level. These antibodies reduce the effectiveness of a repeat dose and increase the risk of an anaphylactic reaction. It should therefore not be readministered in the period between 5 days and a minimum of 2 years following initial treatment. Frequently used thrombolytic regimens are given in Fig. 30.7.

Angioplasty

This may be attempted if the patient has contraindications to thrombolysis but only when rapid access to a catheterization laboratory is possible. It may also be attempted on a coronary artery that remains occluded despite thrombolytic therapy.

Prophylactic therapy in the acute phase
Aspirin

Aspirin therapy 150 mg should be prescribed early. This

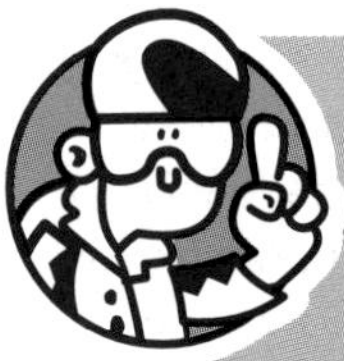

If the first ECG does not show diagnostic changes despite a strong history, then frequent or continuous ECG recordings should be obtained.

leads to a 29% reduction in deaths or 24 lives saved in 1000 treated. Contraindications include:

- Known hypersensitivity.
- Bleeding peptic ulcer.
- Blood dyscrasias
- Severe hepatic disease.

ß-Blockers

The intravenous adminstration of ß-Blockers in the acute phase potentially limits infarct size, reduces the risk of fatal arrhythmias, and relieves pain. There is a 15% reduction in mortality at 1 week. It is particularly appropriate when the patient has a tachycardia (in the absence of heart failure), relative hypertension, or pain unresponsive to opioids.

Angiotensin-converting enzyme inhibitors

Angiotensin-converting enzyme (ACE) inhibitors are of definite value in patients with clinical symptoms or signs of heart failure, or impaired left ventricular function echocardiographically. Opinions differ as to the best time to initiate treatment—whether acutely or after a few days. The benefits appear to be a class effect, and doses should be titrated to the target dose (Fig. 30.8).

Complications of myocardial infarction

A summary of the complications that may occur in MI is given in Fig. 30.9.

Pump failure and shock

Left ventricular failure (LVF) during the acute phase of MI associated with a poor prognosis. Repeated examinatio of the heart and lungs for signs of incipient heart failure should be practised in all patients (Fig. 30.10).

Contraindications to thrombolytic therapy	
contraindications	stroke major surgery, trauma, or head injury within 3 weeks gastrointestinal bleed within the last week known bleeding disorder dissecting aneurysm
relative contraindications	transient ischaemic attack in the preceding 6 months warfarin therapy pregnancy non-compressible punctures traumatic resuscitation refractory hypertension (SBP >180 mmHg) recent retinal laser treatment

Fig. 30.6 Contraindications to thrombolytic therapy. (SBP, systolic blood pressure.)

Frequently used thrombolytic regimens		
Drug	**Initial treatment**	**Heparin treatment**
streptokinase	1.5 million units i.v. over 30–60 minutes	none
anistreplase	30 units i.v. over 3–5 minutes	none
alteplase	15 mg i.v. bolus 0.75 mg/kg i.v. over 30 minutes 0.5 mg/kg i.v. over 60 minutes total dosage not to exceed 100 mg	i.v. for 48 hours determined by the APTT

Fig. 30.7 Frequently used thrombolytic regimens. (APTT, activated partial thromboplastin time.)

General measures include monitoring for arrhythmias, and checking for electrolyte abnormalities and for the diagnosis of concomitant conditions such as valvular dysfunction or pulmonary disease.

Chest X-rays and echocardiography for assessing ventricular function, mitral regurgitation, and ventricular septal defects may be of help.

The management of heart failure is described in pp 211–215. Cardiogenic shock is defined as a systolic blood pressure less than 90 mmHg in association with signs of circulatory deterioration expressed as peripheral vasoconstriction, low urinary output (<20 mL/hour), and mental confusion and dulling.

Other causes of hypotension should be excluded such as hypovolaemia, vasovagal reactions, electrolyte disturbance, drugs, or arrhythmias. Ventricular function should be evaluated by echocardiography, and haemodynamics measured with a balloon flotation catheter. Inotropic agents are of value. Low-dose dopamine (2.5 µg/kg/min) may be given to improve renal function, and additional administration of dobutamine (5–10 µg/kg/min) should be considered. Correction of acidosis is important.

Emergency percutaneous transluminal coronary angioplasty (PTCA) or surgery should be considered.

Cardiac rupture and mitral regurgitation
Free wall rupture, if acute, is usually fatal within minutes. If subacute, there is haemodynamic deterioration with hypotension and signs of cardiac tamponade. Immediate surgery should be considered.

Ventricular septal defect (VSD) occurs in 1–2% of all infarctions, appearing early after MI. Without surgery the mortality is 54% within the first week and 92% within the first year. It should be suspected if there is clinical deterioration and a loud pansystolic murmur. Treatment is by surgical closure of the defect and bypass grafts as necessary. Predictors of poor postoperative outcome are:
- Cardiogenic shock.
- Posterior location.
- Right ventricular dysfunction.
- Age.
- Long delay between septal rupture and surgery.

Mitral regurgitation
The incidence of moderately severe or severe mitral regurgitation is about 4% and the mortality without surgery is high at about 24%. Valve replacement is the procedure of choice in papillary muscle dysfunction and rupture.

Arrhythmias and conduction disturbances
These are extremely common in the early period following MI. Often, however, the arrhythmias are

Treatment regimens for angiotensin-converting enzyme inhibitors		
Drug	**Initial dose**	**Target dose**
enalapril	2.5 mg	20 mg o.d.
lisinopril	2.5 mg	10 mg o.d.
captopril	6.25 mg	50 mg t.d.s.
ramipril	2.5 mg	5 mg b.d.
trandolapril	0.5 mg	4 mg o.d.

Fig. 30.8 Treatment regimens for angiotensin-converting enzyme inhibitors.

Complications of myocardial infarction		
Complication	Interval	Mechanism
sudden death	usually within hours	often ventricular fibrillation
arrhythmias	first few days	–
persistent pain	12 hours to a few days	progressive myocardial necrosis (extension of MI)
angina	immediate or delayed (weeks)	ischaemia of non-infarcted muscle
cardiac failure	variable	ventricular dysfunction following muscle necrosis; arrhythmias
mitral incompetence	first few days	papillary muscle dysfunction, necrosis or rupture
pericarditis	2–4 days	transmural infarct with inflammation of the pericardium
cardiac rupture and ventricular septal defects	3–5 days	weakening of wall following muscle necrosis and acute inflammation
mural thrombus	one week or more	abnormal endothelial surface following infarction
ventricular aneurysm	4 weeks or more	stretching of newly formed collagenous scar tissue
Dressler's syndrome	weeks to months	autoimmune
pulmonary emboli	1 week or more	deep venous thrombosis in lower limbs
late ventricular arrhythmias	–	–

Fig. 30.9 Complications of myocardial infarction.

The Killip classification	
Class	Features
1	no crepitations or third heart sound
2	crepitations over less than 50% of lung fields or third heart sound
3	crepitations over 50% of the lung fields
4	shock

Fig. 30.10 The Killip classification.

not hazardous in themselves but are a manifestation of a serious underlying disorder such as continuing ischaemia, vagal overactivity, or electrolyte disturbance that requires attention. Arrhythmias are also discussed on pp.206–211.

Ventricular arrhythmias

Ventricular arrhythmias may present as ventricular ectopics, VT, or ventricular fibrillation.

Ventricular ectopics are almost universal on the first day and require no treatment if the patient is asymptomatic.

Short episodes of VT may be well tolerated and require no treatment. More prolonged episodes may cause hypotension and heart failure. Lidocaine is the drug of first choice. Direct current (DC) cardioversion may be required if haemodynamically significant VT persists.

If ventricular fibrillation occurs, immediate defibrillation should be performed.

Supraventricular arrhythmias

Atrial fibrillation complicates 15–20% of MIs and is often associated with severe left ventricular damage and heart failure; it is usually self limiting. If the heart rate is fast, digoxin is effective in slowing the rate, but amiodarone may be more efficacious in terminating the arrhythmia.

Other supraventricular arrhythmias are rare but are also usually self limiting. They may respond to carotid sinus massage. ß-Blockers may be effective and DC shock should be employed if the arrhythmia is poorly tolerated.

Sinus bradycardia and heart block

Sinus bradycardia is common in the first hour, especially in inferior MI, and usually responds to atropine in 300 mg boluses titrated against response. The administration of unnecessarily large doses of atropine should be avoided.

Atrioventricular (AV) block is common in inferior MI and may respond to atropine, though some patients will need a permanent pacemaker. However, it may take up to 14 days before normal conduction is restored.

Heart block with anterior MI is ominous because it indicates a large infarct. The development of left bundle branch block or bifasicular block may presage complete heart block and is an indication for temporary pacemaker insertion. If complete heart block does occur and persists, a permanent pacemaker will be needed.

Management of the later inpatient course
General management

Patients should be on bed rest for the first 24 hours. If uncomplicated, the patient can then sit out of bed, use a commode, and undertake self care and self feeding. Ambulation can be started the next day up to about 100 m on the flat, and the exercise is gradually built up to climbing stairs within a few days.

Deep venous thrombosis and pulmonary embolism

Deep venous thrombosis (DVT) and pulmonary embolism (PE) may be prevented by subcutaneous heparin when in bed. If they do occur, the patient should be treated initially with intravenous heparin, followed by oral anticoagulation for 3–6 months. Patients are usually started on subcutaneous heparin 5000 μ b.d. or a low molecular weight heparin, e.g. enoxaparin subcutaneously 20 mg once daily after admission to the coronary care unit.

Intraventricular thrombus and systemic emboli

This may be confirmed on echocardiography and treated with intravenous heparin followed by oral anticoagulation for 6 months.

Pericarditis

This may occur within the first few days, causing pain that is sharp in nature and varies with posture and respiration. The diagnosis can be confirmed by a pericardial rub. If troublesome it may be treated with high-dose aspirin, non-steroidal anti-inflammatory drugs (NSAIDs), or steroids.

Late ventricular arrhythmias

When arrhythmias occur late in the course of MI, they are liable to recur and are associated with a high risk of death. If it is probable that the arrhythmia is induced by ischaemia, revascularization should be considered. If this is unlikely, antiarrhythmic agents, e.g. ß-blockers and amiodarone, and electrophysiologically guided treatment may be given. In some cases an implantable defibrillator is indicated.

Rehabilitation

Rehabilitation is aimed at restoring the patient to as full a life as possible, and must take into account physical, physiological, and socio-economic factors. The process should start as soon as possible after hospital admission and should be continued in the succeeding weeks and months. Depression and denial are common. Lifestyle advice should be individualized and include advice on diet, exercise, and stopping smoking.

Secondary prevention
Smoking

Observational studies show that those who stop smoking have a mortality in the succeeding years of less than half that of those who continue to smoke. It is potentially the most effective of all the secondary prevention measures. All smokers should be counselled to stop smoking. Nicotine replacement therapy may be of value.

Diet

A weight-reducing diet should be prescribed to the overweight. Eating fatty fish at least twice a week may reduce the risk of reinfarction and death.

> **Remember the causes of pericarditis by the mnemonic CARDIAC RIND,** i.e. Collagen vascular disease, Aortic aneurysm, Radiation, Drugs (e.g. hydralazine), Infections, Acute renal failure, Cardiac infarction, Rheumatic fever, Injury, Neoplasms, and Dressler's syndrome.

Antiplatelet treatment

Aspirin 75–150 mg daily reduces the risk of reinfarction and death by 25%. There is no clear benefit of oral anticoagulation over antiplatelet therapy, although it may be considered for patients with left ventricular aneurysm, atrial fibrillation, or echocardiographically proven left ventricular thrombus.

ß-Blockers

ß-Blockers reduce the risk of mortality and reinfarction by 20–25%. About 25% of patients have contraindications to ß-blockers because of uncontrolled heart failure, respiratory disease, or other conditions.

Calcium antagonists

Verapamil may prevent reinfarction and death and should be considered in patients in whom ß-blockers are contraindicated because of airways obstruction.

Angiotensin-converting enzyme inhibitors

Provided there are no contraindications, ACE inhibitors are of potential benefit to all those after MI. However, patients at low risk gain only marginal benefit and they are often reserved for people with clinical signs of heart failure, people with low ejection fraction on echocardiography, or people with anterior MI.

Lipid-lowering agents

There are clear benefits from treatment with HMG-CoA reductase inhibitors, or statins, if total cholesterol is above 4.8 mmol/L after dietary measures have been tried. The risk of subsequent major coronary heart disease events is lowered by about 30%. All subgroups of patients appear to benefit from treatment.

ARRHYTHMIAS

Arrhythmias are usually secondary to IHD, particularly after MI. Ventricular ectopic beats are extremely common in the first 24 hours following an MI, but any arrhythmia including conduction disturbances may occur.

Other causes include drugs, cardiomyopathy, myocarditis, thyroid dysfunction, and electrolyte disturbances.

Clinical features

Arrhythmias may present with palpitations (Chapter 3), dizziness, angina, shortness of breath (Chapter 2), syncope, cardiac arrest, or sudden death; they may also be symptomless. The history should focus on symptoms and possible underlying aetiologies.

Investigations

An ECG with a long rhythm strip will allow diagnosis of the arrhythmia, if present at the time of the test. For infrequent symptoms, 24-hour Holter monitoring (with a diary of events) may catch and record the rhythm disturbance. Other routine investigations should include FBC, U&Es, calcium, magnesium, thyroid function tests (TFTs), and a CXR. An echocardiogram should be considered if an underlying cause is not evident, to look for cardiomyopathy or valve disease.

Finally electrophysiological studies may reveal an arrhythmogenic focus, and response to treatment may be assessed, but this is only available in specialized centres.

Supraventricular arrhythmias
Sinus tachycardia

There is usually an underlying cause, which should be treated on its own merits. Also see p.16.

Atrial fibrillation

This is an irregular, chaotic atrial rhythm at a rate of 300–600 beats per minute (bpm). It is transmitted to the ventricles via the AV node at different intervals leading to an irregular heart rate, dependent on the speed of conduction and refractoriness down the AV node. The incidence rises with age and is over 10% in the very elderly.

Common causes include:
- IHD.
- Mitral valve disease.
- Hyperthyroidism.
- Hypertension.
- Cardiomyopathy.
- Pericarditis.
- Pneumonia.
- Bronchial carcinoma.
- Atrial myxoma.
- Endocarditis.
- Infiltrative diseases of the heart, e.g. sarcoidosis.

Clinically, there is an irregularly irregular pulse and the apical rate is greater than the rate at the radial artery. The first heart sound is of variable intensity.

The ECG shows absent p waves and irregular narrow complex QRS complexes (unless there is associated bundle branch block) (Fig. 30.11).

Treatment
The ventricular rate can usually be controlled with digoxin. If not, a ß-blocker or verapamil can be added if left ventricular function is good. Other classes of drugs may sometimes be required. Patients should be anticoagulated to reduce the risk of emboli. If the patient has contraindications to warfarin, aspirin should be considered.

If the atrial fibrillation is of recent onset, DC cardioversion or intravenous flecainide to restore sinus rhythm may be attempted. If after more than 2 days, the patient should be 'warfarinized' for at least 1 month before cardioversion. If this is unsuccessful, the aim is control of the ventricular rate.

If the atrial fibrillation is paroxysmal, drugs such as amiodarone or sotalol may maintain the patient in sinus rhythm.

Atrial flutter
This is due to a regular circus movement of continuous atrial depolarization. As the AV node cannot conduct that fast, it is usually transmitted with a degree of block.

The causes and treatment are similar to those for atrial fibrillation.

The ECG shows a 'sawtooth' appearance to the baseline at 300 bpm due to flutter or F waves (Fig. 30.12). The ventricular rate is usually divisible into this, e.g. 150 bpm in 2:1 block, or 100 bpm in 3:1 block.

Paroxysmal supraventricular tachycardias
This is normally due to the presence of a second pathway between the atria and ventricles. An impulse is conducted normally through one AV connection and is

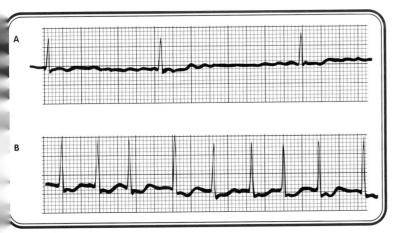

Fig. 30.11 ECG of atrial fibrillation with a slow ventricular rate (A), and fast ventricular rate (B).

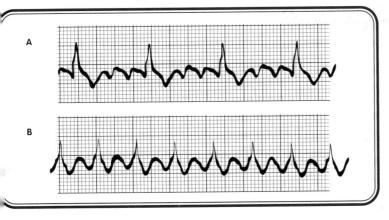

Fig. 30.12 ECG of atrial flutter. (A) Atrial flutter with 4:1 block. (B) Atrial flutter with 2:1 block.

then reconducted retrogradely up the other, causing a premature atrial contraction. This is then conducted down the first AV connection. On each occasion, the ventricle also depolarizes, giving rise to a fast ventricular rate. The refractory period for an accessory pathway may be shorter than the AV node, leading to ventricular rates exceeding 200 bpm.

Management
Initially, try vagal stimulation, which can be achieved in the following ways:
- Valsalva manoeuvre: ask the patient to blow against resistance for about 15 seconds, as if straining at stool. The tachycardia usually terminates in the relaxation (parasympathetic) phase.
- Carotid sinus massage: massage of the carotid artery at the level of the thyroid cartilage.
- Diving reflex: the patient holds his breath while the face is wetted with cold water.
- Vomiting: this may be induced if the patient gives a clear history of termination by vomiting.
- Eye pressure: this should not now be done as it may cause retinal detachment.

Drug treatment
Intravenous adenosine is the treatment of choice. Digitalization or intravenous ß-blockers may also be effective. Intravenous verapamil may be useful for

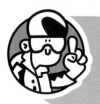
If the heart rate is 150 bpm, always consider atrial flutter with 2:1 block as the diagnosis (Fig. 30.12B).

patients without MI or valvular disease. If the arrhythmia is poorly tolerated, synchronized DC shock usually provides rapid relief.

U&Es should be checked for hypokalaemia and corrected.

If the patient is already on digoxin, the levels should be checked to exclude toxicity.

Ventricular tachycardia
This is defined as three or more consecutive ventricular extrasystoles with a rate greater than 120 bpm (Fig. 30.13)

Treatment
If there is circulatory collapse, the patient should be the treated with synchronized DC cardioversion. If conscious, the patient will require a brief anaesthetic. Electrolyte abnormalities should be corrected.

Drug treatment is also used for prophylaxis of recurrent attacks. The most common setting is after MI; lidocaine is the preferred therapy for emergency use. Other options include amiodarone or procainamide.

Torsade de pointes ('twisting of the points')
This is a special form of VT, which tends to occur in the presence of a long QT interval. It may progress to ventricular fibrillation and is often refractory to treatment, which is with intravenous magnesium sulphate. Antiarrhythmics may further prolong the QT interval and worsen the condition. Overdrive pacing may be effective.

Ventricular fibrillation
This is an emergency and requires immediate DC cardioversion with cardiopulmonary resuscitation (Fig. 30.14).

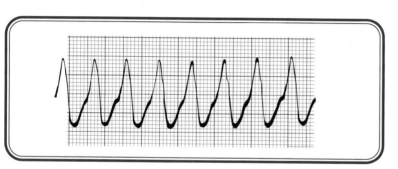

Fig. 30.13 ECG of ventricular tachycardia.

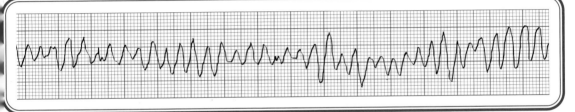

Fig. 30.14 ECG of ventricular fibrillation. Coordinated activity of the ventricles ceases. The ECG shows irregular waves of no defined shape. In this trace there are short periods suggestive of ventricular flutter.

Before carotid sinus massage:
- Always check that there are two carotid pulses.
- Never massage both carotids at the same time.

Listen for carotid bruits first—don't massage if one is present as it may cause a cerebral embolus.

A favourite exam question is how to distinguish VT from SVT with aberrant conduction. The following features suggest VT:
- Fusion or capture beats (these are pathognomonic).
- Different QRS morphology to that in sinus rhythm.
- QRS duration >0.14 seconds with RBBB configuration or >0.16 seconds with LBBB configuration.
- QRS axis: left axis deviation with RBBB morphology, or extreme left axis deviation (northwest axis) with LBBB morphology.
- Concordance in the chest leads (all complexes have similar polarities).

Bradycardias

Sinus bradycardia
For notes on sinus bradycardia, see p.16.

Heart block
All negatively chronotropic drugs should be stopped. If the patient is symptomatic, atropine can be tried. If this fails, consider temporary pacing. If the patient remains symptomatic or has second or third degree block, permanent pacing may be required.

Sick sinus syndrome
This is due to dysfunction of the sinus node and can lead to periods of sinus bradycardia with periods of asystole, and tachycardia. Atrial pacing is the treatment of choice if there is no AV conduction defect. Otherwise dual chamber pacing (atria and ventricles) is the treatment of choice.

First degree heart block
The ECG shows a long PR interval (more than 0.2 seconds) (Fig. 30.15).

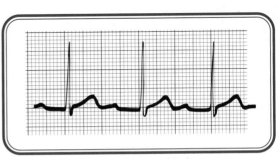

Fig. 30.15 ECG of first degree heart block.

Second degree heart block
In Wenckebach (Mobitz type I) heart block there is progressive widening of the PR interval, culminating in

In complete heart block, work out the atrial rate and the ventricular rate separately by marking them on a piece of paper. They should both be regular but at different rates.

non-conduction through the AV node. The cycle then continues (Fig. 30.16).

Mobitz type II heart block is intermittent failure of AV conduction (Fig. 30.17).

Third degree or complete heart block
Here, there is dissociation between the atria and ventricles (Fig. 30.18).

Antiarrhythmic drugs
Traditionally, antiarrhythmics are classified according to their effects on the action potential (Vaughn Williams classification; Fig. 30.19). However, this is now of less clinical relevance than a classification based on the site of action in the heart—supraventricular, ventricular, and both. Some examples of antiarrhythmic drugs are given below.

Supraventricular arrhythmias
Adenosine
Adenosine is used for terminating paroxysmal supraventricular tachycardia (SVT). The half-life is 8–10 seconds but is longer if the patient is on dipyridamole. It can cause flushing and bronchospasm.

Verapamil
Verapamil should not be used for wide complex tachycardias unless a supraventricular origin has been established beyond doubt. It should not be used with ß-blockers.

Supraventricular and ventricular arrhythmias
Amiodarone
Amiodarone should only be used when other drugs are ineffective or contraindicated, and usually under hospital supervision. It can be used orally or intravenously for rapid effect. The half-life is several weeks. It may therefore take some weeks to achieve steady-state plasma concentration.

Side effects include hypo- and hyperthyroidism and liver dysfunction. TFTs and liver function tests (LFTs) should therefore be checked at baseline and every 6 months. It may also cause pneumonitis, corneal microdeposits (which are reversible on stopping treatment), and photosensitivity.

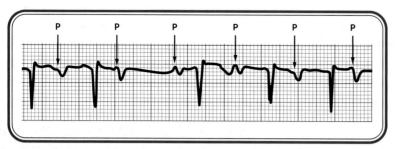

Fig. 30.16 ECG of Wenckebach heart block.

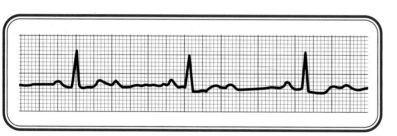

Fig. 30.17 ECG of Mobitz type II heart block showing two p waves for each QRS complex (i.e. 2:1 block).

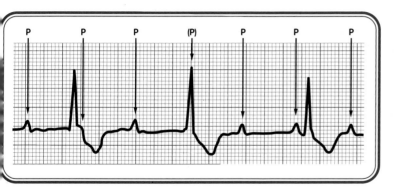

Fig. 30.18 ECG of complete heart block.

β-Blockers
β-Blockers act mainly by attenuating the effects of the sympathetic nervous system on automaticity and conductivity within the heart.

Disopyramide
Disopyramide may be used intravenously to control arrhythmias after MI. It is negatively inotropic and has antimuscarinic side effects.

Flecainide
Flecainide is useful for symptomatic ventricular arrhythmias and paroxysmal atrial fibrillation. It has been shown to increase mortality in patients treated for symptomatic ventricular ectopics after MI, and is therefore contraindicated in patients with IHD.

Procainamide
Procainamide is used for ventricular arrhythmias and paroxysmal atrial fibrillation. It can cause a syndrome resembling systemic lupus erythematosus (SLE) with prolonged use.

Propafenone and quinidine
Propafenone and quinidine are also useful for ventricular and some supraventricular arrhythmias.

Ventricular arrhythmias
Bretylium
Bretylium is only used as an antiarrhythmic drug in resuscitation. It can cause severe hypotension, nausea, and vomiting.

Lidocaine
Lidocaine is used commonly for VT after an MI but it can only be given intravenously. The dose should be decreased with cardiac or liver failure to avoid convulsions, depression of the central nervous system, or depression of the cardiovascular system.

Mexiletine
Mexiletine has a similar action to lidocaine. It is negatively inotropic.

HEART FAILURE

Heart failure occurs when the heart is unable to maintain sufficient cardiac output to meet the demands of the body, despite the presence of normal filling pressures. The incidence rises with age and is present in over 1% of the over-65s. It is classified by its severity (Fig. 30.20). The mortality in severe heart failure is about 50% at 1 year.

The Vaughn Williams classification of antiarrhythmic drugs	
Class	**Features**
Ia,b,c	membrane stabilizing drugs (e.g. quinidine, lidocaine and flecainide, respectively)
II	β-blockers
III	amiodarone, bretylium, sotalol
IV	calcium channel blockers (excluding dihydropyridines, e.g. nifedipine)

Fig. 30.19 The Vaughn Williams classification of antiarrhythmic drugs.

Causes of heart failure

High output failure

The heart maintains a normal or increased cardiac output in the face of grossly elevated requirements. It is then unable to meet these requirements. Conditions causing this include:

- Thyrotoxicosis.
- Nephritis.
- Anaemia.
- AV shunts.
- Beriberi.
- Fever.
- Paget's disease.
- Pregnancy.

True heart failure

True heart failure is due primarily to an abnormality of the heart, when the cardiac output at rest is low or normal, but low on exercise. Causes include the following:

- Myocardial disease: ischaemia and infarction; structure, e.g. hypertrophic obstructive cardiomyopathy, hypertension; fibrosis, e.g. infections, immunological reactions, small vessel disease; others, e.g. thyroid disease, beriberi, amyloidosis, sarcoidosis, heavy metals, alcohol.
- Drugs, e.g. antiarrhythmics, calcium antagonists, ß-blockers.
- Arrhythmias, e.g. atrial fibrillation.
- Volume overload, e.g. aortic and mitral regurgitation.
- Outflow obstruction, e.g. aortic stenosis.
- Restricted filling, e.g. constrictive pericarditis or tamponade, restrictive cardiomyopathy.

The New York Heart Association classification of heart failure	
Class	**Features**
I	no limitation of physical activity
II	slight limitation of physical activity
III	marked limitation of physical activity
IV	inability to carry out any physical activity without discomfort

Fig. 30.20 The New York Heart Association classification of heart failure.

Clinical features

Left heart failure

Symptoms include:

- Exertional dyspnoea.
- Orthopnoea.
- Paroxysmal nocturnal dyspnoea.
- Fatigue.
- Wheeze.
- Cough
- Haemoptysis.

Signs include:

- Tachypnoea.
- Tachycardia.
- Pulsus alternans (alternating large and small pulse pressures)
- Peripheral cyanosis.
- Cardiomegaly.
- A third heart sound.
- Functional mitral regurgitation secondary to dilatation of the mitral annulus.
- Basal crepitations.
- Pleural effusions.

Right heart failure

This may occur secondary to chronic lung disease, multiple pulmonary emboli, pulmonary hypertension, right-sided valve disease, left-to-right shunts, or isolate right ventricular cardiomyopathy. It is most commonly associated secondary to LVF, in which case the term congestive cardiac failure is used.

Symptoms include:

- Fatigue.
- Nausea.
- Wasting.
- Swollen ankles.
- Abdominal discomfort.
- Anorexia.
- Breathlessness.

The signs include:

- A raised jugulovenous pressure (JVP).
- Smooth hepatomegaly.
- Liver tenderness.
- Pitting oedema.
- Ascites.
- Functional tricuspid regurgitation.

- Tachycardia.
- Right ventricular third heart sound.

Investigations

The cause for the heart failure must always be sought as heart failure itself is an inadequate diagnosis. After the history and examination, investigations include the following:

- FBC: anaemia.
- U&Es: e.g. for hypokalaemia with diuretics.
- LFTs: liver congestion.
- Echocardiography: left ventricular function and valves.
- TFTs.
- Cardiac enzymes: if acute onset, to exclude MI.
- ECG: IHD, arrhythmias, and left ventricular hypertrophy.
- CXR: cardiomegaly, alveolar oedema, bat's wings shadowing, prominent upper lobe vessels, Kerley B lines, pleural effusions.

Other investigations to consider are:

- Exercise testing: functional severity and prognosis.
- Cardiac catheterization.
- Nuclear techniques: ejection fraction, cardiac function, prognosis.

Management

The aims of management are to relieve symptoms and to improve the prognosis. The cause of the heart failure should be sought and treated appropriately, e.g. valve lesions. Exacerbating factors such as anaemia and hypertension should be treated. Check the patient's drugs as some may cause fluid retention, e.g. non-steroidal anti-inflammatory drugs (NSAIDs). Patients should be advised to maintain an optimal weight, avoid excessive salt intake and large amounts of alcohol, and stop smoking.

Drug treatment

Diuretics relieve the symptoms of heart failure, and ACE inhibitors improve symptoms and prognosis. They reduce the risk of MI and increase survival. Treatment is best planned as a stepped care plan.

Step 1

If the heart failure is mild, start a thiazide diuretic, e.g. bendrofluazide 2.5 mg o.d. Many patients are started on a loop diuretic from the outset, e.g. frusemide 20–40 mg daily. Diuretics increase the excretion of sodium and water, and, by reducing the circulatory volume, they decrease the preload and oedema. Loop diuretics have a thiazide-like action on the early distal tubule but more importantly they inhibit sodium and chloride reabsorption in the thick ascending loop of Henle. This segment has a high capacity for absorbing sodium and chloride, and so drugs which act on this site produce a diuresis that is much greater than that of other diuretics. Side effects include hyperglycaemia, hyperuricaemia, hypotension, and hypokalaemia.

Step 2

An ACE inhibitor should be commenced at the same time if there are no contraindications. The dose should be increased to the maximum tolerated dose (Fig. 30.8). As the name suggests, ACE inhibitors inhibit the conversion of angiotensin I to angiotensin II. To avoid dangerous hyperkalaemia, any potassium-sparing diuretic should be omitted from the diuretic regimen before introducing an ACE inhibitor, changing to the loop diuretic alone. Potassium supplements should be discontinued.

Profound first dose hypotension may occur when ACE inhibitors are introduced to patients with heart failure who are already on a high dose of a loop diuretic, e.g. frusemide 80 mg o.d. or higher. Temporary withdrawal of the loop diuretic reduces the risk but may cause severe rebound pulmonary oedema. The ACE inhibitor should therefore be started at a very low dosage with the patient recumbent and under close medical supervision, and with facilities to treat profound hypotension.

Patients with severe heart failure should start ACE inhibitors in hospital. Initiation in hospital is also recommended for patients with mild to moderate heart failure and the conditions given in Fig. 30.21.

Alternative step 2

The contributions of venodilators such as ISMN, which will reduce preload, and arterial dilators such as hydralazine, which will reduce afterload, have been shown to be of prognostic benefit in people with heart failure but are inferior to ACE inhibitors in this respect. They may be prescribed to patients in whom ACE inhibitors are contraindicated.

Recommendations for inpatient initiation of ACE inhibitors
• frusemide 80 mg o.d. or more • hypovolaemia (check for diarrhoea and vomiting) • hyponatraemia (plasma sodium <130 mmol/L) • systolic blood pressure <90 mmHg • unstable heart failure • renal impairment: plasma creatinine >150 mmol/L • high-dose vasodilator therapy • age 70 years or more

Fig. 30.21 Recommendations for inpatient initiation of angiotensin-converting enzyme (ACE) inhibitors. ACE inhibitors are contraindicated in people with known or suspected bilateral renal artery stenosis, in aortic stenosis, or outflow tract obstruction, pregnancy, and porphyria. Common side effects include a dry cough, hypotension, dizziness, and headache.

Step 3

This next stage is to increase the dose of loop diuretic. For patients with intractable heart failure, very high doses of frusemide may be needed—up to 1 g per day.

Step 4

The addition of digoxin for its inotropic effect has been shown to reduce hospital admissions and symptoms, although not mortality. It is of particular benefit in patients with atrial fibrillation. They should be used with caution in the elderly who are particularly susceptible to digoxin toxicity.

Common toxic effects are anorexia, nausea, and vomiting. They may also cause almost any supraventricular or ventricular arrhythmia, and heart block. These unwanted effects depend both on the plasma digoxin concentration and on the sensitivity of the conducting system or myocardium, which is often increased in heart disease.

Hypokalaemia predisposes to toxicity and serum potassium should be monitored. Renal function is the most important determinant of digoxin dosage. Typical maintenance doses are 125–250 mg daily although lower doses may be needed if there is renal impairment. Toxicity can often be managed by discontinuing therapy and correcting hypokalaemia if appropriate. Digoxin-specific antibody fragments are available for the reversal of life-threatening overdosage.

Step 5

Traditionally, β-blockers are contraindicated in patients with heart failure because of their negative inotropic effect. However, carvedilol, which is a β-blocker with additional arteriolar vasodilating action, may be of benefit if heart failure is severe.

Step 6

If heart failure is intractable, the addition of metolazone, a powerful thiazide diuretic, produces a profound diuresis acting synergistically with loop diuretics.

Angiotensin II antagonists are being increasingly used in patients with heart failure. They should be considered if there are contraindications to ACE inhibitors.

Other drug options

Other drug options to consider are phosphodiesterase inhibitors such as enoximone and milrinone, which increase myocardial contraction and are vasodilators. Sustained haemodynamic benefit has been shown after administration but as yet there is no conclusive evidence of any beneficial effect on survival.

Bed rest may promote diuresis. Prophylaxis for DVT should be given with subcutaneous heparin. It may sometimes help giving frusemide intravenously, either as a slow bolus or continuous intravenous infusion. As a last resort, β-adrenergic agonists, dopamine and dobutamine produce a positive inotropic effect but must be given intravenously. They may be useful for acute exacerbations of heart failure but may induce 'inotrope dependence' making it difficult to wean the patient off them.

For patients with severe heart failure, heart transplantation should be considered. This can dramatically improve the quality of life; 5 year survival over 70%.

Acute heart failure

This is an emergency characterized by acute breathlessness, wheezing, anxiety, and sweating. There may be pink frothy sputum, as well as signs of pulmonary oedema. If severe, the management (listed below) should begin before investigations are performed.

- Sit the patient upright.
- Give high-concentration oxygen unless there is coexisting chronic hypercapnia due to long-standing respiratory failure. It may even be necessary to ventilate the patient.

- Give intravenous frusemide or bumetanide. These cause an immediate vasodilatation, as well as their more delayed diuresis.
- Give 5 mg intravenous diamorphine slowly unless there is liver failure of chronic obstructive pulmonary disease. This causes sedation, relieves dyspnoea, and causes vasodilatation. It should be given with an antiemetic.
- Give intravenous venodilators, e.g. ISDN, if systolic blood pressure is greater than 100 mmHg. This will reduce preload.
- Load the patient with digoxin, orally or intravenously, if in fast atrial fibrillation. Other arrhythmias should be treated appropriately.
- Consider giving intravenous aminophylline 5 mg/kg intravenously over 10 minutes. This is positively inotropic and causes vasodilatation and bronchodilation. It is usually reserved only for those patients with bronchospasm.
- Intravenous inotropic agents may be of value if there is hypotension. If signs of renal hypoperfusion are present, dopamine is recommended intravenously at 2.5–5 µg/kg/min. If pulmonary congestion is dominant, dobutamine is preferred at 2.5 µg/kg/min increasing gradually to 10 µg/kg/min if needed.

YPERTENSION

ne prevalence of hypertension differs depending on ood pressure cut-off points, age, sex, and race. It creases with age, and is more common in men and fro-Caribbeans. About 20% of the UK adult population ave blood pressures above 160/95 mmHg. The risk of orbidity and mortality rises continuously with increasing ood pressure, and marginal risk is greater at higher ood pressures. Similarly, the lower the blood pressure chieved with treatment, the lower the risk of omplications of hypertension. However the benefit of wering diastolic blood pressure to below 90 mmHg is inimal in uncomplicated hypertension in young or iddle-aged patients.

Definitions of hypertension differ but whatever the ood pressure thresholds used, the mean of several ood pressure measurements should be taken over ne, as an isolated reading predicts cardiovascular risk ly very poorly. Blood pressure should be taken sitting lying after 2–3 minutes rest. The bladder cuff should cover at least 80% of the arm circumference, otherwise, in obese patients, artificially high readings are observed. The dial or mercury column should fall at 2 mm per second, i.e. slowly, and be read to the nearest 2 mm. The diastolic pressure is recorded at the disappearance of sounds, i.e. phase V.

Aetiology

In over 90% of people, the diagnosis of hypertension is idiopathic ('essential'), i.e. no cause can be found. Genetic influences on blood pressure regulation have been suggested by family studies. A number of environmental factors are also associated with the developments of hypertension. These include obesity, alcohol, dietary sodium intake, dietary potassium, and smoking.

Vegetarians have less hypertension than meat eaters, though it is difficult to know whether the blood pressure differences are due to diet *per se* or other causes. It is not clear whether psychological factors play a significant part in long-term blood pressure regulation, though there is no doubt that emotional factors can induce pronounced but transient variations in blood pressure.

Obesity
There is a continuous linear relationship between excess body fat and blood pressure levels.

Alcohol
Increasing alcohol consumption is related to higher blood pressure levels, and the effects are additive to those of obesity.

Dietary sodium intake
Salt intake has a small effect on population blood pressure levels. Salt restriction may reduce systolic blood pressure by 3–5 mmHg in hypertensives and is most clear-cut in older subjects and those with more severe hypertension.

Dietary potassium
Dietary sodium and potassium intake are generally inversely related. Dietary potassium may have a blood pressure lowering effect, and estimates of dietary sodium/potassium ratios are more strongly associated with blood pressure levels than either of the cations independently.

Smoking

This leads to an acute elevation in blood pressure, which subsides within 15 minutes of finishing a cigarette. Regular smokers actually have slightly lower blood pressures than non-smokers, although the small potential benefit is greatly outweighed by the increased cardiovascular risk.

Secondary hypertension

A definite underlying cause for hypertension is commoner in younger people, and should be looked for specifically in the under-35s:

- Renal disease: chronic glomerulonephritis, chronic pyelonephritis, renal artery stenosis, polycystic kidney disease, and polyarteritis nodosa. Although it only accounts for 1% of all hypertension, the diagnosis of renal artery stenosis is important as it is the commonest curable cause.
- Endocrine disease: Cushing's and Conn's syndromes, phaeochromocytoma, and acromegaly.
- Pregnancy-induced hypertension and pre-eclampsia: associated with oedema and proteinuria.
- Coarctation of the aorta.
- Drugs: oestrogen-containing oral contraceptive pill, NSAIDs, steroids, sympathomimetics in cold cures, carbenoxolone, and liquorice.

History

Patients with hypertension are usually asymptomatic. The history should concentrate on environmental predisposing factors, associated cardiovascular risk factors, and the symptoms of underlying secondary causes. For example, patients with phaeochromocytoma may have symptoms of panic, headache, sweating, nausea, tremor, and pallor. Accelerated hypertension may lead to symptoms secondary to heart failure, renal failure, headaches, nausea and vomiting, visual impairment, or fits.

Examination

The clinical approach to the patient with hypertension is summarized in Fig. 30.22. Apart from the blood pressure itself, the examination should focus on complications of hypertension or underlying secondary causes. The patient should be examined for left ventricular hypertrophy (displaced apex beat), coarctation of the aorta (difference in blood pressure in the arms, weak femoral pulses, radiofemoral delay), renal bruits for possible underlying renal artery stenosis, and palpable kidneys, e.g. in polycystic kidney disease. There may be retinopathy, classified by the Keith–Wagener changes (Fig. 30.23).

Clinical evaluation of the patient with hypertension	
causes of hypertension	drugs causing hypertension? paroxysmal features? (phaeochromocytoma) present, past or family history of renal disease? general appearance? (Cushing's syndrome) radiofemoral delay? (coarctation) kidney(s) palpable? (polycystic, hydronephrosis, neoplasm) abdominal or loin bruit? (renal artery stenosis)
contributory factors	overweight? alcohol intake?
complications	cerebrovascular disease left ventricular hypertrophy or cardiac failure ischaemic heart disease fundal haemorrhages and exudates (accelerated phase)
contraindications to drugs	gout, diabetes (thiazides) asthma, heart failure, heart block (ß-blockers) heart failure, heart block (verapamil)
cardiovascular risk	assessment of other cardiovascular risk factors

Fig. 30.22 Clinical evaluation of th patient with hypertension. Look for the 'five Cs'.

Investigation policy

The minimum tests include urinalysis and serum biochemistry for evidence of renal disease, and ECG for evidence of left ventricular hypertrophy or ischaemia.

Consideration should also be given to the following:
- CXR: cardiac size and signs of heart failure.
- Serum lipids: cardiovascular risk.
- Echocardiography: left ventricular hypertrophy and left ventricular function.

Further invesigations are warranted in young patients where a secondary cause is more likely, in patients with rapidly rising blood pressure or severe hypertension, in patients with hypertension resistant to treatment, and in patients with deranged U&Es. These investigations include urinary vanillylmandelic acids for phaeochromocytoma and an intravenous urogram (IVU) for evidence of renal artery stenosis. If this is abnormal, renal arteriography is indicated.

Further investigations depend on clinical suspicion, e.g. aortography for coarctation of the aorta.

Management of hypertension

For secondary hypertension, treatment of the underlying condition may sometimes be indicated, e.g. treatment of an underlying endocrine condition or surgical correction of aortic coarctation. In renovascular hypertension, drug treatment may effectively control blood pressure. It is therefore reasonable to consider angioplasty or surgery only for young patients who are more likely to have fibromuscular hyperplasia compared to atherosclerosis, patients with severe hypertension, or patients whose blood pressure is difficult to control medically. Surgery may also be

The Keith–Wagener classification of retinopathy	
Grade	**Features**
I	arterial narrowing and increased tortuosity
II	arteriovenous nipping
III	haemorrhages and soft exudates
IV	grades I–III and papilloedema

Fig. 30.23 The Keith–Wagener classification of retinopathy.

indicated where progressive renal failure in a hypertensive patient is due either to bilateral renal artery stenosis or stenosis of an artery to a single kidney.

An algorithm of the decision making process in patients with hypertension is given in Fig. 30.24. The aim is to reduce blood pressure to below 160/90 mmHg.

Accelerated hypertension

Malignant hypertension or very severe hypertension (diastolic blood pressure over 140 mmHg) requires urgent treatment in hospital. Treatment is normally given orally with β-blockers or calcium antagonists to reduce diastolic blood pressure to 100–110 mmHg within the first 24 hours. Over the next few days, further antihypertensives should be given to lower blood pressure further.

Very rapid falls in blood pressure should be avoided because the reduction in cerebral perfusion may lead to cerebral infarction, blindness, worsening renal function, and myocardial ischaemia. Parenteral antihypertensive drugs are rarely required.

In moderate to severe hypertension, i.e. diastolic blood pressure over 110 mmHg or in patients with vascular complications, drugs are best added 'stepwise' until control has been achieved. An attempt can then be made to 'step down' treatment under supervision. Monotherapy controls blood pressure in only 30–50% of patients, and most patients therefore need two or more drugs. In uncomplicated mild hypertension, drugs may be substituted rather than added.

A good 'stepped care' plan is given in Fig. 30.25.

Drug treatment
Thiazides

Thiazides lower blood pressure mainly by lowering body sodium stores. Initially blood pressure falls because of a decrease in blood volume, venous return, and cardiac output. Gradually the cardiac output returns to normal but the hypotensive effect remains because the peripheral resistance decreases. Side effects include impaired glucose tolerance and gout. Low doses (bendrofluazide 2.5 mg) cause little biochemical disturbance without loss of the antihypertensive effect. Higher doses are never needed, nor usually are potassium supplements. Thiazides are better tolerated in women than men, and are more effective in the elderly.

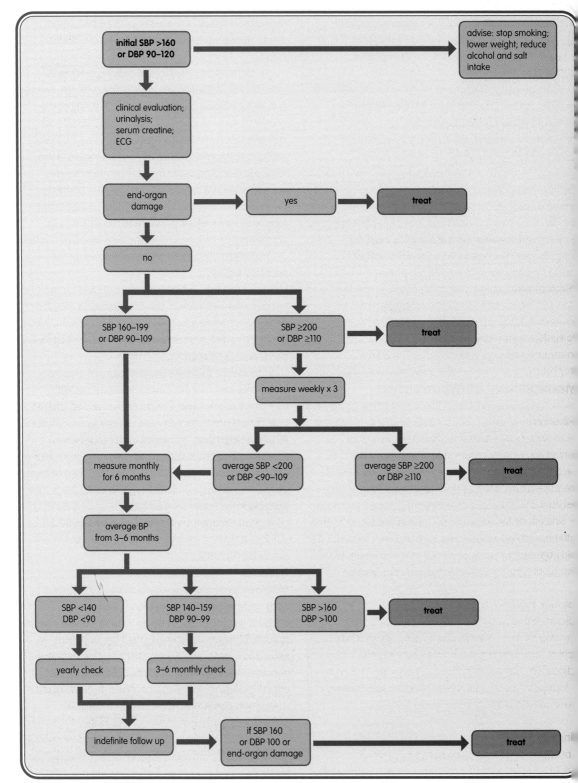

Fig. 30.24 Algorithm for making decisions in systolic and diastolic hypertension. (BP, blood pressure; DBP, diastolic blood pressure; SBP, systolic blood pressure.)

Stepped care plan for management of hypertension	
Step	**Measures**
0	non-drug treatment: weight reduction, alcohol reduction, moderate salt restriction, stop smoking
1	women, and men over 60 years—bendrofluazide 2.5 mg men under 60 years—bendrofluazide 2.5 mg or β-blocker, e.g. atenolol 50 mg
2	bendrofluazide 2.5 mg + atenolol 50 mg
3	add ACE inhibitor, e.g. enalapril 2.5–40 mg (alternatives: dihydropyridine calcium antagonist, e.g. amlodipine 5–10 mg o.d., selective α-blocker, e.g. doxazosin 1–8 mg b.d., angiotensin II antagonist, e.g. losartan 50–100 mg o.d.)
4*	substitute frusemide 40–80 mg for thiazide exclude non-compliance, drug interactions, secondary hypertension consider referral for detailed investigation
5*	non-urgent: try other step 3 drugs urgent: minoxidil (men only–causes hirsuitism)

Fig. 30.25 Stepped care plan for the management of hypertension. *Steps 4 and 5 require detailed investigation and intensive biochemical monitoring, best performed in a specialist clinic. Drugs may also be chosen with concomitant conditions in mind. For example, ß-blockers and calcium antagonists may be used early for patients with angina; ACE inhibitors are a sensible first choice in DM because they may delay the progression of nephropathy.

Potassium-sparing diuretics

Potassium-sparing diuretics may be used for the prophylaxis or treatment of diuretic-induced hypokalaemia (Fig. 30.26).

β-Blockers

β-Blockers initially produce a fall in blood pressure by decreasing cardiac output. With continued treatment the cardiac output returns to normal but the blood pressure remains low because the peripheral resistance is 'reset' at a lower level.

Side effects include negative inotropism, provocation of asthma, and heart block. Less serious side effects include cold hands and fatigue. β-blockers are more effective in young patients and less effective in black patients.

Calcium antagonists

Calcium antagonists work in different ways. The dihydropyridines, e.g. nifedipine, may cause a reflex tachycardia, flushing, headache oedema, and indigestion. The oedema does not respond to diuretics. Verapamil cannot be used with a β-blocker. It may cause constipation.

Minoxidil

Minoxidil is a potent vasodilator and decreases peripheral resistance. It may cause a reflex tachycardia, which can be prevented by combination with a β-blocker. It may also cause fluid retention, which is prevented by combination with a diuretic.

ACE inhibitors

ACE inhibitors are well tolerated and more effective in younger patients. They cause a persistent dry cough in 20% of women and 10% of men. Renal function should be checked before starting treatment and when dose titration is complete.

α-Blockers

α-Blockers reduce both arteriolar and venous resistance, and maintain a high cardiac output.

Indications for a potassium-sparing diuretic in prophylaxis or treatment of diuretic induced hypokalaemia

- digoxin treatment
- chronic liver disease
- history of arrhythmia or antiarrhythmic treatment
- severe or unstable angina
- Conn's syndrome and other states of mineralocorticoid excess
- severe hypokalaemia, i.e. serum potassium <3.0 mmol/L

Fig. 30.26 Indications for use of a potassium-sparing diuretic for prophylaxis or treatment of diuretic induced hypokalaemia.

Methyldopa

Methyldopa stimulates α_2-receptors in the medulla and reduces sympathetic outflow. In 20% of patients, it causes a positive Coombs' test and, rarely, haemolytic anaemia. Drug-induced hepatitis with fever may also occur.

Hypertension in pregnancy

Good blood pressure control in pregnancy is important—oral methyldopa is safe. ß-Blockers are effective and safe in the third trimester but may cause intrauterine growth retardation when used earlier in pregnancy. Hydralazine may also be used.

Age and hypertension

Factors relating to hypertension associated with advancing age are summarized in Fig. 30.27.

Follow up

Of patients, 25–50% default or discontinue treatment, so an effective recall system is needed. When the blood pressure is satisfactorily controlled, it should be checked once every 3 months. More frequent checks are needed during dose titration if the control is borderline, if compliance is a problem, or if the treatment regimen is complex. On routine visits, the blood pressure and weight should be measured, and the patient should be asked about side effects. The urine should be checked for protein and glucose yearly.

Apart from this, routine re-examination or investigation is unnecessary, and should only be performed if there is a special indication, e.g. variable or borderline blood pressure control, or at the onset of new symptoms.

Prognosis

Patients with untreated malignant hypertension have a 90% mortality in 1 year, and treatment is therefore life saving. The risk of hypertension in other cases depends on the level of blood pressure, the presence of complications, e.g. cardiac or renal failure, and the presence of other cardiovascular risk factors, e.g. male sex, smoking, diabetes, and older age. Those at highest risk gain most benefit from treatment.

VALVULAR HEART DISEASE

Mitral stenosis (see p. 21)

The cause of mitral stenosis is usually rheumatic fever

although only about half of all patients give a positive history. It is four times more common than mitral regurgitation, and is commoner in women than men.

Progressive stenosis of the mitral valve, via thickening of the cusps and fusion of the commissures, results in a pressure gradient between the left atrium and the left ventricle. As the stenosis worsens, ventricular filling becomes impaired, and this is compounded by fibrosis of the subvalvar apparatus leading to left atrial dilatation and hypertrophy, atrial fibrillation and thrombosis. Pulmonary congestion may ensue, and an increase in pulmonary artery pressure may lead to right heart failure.

Management

Anticoagulation is indicated in patients with atrial fibrillation although some would anticoagulate all patients with mitral stenosis. The risk of emboli is greater with a large left atrium or left atrial appendage.

Pulmonary congestion is treated with diuretics, and digoxin is used to control the ventricular rate in atrial fibrillation. It may be necessary to add in other rate-controlling drugs such as ß-blockers or verapamil.

If symptoms persist the patient should be considered for mitral valvotomy or valve replacement. If the valve is not calcified and the leaflets are pliable, balloon valvuloplasty may be attempted.

All patients should receive antibiotic prophylaxis before dental and surgical procedures to avoid subacute bacterial endocarditis.

Mitral regurgitation

The incidence of mitral regurgitation is equal in men and women. It is usually secondary to rheumatic fever, floppy prolapsing mitral valve leaflets, papillary muscle dysfunction, rupture after an inferior MI or

---

Age and hypertension—factors associated with advancing age

- greater likelihood of hypertension (>50%)
- greater damage when hypertensive
- disatolic threshold for treatment 90 mmHg
- as much or more benefit from treatment
- no increase in treatment side effects
- elderly should be offered treatment unless suffering other life-shortening illness
- erect pressures should be measured

Fig. 30.27 Age and hypertension—factors associated with advancing age.

cardiomyopathy, or secondary to ventricular dilatation or dysfunction. Less common causes include congenital malformations, which may be associated with an ostium primum atrial septal defect, infective endocarditis, rupture of the chordae tendineae, cardiomyopathy, rheumatoid arthritis, or left atrial tumour interfering with mitral valve closure.

The circulatory changes depend on the speed of onset and severity of mitral regurgitation. Acute regurgitation may lead to acute pulmonary oedema whereas chronic regurgitation allows for compensatory left ventricular and atrial dilatation. (Also see p. 22.)

Management
Diuretics are used for pulmonary congestion, and vasodilators are helpful in acute regurgitation. Digoxin and anticoagulants are given to patients in atrial fibrillation. Antibiotic prophylaxis is needed prior to dental and surgical procedures.

Mitral valve replacement is indicated if symptoms are severe and uncontrolled by medical treatment, or if pulmonary hypertension develops. Good results are achieved if left ventricular function is preserved, and early referral may allow repair of the valve rather than replacement.

Mitral valve prolapse
This is due to prolapse of the mitral valve leaflets into the left atrium during ventricular systole. Prolapse is common in floppy valves and myocardial disease, and should be distinguished from benign mitral prolapse syndrome. It may affect up to 15% of the population and three times commoner in women. Pathologically, there is an increase in the zona spongiosa of the valve leaflets.

Clinical signs and symptoms
Is often asymptomatic and found incidentally. An apical midsystolic click is heard, associated with a late systolic murmur if the valve is regurgitant. It may be associated with palpitations and atypical chest pains, though the latter is more common in people aware of their condition. Systemic emboli and syncope are rare.

Investigations
Electrocardiography
The ECG may show inferolateral ST/T segment changes. Arrhythmias may be confirmed by Holter monitoring.

The commonest rhythm disturbance is ventricular extrasystoles.

Echocardiography
Echocardiography is diagnostic.

Management
Patients should receive endocarditis prophylaxis. Treatment is only indicated for complications, e.g. antiarrhythmic drugs for significant rhythm disturbances, or anticoagulants for emboli.

Aortic stenosis
The commonest cause of aortic stenosis is a calcified bicuspid valve, and this is more common in men. In younger patients the cause may be congenital or due to rheumatic fever but in older patients it may be due to senile degenerative calcification, which is commoner in women. Aortic stenosis tends to progress gradually causing obstruction to the left ventricular outflow with resultant hypertrophy. Ventricular dilatation and heart failure are late complications. Conduction defects may result from calcification extending into the ventricular system. (Also see p. 23.)

Management
Valve replacement is indicated for severe stenosis because of the risk of sudden death, or for symptomatic aortic stenosis. Drugs do not alter the progression of the disease though diuretics and digoxin can be given for heart failure

Aortic regurgitation
The more common causes include cusp malformation (e.g. bicuspid valve) and cusp erosion (e.g. infective endocarditis). (Also see p. 24.)
Other causes include:
- Cusp distortion (e.g. senile calcification and rheumatic fever).
- Loss of support (e.g. VSD).
- Aortic wall disease due to inflammation (e.g. syphilis).
- Ankylosing spondylitis.
- Reiter's syndrome.
- Psoriatic arthropathy.
- Aortic wall disease due to dilatation (e.g. hypertension with or without dissection).
- Chronic regurgitation causes left ventricular dilatation and hypertrophy.

Management
Valve replacement is indicated for symptomatic patients. In the meantime, diuretics and digoxin may be given to control symptoms of heart failure. The prognosis is good while ventricular function is good but death usually occurs within 2–3 years after the onset of ventricular failure.

Tricuspid regurgitation
This may be functional secondary to right heart failure, commonly as a result of pulmonary hypertension. It may also be rheumatic in association with mitral valve disease, or due to endocarditis in drug addicts.

MISCELLANEOUS CARDIOVASCULAR CONDITIONS

Congenital heart disease
Ventricular septal defect
VSD is the most common congenital heart lesion, accounting for about one-third of all malformations. Blood moves from the high pressure left ventricle to the right ventricle. If the defect is large, pulmonary flow increases leading to obliterative pulmonary vascular changes and an increase in pulmonary vascular resistance. The pulmonary arterial pressure may then equal the systemic pressure reducing or reversing the shunt, and central cyanosis may develop (Eisenmenger's syndrome).

Clinical features
A small defect (maladie de Roger) may cause no symptoms but there is a loud pansystolic murmur at the left sternal edge; it may close spontaneously. Larger VSDs produce dyspnoea and fatigue, and the pulse volume may be decreased. The apex beat is prominent due to left ventricular hypertrophy, and there may be a left parasternal heave if there is right ventricular hypertrophy (RVH) with pulmonary hypertension. There is a thrill at the left sternal edge as well as a pansystolic murmur in the same place. A mitral diastolic flow murmur implies a large shunt.

Investigation
Electrocardiography
There may be no changes in small VSDs. There may be features of right and left ventricular hypertrophy.

Chest X-ray
This may be normal in small VSDs. Prominent pulmonary arteries are present in pulmonary hypertension. There may be left atrial and ventricular enlargement.

Echocardiography
This is diagnostic if the defect can be imaged. Doppler studies identify abnormal flow across the septum

Cardiac catheterization
There is a step-up in oxygen saturation at the right ventricular level due to shunting of oxygenated blood from the left ventricle to the right ventricle. Left ventricular angiography produces opacification of the right ventricle through the defect.

Management
Antibiotic prophylaxis should be advised to prevent endocarditis. Moderate and large defects should be closed surgically to prevent pulmonary hypertension and Eisenmenger's syndrome.

Atrial septal defect
Atrial septal defect (ASD) accounts for 10% of congenital heart defects, and is more common in women than men. There are two types: ostium secundum (the more common type) and ostium primum. The communication between the atria allows for left-to-right atrial shunting. Atrial arryhthmias are common. In ostium primum defects, there may be involvement of the mitral and tricuspid valves producing regurgitation.

Clinical features
Most patients are asymptomatic; a few have dyspnoea and weakness. The patient may have palpitations secondary to atrial arrhythmias, and right heart failure may develop later in life. Auscultation reveals wide, fixed splitting of the second heart sound. The increased right heart output gives rise to a pulmonary systolic flow murmur. There may be a tricuspid diastolic flow murmur with large defects. There may be a left ventricular heave of RVH.

Investigations
Electrocardiography
There may be evidence of atrial arrhythmias, e.g. atrial fibrillation. In ostium secundum defects there is right bundle branch block (RBBB), right axis deviation and

RVH. In ostium primum defects, there is RBBB, left axis deviation, and RVH.

Chest X-ray
Pulmonary arteries are prominent and the lung fields are plethoric. The right atrium and ventricles are enlarged.

Echocardiography
This shows dilatation of the right-sided cardiac chambers. Doppler studies allow visualization of the left-to-right shunt across the atrial septum.

Cardiac catheterization
There is a step-up in oxygen saturation at the right atrial level due to shunting of oxygenated blood from the left atrium to the right atrium. The catheter can be directed across the defect into the left atrium.

Management
The defect should be closed surgically if the pulmonary/systemic flow ratio is greater than 2:1.

Patent ductus arteriosus

Patent ductus arteriosus (PDA) accounts for about 10% of congenital heart defects and is more common in women. The ductus arteriosus connects the pulmonary artery to the descending aorta but it should close off at birth. The condition is sometimes associated with maternal rubella. Because the aortic pressure is higher than the pulmonary artery pressure throughout the cardiac cycle, the PDA produces continuous shunting from the aorta to the pulmonary artery, leading to increased pulmonary venous return to the left heart and an increased left ventricular volume load.

Clinical features
There are usually no symptoms. Large defects lead to left ventricular failure with dyspnoea. The pulse is collapsing. There may be left ventricular hypertrophy. There is a continuous 'machinery' murmur with systolic accentuation loudest in the first or second left intercostal space.

Investigations
Electrocardiography
This is normal or shows features of left atrial and left ventricular hypertrophy.

Chest X-ray
The aorta and pulmonary arteries are prominent. The lung fields are plethoric.

Echocardiography
There is dilatation of the left-sided cardiac chambers. Doppler studies identify the abnormal flow across the ductus.

Cardiac catheterization
There is a step-up in oxygen saturation at pulmonary artery level. The catheter can sometimes be passed across the ductus into the descending aorta.

Management
Indomethacin given within the first few days of birth may stimulate duct closure by inhibiting prostaglandin synthesis. If this fails, the duct can be ligated surgically or with an umbrella occlusion device. Antibiotic prophylaxis is advised.

Pulmonary stenosis

This accounts for about 7% of defects.. It may be valvar or subvalvar (infundibular).

Clinical features
If very severe there is peripheral cyanosis. There is a pulmonary systolic thrill and murmur, louder on inspiration. The second heart sound is widely split due to a delayed P_2. There may be signs of right heart failure. In severe stenosis, the pulse volume is small and P_2 is soft or absent

Investigations
Electrocardiography
Electrocardiography may exhibit features of right atrial hypertrophy (p pulmonale) and RVH.

Chest X-ray
There may be poststenotic dilatation of the pulmonary artery and pulmonary oligaemia.

Echocardiography
This will confirm the diagnosis if adequate views are obtainable. Doppler studies can be used to measure the gradient across the valve.

Management
For severe pulmonary stenosis, balloon valvuloplasty or valvotomy is indicated.

Coarctation of the aorta

This accounts for 5–7% of congenital heart defects. It is twice as common in men, and is associated with Turner's syndrome, Marfan's syndrome and berry aneurysms. There is a narrowing of the aorta at or just distal to the ductus arteriosus; the vast majority are distal to the origin of the left subclavian artery. The condition is a cause of secondary hypertension. It encourages the formation of a collateral arterial circulation involving the intercostal arteries. In 80% of patients there is an associated bicuspid aortic valve.

Clinical features

The condition is often asymptomatic. When present, symptoms include headache, intermittent claudication, stroke, and endocarditis. On examination the femoral pulses are weak or absent, and there is radiofemoral delay. The upper limbs may be hypertensive or have unequal blood pressure, and the lower limbs have a low pressure. There may be features of LVH. There is a mid- or late systolic murmur over the upper praecordium or back due to turbulent flow through the coarctation. Collateral murmurs may be heard over the scapulae and there may be an aortic systolic murmur of an associated bicuspid valve.

Investigation

Electrocardiography
There may be LVH.

Chest X-ray
Tortuous and dilated collaterals may erode the undersurface of the ribs to produce 'rib notching'. There is a double aortic knuckle due to stenosis and poststenotic dilatation. There may be cardiomegaly.

Aortography
This confirms the diagnosis.

Management

Antibiotic prophylaxis should be advised. Treatment is by surgical resection.

Fallot's tetralogy

This represents 6–10% of cases of congenital heart disease. The four features comprising the tetrad are as follows:
- VSD.

- Right ventricular outflow obstruction (pulmonary stenosis—infundibular or valvar).
- The aorta is positioned over the ventricular septum ('overriding aorta').
- RVH.

Because there is right ventricular outflow obstruction, the shunt through the VSD is from right to left. This results in central cyanosis.

Clinical features

Children may present with deep cyanosis and syncope. Squatting helps to decrease the right-to-left shunt by increasing systemic resistance. Signs include cyanosis and finger clubbing. There is a parasternal heave and systolic murmur in the pulmonary area (second left intercostal space), P_2 is soft or absent, and there may be growth retardation.

Investigation

Electrocardiography
Features of right atrial and ventricular hypertrophy are present.

Chest X-ray
The heart is boot shaped ('coeur en sabot'). The pulmonary artery is small and the lung fields are oligaemic.

Echocardiography
This can be diagnostic but it may be necessary to proceed to cardiac catheterization studies to confirm the diagnosis.

Management

This is by total surgical correction. There are palliative procedures for the very young as holding measures, e.g. the Blalock shunt, which is anastamosis of a subclavian artery to a pulmonary artery to increase pulmonary blood flow.

Cardiomyopathy

Cardiomyopathy is a disorder of heart muscle. They are classified into three types as hypertrophic, dilated, and restrictive. Fig. 30.28 gives a classification.

Hypertrophic cardiomyopathy

Hypertrophic cardiomyopathy (HCM) follows an

autosomal dominant inheritance although half of all cases occur sporadically. There is asymmetrical left ventricular hypertrophy, which leads to symptoms of dyspnoea, angina, palpitations, and syncope. On examination, there is a jerky pulse, the apex beat has a double impulse, there may be third and fourth heart sounds, and there is a late systolic murmur best heard at the left sternal edge. There may also be associated mitral regurgitation.

HCM may be complicated by atrial fibrillation, systemic emboli, heart failure, and sudden death, the risk of which is probably increased by strenuous exercise.

Investigation

Electrocardiography
Electrocardiography shows left ventricular hypertrophy, and sometimes left bundle branch block.

Echocardiography
Echocardiography shows asymmetrical septal hypertrophy and systolic anterior movement of the mitral valve.

24-Hour ECG monitoring
This may identify silent arrhythmias.

Cardiac catheterization
This shows a small left ventricular cavity with obliteration in systole. There is a systolic gradient within the ventricle.

Management
β-Blockers help with symptoms and are useful for angina or dysrhythmias. Some treat dysrhythmias prophylactically with amiodarone. The patient should be anticoagulated if there is atrial fibrillation. If medical treatment is ineffective, the patient should be considered for septal myectomy or myotomy or cardiac transplantation.

Dilated (congestive) cardiomyopathy
The ventricles are dilated and contract poorly. Clinically, there are usually signs of right and left heart failure, cardiomegaly, and atrial fibrillation with emboli. More dangerous arrhythmias and conduction defects occur.

There are a number of possible heterogeneous causes, which include infiltrative disorders, collagen diseases, infective, toxic, metabolic, and genetic conditions. Echocardiography shoes a globally hypokinetc and dilated heart. Coronary arteriography is usually normal.

Management
Heart failure should be treated in the usual manner with diuretics and ACE inhibitors. Any underlying condition is treated as appropriate. Some prescribe anticoagulants to reduce the risk of emboli. The mortality is 40% at 2 years. Patients should be considered for cardiac transplantation.

Restrictive cardiomyopathy
This is due to endomyocardial stiffening and includes fiboplastic and infiltrative conditions in Fig. 30.28. The commonest cause in the UK is amyloidosis.

Pericarditis
Symptoms of pericarditis include a sharp retrosternal pain relieved by sitting forward. It may radiate to the left arm, or inferiorly. It is worse on lying down, with inspiration and coughing. There may be a 'scratchy' friction rub on examination.

The causes of pericarditis are given in Fig. 30.29.

Investigations
In addition to ECG and CXR (below), the following investigations should be performed:
- Blood and sputum culture for bacteria.
- Viral titres and viral culture from throat swabs and stools.
- Autoantibodies if there is evidence of connective tissue disease.
- TFTs.

Electrocardiography
This shows concave upwards ST segments; T wave inversion may also occur.

Chest X-ray
This is usually normal. If there is an associated pericardial effusion, the heart appears large and globular.

Management
The underlying cause is treated. NSAIDs (e.g. indomethacin 25–50 mg 6–8 hourly or aspirin 600 mg 6 hourly) relieve pain.

Clinical features of an associated pericardial effusion include signs of left and right heart failure. Pericardial tamponade means that the intrapericardial pressure increases, with reduced cardiac filling and hypotension. Clinically there is tachycardia, pulsus paradoxus, Kussmaul's sign (the JVP increases on inspiration), and muffled heart sounds. The CXR shows a globular heart. The ECG may show a changing axis and low amplitude QRS complexes. Echocardiography is diagnostic. Management is by pericardiocentesis.

Constrictive pericarditis

This is usually idiopathic or secondary to tuberculosis, although it may follow any cause of pericarditis. The heart is encased within a non-expansile pericardium. Clinically the signs are of right heart failure with ascites, hepatomegaly, and a raised JVP. There may be pulsus paradoxus, hypotension, and auscultation reveals a pericardial 'knock' due to an abrupt end to ventricular filling. The CXR may show pericardial calcification. Management is by pericardiectomy if constriction is severe.

Infective endocarditis

Infective endocarditis is an illness caused by microbial infection of the cardiac valves or endocardium. The annual incidence in the UK is about 7 in 10 000. It follows invasion of the bloodstream by micro-organisms from the mouth, gastrointestinal and genitourinary tracts, respiratory tract, or the skin. Platelets adhere to endothelial breaks and form 'vegetations', which are then colonized by circulating bacteria. Common sites of infection are bicuspid aortic valves and mitral valves with prolapse and regurgitation.

Prosthetic valve endocarditis is becoming increasingly important and may occur early postoperatively or late; 50% of patients have no previously known valve disease. In this group, endocarditis tends to follow a more acute course.

Streptococcus viridans is the commonest pathogen; others include *Strep. faecalis, Staphylococcus aureus,* and *Staph. epidermidis,* especially in drug addicts.

Clinical features

The diagnosis should be suspected in a patient with fever and changing heart murmurs. The clinical features are:

- Infection: malaise and lassitude, sweats, myalgia, arthralgia, weight loss, finger clubbing, anaemia, and splenomegaly. Fever is often low grade.

Causes of cardiomyopathy	
Cause	**Examples**
toxic	alcohol, cyclophosphamide, corticosteroids, lithium, phenothiazines
metabolic	thiamine deficiency, pellagra, obesity, porphyria, uraemia
endocrine	thyrotoxicosis, acromegaly, myxoedema, Cushing's disease, diabetes mellitus
collagen diseases	SLE, PAN
infiltrative	amyloidosis, haemochromatosis, neoplastic, sarcoidosis, mucopolysaccharidosis, Whipple's disease
infective	viral, rickettsial, mycobacterial
genetic	hypertrophic cardiomyopathy, muscular dystrophies
fibroplastic	endomyocardial fibrosis, Loeffler's endomyocardial disease, carcinoid
miscellaneous	ischaemic heart disease, postpartum

Fig. 30.28 Causes of cardiomyopathy. (PAN, polyarteritis nodosa; SLE, systemic lupus erythematosus.)

Causes of pericarditis
• idiopathic
• infections—viral (e.g. coxsackie virus B), bacterial (e.g. *Mycobacterium*), parasitic
• neoplastic (e.g. breast, lung, lymphoma)
• connective tissue disease (e.g. SLE, RA)
• uraemia
• myocardial infarction
• Dressler's syndrome following myocardial infarction or cardiac surgery
• radiotherapy
• trauma
• hypothyroidism

Fig. 30.29 Causes of pericarditis. (RA, rheumatoid arthritis; SLE, systemic lupus erythematosus.)

• Heart disease: listen for murmurs. In tricuspid endocarditis the patient may be murmur free. The patient may present with embolic pneumonia, pleurisy or haemoptysis, or later with a raised venous pressure, jaundice and a pulsating liver.
• Embolism: this is the most common cause of death in endocarditis. Most emboli are sterile but large fungal mycelia may embolize.
• Immunological phenomena: examples include vasculitic skin lesions, splinter haemorrhages, Roth spots in the retina, and Osler's nodes.
• Urine: this is normal in uncomplicated endocarditis. There may be mild proteinuria resulting from fever, or haematuria as a result of embolism with infarction.

Investigations

Numerous sets of blood cultures from different sites at different times are the essential investigation. A positive culture confirms the diagnosis. Other investigations are only supportive.

Erythrocyte sedimentation rate and white cell count

The erythrocyte sedimentation rate (ESR) and white cell count are usually raised. There is a normochromic normocytic anaemia.

Chest X-ray

A CXR with right-sided endocarditis may show multiple shadows due to an embolic pneumonia with infarction.

Electrocardiography

The ECG may show changes of MI due to coronary embolism, or conduction defect due to the development of an aortic root abscess.

Echocardiography

Echocardiography may show vegetations or paravalvular abscess formation. A negative echo does not exclude the diagnosis of endocarditis.

Management

Treatment should be started after blood has been taken for culture, but before obtaining confirmation of a positive culture, because valve destruction can occur rapidly and vegetations may grow and embolize.

Prophylaxis

Prophylactic antibiotics should be given before dental procedures for patients with heart valve lesions, septal defects, patent ductus, or prosthetic valves. For dental procedures under local or no anaesthesia, oral amoxycillin 3 g is given 1 hour before the procedure.

Patients who are penicillin allergic or who have received more than a single dose of penicillin in the previous month are given oral clindamycin 600 mg 1 hour before the procedure. For procedures under general anaesthesia, intravenous amoxycillin 1 g is given at induction followed by oral amoxycillin 500 mg 6 hours later.

Patients at special risk, e.g. those with prosthetic valves or who have had endocarditis, are given 1 g intravenous amoxycillin and 120 mg intravenous gentamicin at induction, followed by 500 mg oral amoxycillin 6 hours later.

Patients who are penicillin allergic are given 1 g vancomycin over 100 minutes, then 120 mg intravenous gentamicin at induction. The regimen for patients with upper respiratory tract infection is the same as for dental procedures. For patients undergoing genitourinary or gastrointestinal procedures, the regimen is as for special risk patients undergoing dental procedures under anaesthetic.

Treatment

Patients with endocarditis caused by penicillin-sensitive streptococci, e.g. *Strep. viridans*, are given intravenous benzylpenicillin (or vancomycin if penicillin allergic) plus low dose gentamicin (i.e. 60–80 mg twice daily).

Treatment is for 4 weeks. Gentamicin is stopped after 2 weeks if the organism is fully sensitive to penicillin. Oral amoxycillin may be substituted for benzylpenicillin after 2 weeks.

For patients with endocarditis caused by streptococci with reduced sensitivity to penicillin, e.g. *Strep. faecalis*, intravenous benzylpenicillin (or vancomycin) plus low-dose gentamicin is given for 4 weeks. If the organism is *Staph. aureus*, intravenous flucloxacillin plus either gentamicin or fusidic acid (or vancomycin alone if penicillin allergic) is given for at least 4 weeks. The gentamicin may be stopped after 2 weeks.

Surgery
This is needed for haemodynamic complications with acute severe valvular regurgitation, for valve obstruction by vegetations, for intractable heart failure, cardiac abscess formation, and for resistant infections.

Culture-negative endocarditis
Possible causes of culture-negative endocarditis are given in Fig. 30.30.

Acute rheumatic fever
Acute rheumatic fever is a multisystem disease following a group A, ß-haemolytic, streptococcal infection. The multisystem involvement reflects the generalized vasculitic process of the underlying pathology of the disease. It usually affects children of 5–15 years of age but no age or race is immune. Risk factors include crowding and low socio-economic status.

The diagnosis of acute rheumatic fever is based on clinical findings. The presence of two major or one major and two minor criteria indicates a high probability of rheumatic fever (Fig. 30.31). Evidence of a preceding streptococcal infection greatly strengthens the possibility of rheumatic fever.

Notes on Jones' criteria for rheumatic fever
Carditis (40–50%)
There may be myocarditis (tachypnoea, dyspnoea, pulmonary oedema), endocarditis (listen regularly for transient murmurs—the mitral valve is most commonly affected), or pericarditis (friction rub, effusion). It may be asymptomatic or result in death in the acute stage, and it can lead to heart failure and chronic valvular heart disease.

Arthritis (80%)
This is the most common major criterion and usually presents as migratory joint pain affecting larger joints. The onset is sudden with signs of inflammation and limitation of movement. Symptoms last for 3–6 weeks.

Chorea (10%)
There is a latent period of 2–6 months. Symptoms last for about 6 months. It is commoner in girls. Movements are involuntary, involving mainly the face and limbs and may be unilateral. It is associated with emotional lability.

Revised Jones' criteria for guidance in the diagnosis of rheumatic fever	
major criteria	polyarthritis carditis chorea erythema marginatum subcutaneous nodules
minor criteria	fever arthralgia previous rheumatic fever or rheumatic heart disease raised acute phase reactants (ESR, CRP, WCC) prolonged PR interval in ECG

Fig. 30.31 Revised Jones' criteria for guidance in the diagnosis of rheumatic fever. For a diagnosis of rheumatic fever there must also be supporting evidence of preceding streptococcal infection, i.e. increased antistreptolysin O (ASOT) or other streptococcal antibodies, positive throat culture for group A *Streptococcus*, or recent scarlet fever. (CRP, C reactive protein; ESR, erythrocyte sedimentation rate; WCC, white cell count.)

Possible causes of endocarditis in the event of negative culture
• *Coxiella burnetii* (Q fever) • fungi, e.g. aspergillus, histoplasma • partially treated bacterial endocarditis • polyarteritis nodosa or SLE • atrial myxoma • non-bacterial endocarditis associated with carcinoma

Fig. 30.30 Possible causes of endocarditis in the event of negative culture (SLE, systemic lupus erythematous).

Erythema marginatum (<5%)

This is a painless rash appearing as large, pink macules that spread quickly to give a serpiginous edge with a fading centre.

Subcutaneous nodules (rare)

These are round, firm, and painless, ranging from 0.5–2 cm. They are mobile and occur mainly over bony prominences.

Fever

This is usually low grade.

Management

This is bed rest for 2 weeks. Painful joints immobilized. Anti-inflammatory drugs relieve the pain and swelling of joints and possibly the later development of valvular heart disease. Treatment is usually for 12 weeks, or longer for severe carditis.

Aspirin 80–100 mg/kg/day or corticosteroids in severe carditis are the drugs of choice. Diazepam is given to control choreiform movements. Intramuscular penicillin G is given in the acute stages, and is followed by oral penicillin for 5 years in those patients without carditis, and probably indefinitely for those with cardiac involvement.

Atrial myxoma

These are rare, benign, primary tumours usually in the left atrium, which are twice as common in women than men. They present with vague symptoms, e.g. fever, weight loss, general malaise, atrial fibrillation, left atrial obstruction, or systemic emboli. Auscultation may reveal a 'tumour plop'. They are diagnosed by echocardiography and treatment is by surgical excision.

31. Respiratory Diseases

ASTHMA

Diagnosis

Asthma is a disease of the [air]ways characterized by an increased responsivenes[s of the] tracheobronchial tree to many different stimuli. It [is manifeste]d by paroxysms of shortness of breath, cou[gh, and whee]zing. These symptoms may resolve [spontaneously o]r be relieved by treatment.

Asthma is episodic [with acute exacerb]ations interspersed by symptom-free periods. [Ty]pically, most attacks are short (minutes to hours), and clinically the patient appears to recover completely after an attack.

In more severe asthma, patients can experience some degree of airway obstruction daily with accompanying symptoms.

Incidence

Asthma is very common and occurs in about 5% of the population in most Western countries. Bronchial asthma occurs at all ages but peaks in childhood and is more common in boys. However, in adult asthma, the sex ratio is about equal by the age of 30 years.

Aetiology

It is helpful to classify asthma by the main factors associated with acute episodes, i.e. into allergic asthma and intrinsic asthma.

Allergic asthma is often associated with a personal or family history of allergy such as hay fever, urticaria, and eczema. There may also be increased levels of immunoglobulin (Ig) E in the serum, and a positive response to provocation tests, e.g. methacholine challenge.

Intrinsic (or idiosyncratic) asthma is a term used to define those patients presenting with no personal or family history of allergy, with negative skin tests, and with normal serum levels of IgE. Many develop typical symptoms following an upper respiratory infection, which, after several days, leads to paroxysms of wheezing and shortness of breath that can last for months.

In general, asthma that occurs in childhood, or early adult life, tends to have a strong allergic component, whereas asthma that develops late tends to be non-allergic.

Despite this, many patients do not fit into either category but fall into a group with a mixture of allergic and non-allergic features.

Pathophysiology

Many theories have been proposed to explain the increased airway reactivity of asthma but the basic mechanism remains unknown.

The most popular hypothesis is that of airway inflammation. This is based on the observation that increased numbers of mast cells, epithelial cells, neutrophils, eosinophils, and lymphocytes have been found in the bronchoalveolar lavage fluid of patients with asthma. Along with these cellular components of inflammation a variety of inflammatory mediators such as histamine, bradykinin, the leukotrienes C, D, and E, and platelet-activating factor; prostaglandins E_2 and $F_{2\alpha}$ have also been found.

The clinical features of asthma probably derive from an interaction between the normally resident and infiltrating inflammatory cells in the airways, and the surface epithelium. These produce an intense immediate inflammatory reaction involving bronchoconstriction, vascular congestion, and oedema formation—the pathological hallmarks of asthma. Leukotrienes, in addition to evoking contraction of airway smooth muscle and mucosal oedema, may also account for other typical features of asthma, such as increased mucus production and impaired mucociliary transport.

A number of factors interact with normal airway responsiveness and provoke acute episodes and include the following:
- Allergens, e.g. house dust, mites, and animal dander.
- Drugs, e.g. β-blockers.
- The environment, e.g. climatic conditions and air pollution.
- Occupations, e.g. exposure to industrial chemicals, drugs, metals, dusts.
- Infections, e.g. viral and bacterial.

- Exercise.
- Emotion.

Clinical features of asthma

The symptoms of asthma consist of a triad of shortness of breath, cough, and wheezing. In its most typical form, asthma is an episodic disease, and all three symptoms coexist.

At the onset of an attack, patients experience a sense of constriction in the chest, often with a non-productive cough. Respiration becomes audibly harsh, wheezing in both phases of respiration becomes prominent, expiration becomes prolonged, and patients frequently have both tachypnoea and a tachycardia. If the attack is severe or prolonged, there may be a loss of breath sounds, and wheezing becomes either very high-pitched or inaudible. Accessory muscles of respiration can be seen and pulsus paradoxus often develops.

Less typically, a patient with asthma may present with intermittent episodes of non-productive cough or shortness of breath on exertion. These patients often have a normal physical examination but may wheeze after repeated forced exhalations or may show evidence of airways obstruction with spirometry. Occasionally a provocation test may be required to make the diagnosis of airway hyperresponsiveness.

Confirming the diagnosis of asthma

Diagnosing asthma is usually not difficult, especially if the patient is seen during an acute attack. In addition the history of episodic symptoms and a history of eczema, hay fever, or urticaria is valuable. Nocturnal symptoms, e.g. awakening short of breath or wheezing, are very common features.

Investigations

The diagnosis of asthma is established by demonstrating reversible airways obstruction. Reversibility is traditionally defined as a 15% or greater increase in the forced expiratory volume in 1 second (FEV_1) following two puffs of a β_2-agonist. Once the diagnosis is confirmed, peak expiratory flow rates (PEFRs) at home, or the FEV_1 in the clinic, can be used to monitor the course of the illness and the effectiveness of therapy. Sputum and blood eosinophilia and measurement of serum IgE levels may be helpful but are not specific for asthma. Similarly, a chest X-ray (CXR) showing hyperinflation is also not diagnostic of asthma.

Differential diagnosis

In a small minority of patients the diagnosis can cause some difficulty and the following differential diagnoses for wheezing and shortness of breath should be considered:

- Upper airway obstruction: tumour or laryngeal oedema.
- Endobronchial disease, e.g. foreign body aspiration, neoplasm, bronchial stenosis.
- Left ventricular failure.
- Carcinoid tumours.
- Recurrent pulmonary emboli.
- Chronic bronchitis.
- Eosinophilic pneumonias.
- Systemic vasculitis with pulmonary involvement.

Management of asthma

The elimination of the causative agent from the environment of an allergic asthmatic is the most successful means available for treating this condition.

The treatments available for asthma can be divided into two general categories:

- Drugs that inhibit smooth muscle contraction, e.g. β_2-agonists, methylxanthines (or theophylline derivatives), anticholinergics.
- Drugs that prevent or reverse inflammation, e.g. corticoidsteroids and mast cell-stabilizing agents.

Inhibitors of mediator synthesis and mediator–receptor antagonists, e.g. leukotriene antagonists, are currently undergoing clinical trials.

In clinical practice the two most common settings in which patients require treatment are emergency treatment of acute severe asthma and chronic therapy.

Chronic therapy

This is aimed at achieving a stable, asymptomatic state with the best pulmonary function possible. The first step is to educate patients to function as partners in their management. The severity of the illness needs to be assessed and monitored with objective measures of lung function. Asthma triggers should be avoided or controlled, and plans should be made for both chronic management and treatment of exacerbations. Regular follow-up care is mandatory.

Drug therapy should be kept as simple as possible and infrequent symptoms require only the use of an inhaled β_2-agonist on an 'as needed' basis.

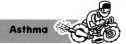

When features such as nocturnal wakenings and worsening daytime symptoms develop, inhaled steroids or mast cell-stabilizing inhalers should be added. If symptoms do not improve, the dose of inhaled steroids can be increased. Severe asthma can be treated with long-acting inhaled β_2-agonists, sustained-release theophylline, and antimuscarinic agents, e.g. ipratropium.

Some patients with severe recurrent symptoms need oral steroids in a single daily dose. Once control is reached and sustained for several weeks, a step-down reduction in therapy should be undertaken, beginning with the most toxic drug, to find the minimum amount of treatment needed to keep the patient well. The PEFR should be monitored and treatment adjusted accordingly, particularly when corroborated by the patient's symptoms. This stepped–care management of chronic adult asthma is illustrated in Fig. 31.1.

Emergency treatment

Emergency treatment of acute asthma is one of the most common emergencies seen in ordinary medical practice and its life-threatening nature can be underestimated by the less experienced.

Features indicating severe airway obstruction include the presence of pulsus paradoxus, the use of accessory muscles, and marked hyperinflation of the thorax with absent breath sounds. Failure of these signs to remit promptly after aggressive therapy requires objective monitoring of the patient using measurements of arterial blood gases (ABGs) and the PEFR or FEV_1.

A checklist for the assessment and treatment of these patients is shown in Fig. 31.2.

Generally, there is a direct correlation between the severity of the obstruction with which the patient presents and the time it takes to resolve it. When the

Step	Measures
\multicolumn{2}{c}{**Stepped-care plan for the management of chronic asthma**}
1	occasional relief bronchodilators inhaled short-acting β_2-stimulant as required (up to once daily)
2	add regular inhaled preventive therapy either regular standard-dose inhaled corticosteroid or regular cromoglycate or nedocromil (but change to inhaled corticosteroid if control not achieved)
3	add high-dose inhaled corticosteroids or long-acting inhaled β_2-stimulant (e.g. salmeterol) or modified-release theophylline or trial of regular cromoglycate or nedocromil if not tried at step 2
4	high-dose inhaled corticosteroids plus regular bronchdilators plus sequential therapeutic trial of one or more of the following: • inhaled long-acting β_2-stimulant • modified-release oral theophylline • inhaled ipratropium • modified-release oral β_2-stimulant • high-dose inhaled bronchodilators • cromoglycate or nedocromil
5	add regular corticosteroid tablets (prednisolone) (note these patients should normally be referred to an asthma clinic)
stepping down	review treatment every 3–6 months if control achieved stepwise reduction may be possible if treatment started recently at step 4 or 5 (or contained corticosteroid tablets) reduction may take place after short interval for other patients a 1–3 month or longer period of stability needed before slow stepwise reduction attempted

Fig. 31.1 Stepped-care plan for the management of chronic asthma. Treatment is started at the step most appropriate initial severity, and a 'rescue' course of prednisolone can be given at any time and with any step to cover an exacerbation. Move up the step ladder if relief bronchodilators are needed frequently or night-time symptoms occur. Check compliance and inhaler technique, and consider the use of spacer devices.

PEFR falls by more than 20% of its previous value, if the magnitude of the pulsus paradoxus is increasing, and if serial measures of ABGs show that the partial pressure of carbon dioxide (pCO_2) is within the normal range or

Assessment and treatment of acute severe asthma	
Tasks to consider	Comment
assessment	clinical features indicating severity: • patient unable to speak sentences • respiratory rate >25/min • heart rate >110/min • peak flow <40% predicted (or <200 mL) • inspiratory fall in systolic BP >10 mmHg life-threatening features: • silent chest on auscultation • cyanosis • bradycardia • exhaustion or confusion ABG: • respiratory failure (pO_2 <8 kPa) • normal or high pCO_2 • low pH
immediate treatment	oxygen at high concentration high doses of inhaled β_2-agonists (e.g. salbutamol 5 mg via nebulizer) high doses of systemic steroids (prednisolone 30–60 mg or hydrocortisone 200 mg i.v.) intravenous bronchodilators for very severe disease
criteria for hospital admission	any life-threatening features any features of severe attack persisting after initial treatment peak flow still <40% predicted or 200 mL 30 minutes after nebulizer recent worsening of daytime or nocturnal symptoms over days or weeks poor social circumstances
indications for intensive care	respiratory failure despite 60% oxygen hypercapnia (pCO_2 >6 kPa) onset of exhaustion confusion or drowsiness unconscious patient respiratory arrest
further investigation in hospital	CXR for pneumothorax, consolidation, or pulmonary oedema U&Es and serum creatinine FBC ECG in older patients
duration of hospital admission	until symptoms and lung function stable peak flow >75% predicted or best level <25% diurnal variability in peak flow no nocturnal symptoms
treatment changes before discharge	inhaled steroids started 48 hours before discharge nebulizers replaced by inhalers 24–48 hours before inhaler technique should be checked patients needing theophylline require therapeutic drug monitoring
drugs on discharge from hospital	all patients should be discharged taking: • oral steroids for 1–3 weeks • an inhaled anti-inflammatory drug (usually a steroid) • inhaled or nebulized β_2-agonists • oral theophylline, or long-acting β_2-agonist, or inhaled ipratropium if needed

Fig. 31.2 Checklist for the emergency assessment and treatment of asthma. (ABG, arterial blood gases; BP, blood pressue; CXR, chest X-ray; ECG, electrocardiogram; FBC, full blood count; pCO_2, partial pressure of carbon dioxide; pO, partial pressure of oxygen; U&Es, urea and electrolytes.)

elevated, then the patient should be monitored in an intensive care setting and may need assisted ventilation.

CHRONIC BRONCHITIS AND EMPHYSEMA

Definitions
Chronic bronchitis
Chronic bronchitis is a condition associated with excessive mucus production sufficient to cause cough with expectoration for at least 3 months of the year for more than 2 consecutive years.

Simple chronic bronchitis is characterized by mucoid sputum production, while chronic mucopurulent bronchitis is identified by persistent or recurrent purulent sputum in the absence of localized suppurative diseases such as bronchiectasis.

Emphysema
Emphysema is defined as the permanent, abnormal distension of the air spaces distal to the terminal bronchiole with destruction of alveolar septa.

Chronic obstructive pulmonary disease
Chronic obstructive pulmonary disease (COPD) is defined as a condition in which there is chronic obstruction to airflow due to chronic bronchitis with or without emphysema. Although the degree of obstruction may be less when the patient is free from respiratory infection and may improve somewhat with bronchodilators, significant obstruction is always present in these patients.

Pathophysiology
The hallmark of chronic bronchitis is hypertrophy of the mucus-producing glands found in the submucosa of large cartilaginous airways. Quantitation of this anatomical change is based on the ratio of the thickness of the submucosal glands to that of the bronchial wall. In lungs from patients with COPD studied at post-mortem there is goblet cell hyperplasia, mucosal and submucosal inflammatory cells, oedema, peribronchial fibrosis, intraluminal mucus plugs, and increased smooth muscle in small airways.

Inflammation in chronic bronchitis occurs at the alveolar epithelium and differs from the predominantly eosinophilic inflammation of asthma by the predominance of neutrophils and the peribronchiolar location of fibrotic changes.

Emphysema is classified according to the pattern of involvement of the gas-exchanging units (acini) of the lung distal to the terminal bronchiole. With centriacinar emphysema, the distension and destruction are mainly limited to the respiratory bronchioles with relatively less change peripherally in the acinus. Because of the large functional reserve in the lung, many units must be involved in order for overall dysfunction to be detectable. Panacinar emphysema involves both the central and peripheral portions of the acinus, which results, if the process is extensive, in a reduction of the alveolar–capillary gas exchange surface and loss of elastic recoil properties.

When emphysema is severe, it may be difficult to distinguish between the two types because, most often, they coexist in the same lung.

Aetiology of chronic bronchitis and emphysema
Cigarette smoking
Cigarette smoking is the most commonly identified factor associated with both chronic bronchitis during life and extent of emphysema at post-mortem. Prolonged cigarette smoking impairs ciliary movement, inhibits function of alveolar macrophages, and leads to hypertrophy and hyperplasia of mucus-secreting glands. It is probable that smoke also inhibits antiproteases and causes polymorphonuclear leukocytes to release proteolytic enzymes acutely. Inhaled cigarette smoke can produce an acute increase in airways resistance due to vagally mediated, smooth-muscle constriction.

Air pollution
Air pollution with sulphur dioxide and particulate matter is associated with exacerbations of chronic bronchitis, and the incidence and mortality rates for chronic bronchitis and emphysema is probably higher in heavily industrialized urban areas.

Occupation
Occupations exposing workers to inorganic or organic dusts, or to noxious gases, result in a higher prevalence of chronic bronchitis among employees.

Acute respiratory infections
These have been implicated as one of the major factors associated with both the aetiology and progression of COPD.

Familial and genetic factors

Familial aggregation of chronic bronchitis has been well demonstrated. α_1-Antitrypsin (α_1AT) deficiency is a recognized genetic cause of emphysema. Either decreased or absent serum levels of the protease inhibitor α_1AT are found in some patients with early-onset emphysema. Most members of the normal population have two M genes, designated as protease inhibitor type MM, but those with defective (Z and S) genes who are homozygous ZZ or SS have markedly decreased serum levels of α_1AT and develop severe panacinar emphysema in their 20s and 30s.

Clinical features of COPD

The clinical presentation of COPD varies in severity from simple chronic bronchitis without disability to patients with severe disability and chronic respiratory failure. In clinical practice it is common to encounter patients with fully developed COPD, and even though most patients will have features of both chronic bronchitis and emphysema it is useful to categorize patients as having predominant features of one or other. The clinical features of emphysema and chronic bronchitis are summarized in Fig. 31.3.

Management of COPD

The management of patients with COPD is based on knowledge of the degree of obstruction, the extent of disability, and the reversibility of the patient's illness.

The extent of the airways obstruction and the potential to reverse this is key as there is a chance that treatment may be effective in improving the overall disability.

Emphysema, however, is an irreversible process and so the prevention of its progression and the avoidance of acute infections are the main approach to management.

Investigations

History, physical examination, and CXRs hould be supplemented by tests of lung function performed during a chronic stable period. Complete spirometry, lung

	Clinical features which distinguish emphysema from chronic bronchitis		
	Clinical feature	**Emphysema**	**Chronic bronchitis**
history and examination	dyspnoea	constant and progressive	intermittent, mild to moderate
	cough	absent or mild	persistent and severe
	sputum	absent or mild (clear, mucoid)	copious (mucopurulent, purulent)
	body weight	thin	obese
	central cyanosis	absent	present
	plethoric face	absent	present
	barrel chest	present	absent
	percussion note	hyperresonant	normal
	auscultation	decreased breath sounds	wheezes
CXR	bullae	present	absent
	peripheral markings	decreased	increased
	hemidiaphragms	flat	normal
	heart size	normal	large, boot shaped
arterial blood gases	hypoxia	absent or mild	moderate to severe
	hypercapnia	absent	moderate to severe

Fig. 31.3 Clinical features which distinguish emphysema from chronic bronchitis.

volumes, transfer of carbon monoxide, and ABGs should be measured. Also, reversibility should be assessed by spirometry and lung volumes after the administration of bronchodilators.

Treatment of COPD

Treatment strategies for COPD are varied and a multidisciplinary approach to the patient is often required. A treatment plan should consider the following:

- Stopping cigarette smoking.
- Education of the patient about their disease.
- Relief of bronchospasm.
- Chest physiotherapy.
- Treatment of acute exacerbations.
- Treatment of cor pulmonale: if appropriate.
- Home oxygen therapy: when indicated.

A trial of bronchodilator drugs is warranted in all patients with COPD. Although treatment follows a similar pattern to that seen in asthma (Fig. 31.1) there are some differences. Inhaled antimuscarinic bronchodilators, e.g. ipratropium, are considered first choice in COPD, often combined with a short-acting β_2-agonist. Oral theophylline also tends to be used sooner in management than for asthma. Oral corticosteroids or high-dose inhaled steroids play an important role in a small minority of patients (perhaps 10–15%) who respond to a corticosteroid trial. This usually consists of weeks of prednisolone at 30–40 mg/day with appropriate monitoring of the peak flow.

Infective exacerbations of COPD are treated with broad spectrum antibiotics such as amoxycillin, trimethoprim, or tetracycline, aiming to cover the likely pathogens pneumococci and Haemophilus influenzae). Type II respiratory failure often accompanies exacerbations of COPD; controlled oxygen therapy is discussed on p.247.

Long-term administration of oxygen (at least 15 hours daily) may prolong survival in patients with severe COPD with cor pulmonale. Guidelines suggest that this treatment should be provided for patients who fulfil the following criteria:

partial pressure of oxygen (pO_2)< 7.3 kPa; pCO_2 > 6 kPa.

FEV$_1$ < 1.5L and FVC (forced vital capacity) < 2L.

Blood gas measurements should be stable on two occasions at least 3 weeks apart after the patient has received appropriate bronchodilator therapy. Increased

respiratory depression is seldom a problem in patients with stable respiratory failure treated with low concentrations of oxygen, although it may occur during exacerbations.

Patients and relatives should be warned to call for medical help if drowsiness or confusion occur. Oxygen concentrators, rather than cylinders, are more economical for patients requiring oxygen for long periods and are now used routinely.

Less information is available on long-term oxygen in patients with a similar degree of hypoxaemia and airflow obstruction but no hypercapnia. The current UK advice is that these patients should not be denied domiciliary oxygen but the effects of long-term therapy have not yet been fully assessed.

TUBERCULOSIS

Tuberculosis (TB) is caused by bacteria belonging to the *Mycobacterium tuberculosis* complex. The disease usually affects the lungs, although in up to a third of cases other organs are involved. If properly treated, TB caused by drug-susceptible strains is curable in virtually all cases. If untreated, the disease may be fatal within 5 years in more than half of cases. Transmission usually takes place through the airborne spread of droplet nuclei produced by patients with infectious pulmonary TB.

The pathogenic species belonging to the *M. tuberculosis* complex, the most frequent and important agent of human disease, is *M. tuberculosis* itself. Closely related organisms that also infect humans include *M. bovis* (the bovine tubercle bacillus, once an important cause of TB transmitted by unpasteurized milk and currently the cause of a small percentage of cases in developing countries).

M. tuberculosis is a rod-shaped, non-spore-forming, thin, aerobic bacterium measuring 0.5–3 μm.

Mycobacteria, including *M. tuberculosis*, do not stain readily and are often neutral on Gram-staining.

Tuberculosis is more common in asians, patients with diabetes mellitus, the immunosupressed, alcoholics, and vagrants.

However, once stained, the bacilli cannot be decolorized by acid alcohol, a characteristic justifying their classification as acid alcohol-fast bacilli (AAFB).

Clinical manifestations of tuberculosis

TB is usually classified as pulmonary or extrapulmonary. Before human immunodeficiency virus (HIV) infection, 80% of all cases of TB were limited to the lungs, but now two-thirds of HIV-infected patients with TB may have both pulmonary and extrapulmonary disease, or even extrapulmonary disease on its own.

Pulmonary tuberculosis

Pulmonary TB can be classified as primary or postprimary (secondary).

Primary pulmonary tuberculosis

Primary pulmonary TB results from an initial infection with tubercle bacilli. Where TB has a high prevalence, primary disease is often seen in children and is localized to the middle and lower lung zones. The lesion is usually peripheral and associated with hilar or paratracheal lymph node enlargement. In most cases, the lesion heals spontaneously and may later be seen as a small calcified nodule (Ghon's lesion).

Patients with impaired immunity who develop primary pulmonary TB may progress rapidly to clinical illness. This may result from spread of infection by the following:
- Pleural effusion: which may lead to tuberculous empyema.
- Necrosis and acute cavitation of the primary lesion: known as progressive primary TB.
- Bloodstream dissemination: resulting in granulomatous lesions in various organs, or even miliary TB with tuberculous meningitis.

Postprimary pulmonary tuberculosis

Postprimary disease is sometimes termed adult, reactivation, or secondary TB. It results from reactivation of latent infection and is usually localized to the apical and posterior segments of the upper lobes. The extent of lung changes can vary from small infiltrates to extensive cavitation. Widespread involvement of the lung with coalescing lesions produces tuberculous pneumonia.

The pathogenicity of TB varies with a third of untreated patients dying from severe pulmonary TB within weeks or months, while the rest undergo spontaneous remission or proceed along a chronic course often involving lung fibrosis.

Symptoms and signs

Symptoms and signs of early TB are often non-specific and include fever, night sweats, weight loss, anorexia, and lethargy. Most patients eventually develop cough with purulent sputum and this may be associated with haemoptysis. Pleuritic chest pain can develop in patients with subpleural lesions or from muscle strain due to persistent coughing. Clinical examination may be of limited use in pulmonary TB but the following features may be present:
- Crepitations: involved areas during inspiration.
- Rhonchi: partial bronchial obstruction.
- Classical amphoric breath sounds: areas with large cavities.
- Pallor: anaemia.
- Finger clubbing.

Extrapulmonary tuberculosis

This most commonly involves lymph nodes, the pleura, genitourinary tract, bones and joints, meninges, and peritoneum.

Diagnostic tests for tuberculosis

The key to the diagnosis of TB is a high index of suspicion. It should form part of the differential diagnosis in patients with febrile illnesses, cervical lymphadenopathy, or patients with focal infiltrates on the chest X-ray.

The CXR may show the typical picture of upper lobe infiltrates, with or without cavitation. The diagnosis is commonly based on the finding of AAFB by microscopy of a diagnostic specimen such as sputum or tissue, e.g. lymph node biopsy. Laboratory identification depends o either auramine–rhodamine staining and fluorescence microscopy or the more traditional light microscopy of specimens stained with Ziehl–Neelsen dye.

Patients with suspected pulmonary TB normally collect three sputum specimens for AAFB smear and mycobacterial culture and sensitivity. Specimens are inoculated on to Lowenstein–Jensen medium. Most species of mycobacteria, including *M. tuberculosis*, are slow-growing so that 4–8 weeks may be required before growth is detected and antibiotic sensitivity can be assessed.

Other diagnostic tests for pulmonary TB include the following:
- Induced sputum by ultrasonic nebulization of hypertonic saline for patients unable to produce a sputum specimen spontaneously.

- Fibre-optic bronchoscopy with bronchial brushings or transbronchial biopsy of the lesion.
- Bronchoalveolar lavage of a lung segment containing an abnormality.

When extrapulmonary TB is suspected, specimens of involved sites may include the following:

- Cerebrospinal fluid: tuberculous meningitis.
- Pleural fluid and biopsy samples: pleural disease.
- Bone marrow and liver biopsy culture: good diagnostic yield in disseminated (miliary) TB.
- Early morning urine: renal TB.

In all cases specimens are sent for AAFB microscopy and culture.

Treatment

TB is treated in an initial phase using at least three drugs and a continuation phase using two drugs. Treatment requires specialized knowledge, particularly where the disease involves resistant organisms or non-respiratory organs.

Initial phase

Three drugs are used during the initial phase to reduce bacterial numbers rapidly and prevent the emergence of drug-resistant bacteria. The initial phase drugs are continued for 2 months. Where a positive culture for *M. tuberculosis* has been obtained, but sensitivities are not available after 2 months, treatment with a third drug is continued until full susceptibility is confirmed.

Continuation phase

After the initial phase, treatment is continued for a further 4 months with isoniazid and rifampicin; longer treatment may be necessary for meningitis or for resistant organisms.

Recommended drugs for a standard, unsupervised, 6-month regimen include:

- Isoniazid: for 6 months.
- Rifampicin: for 6 months.
- Pyrazinamide: for the first 2 months only.

Immunocompromised patients

Immunocompromised patients may develop TB owing to reactivation of previously latent disease or to new infection. Multiresistant *M. tuberculosis* may be present or the infection may be caused by other mycobacteria, e.g. *M. avium* complex, in which case specialist advice is needed. Culture should always be carried out and the type of organism and its sensitivity confirmed.

Monitoring treatment

Isoniazid, rifampicin, and pyrazinamide are associated with liver toxicity, and therefore hepatic function should be checked before treatment with these drugs. Renal function should also be checked before treatment with antituberculous drugs and appropriate dosage adjustments made. Visual acuity should be tested before ethambutol is used because it can cause loss of visual acuity and visual field defects.

Major causes of treatment failure include incorrect prescribing by doctors and inadequate compliance by patients.

Drug-resistant TB should be treated by a specialist physician. Second-line drugs available for infections caused by resistant organisms, or when first-line drugs cause unacceptable side-effects, include capreomycin, cycloserine, newer macrolides (e.g. azithromycin and clarithromycin), and 4-quinolones (e.g. ciprofloxacin and ofloxacin).

Infection control for tuberculosis

By far the best way to prevent TB is the rapid diagnosis of infectious cases with appropriate treatment until cure. Additional strategies include BCG (Bacillus Calmette–Guérin) vaccination and preventive chemotherapy.

Vaccination

BCG was derived from an attenuated strain of *M. bovis* and was first administered to humans in 1921. Many BCG vaccines are now available worldwide, and all are derived from the original strain, but the vaccines vary in efficacy. The vaccine is safe and rarely causes serious complications.

BCG vaccination induces purified protein derivative (PPD) reactivity, but the magnitude of PPD skin test reactions after vaccination does not predict the degree of protection afforded. Currently vaccination is recommended only for PPD-negative infants and children who are at a high risk of intimate and prolonged exposure to patients with TB and who cannot take prophylactic isoniazid. In the UK, BCG is offered to PPD-negative children at the age of 12 years.

Preventive chemotherapy

A major component of TB control involves contact tracing, skin testing, and the administration of isoniazid to contacts at high risk of active disease.

LUNG CANCER

The term 'lung cancer' is usually reserved for tumours arising from the respiratory epithelium (bronchi, bronchioles, and alveoli). Four major cell types make up 88% of all primary lung neoplasms:

- Squamous (epidermoid) carcinoma.
- Small cell (also called oat cell) carcinoma.
- Adenocarcinoma (including bronchioloalveolar).
- Large cell (also called large cell anaplastic) carcinoma.

The remainder includes undifferentiated carcinomas, carcinoids, bronchial gland tumours, and rarer tumour types, e.g. mesothelioma arising from the pleura. All cell types have different natural histories and responses to therapy, and therefore making a correct histological diagnosis is the mandatory first step to correct assessment and treatment.

Aetiology

The majority of lung cancers are caused by carcinogens and tumour promoters inhaled via cigarette smoking. Overall, the relative risk of developing lung cancer is increased about 13-fold by active smoking and about 1.5-fold by long-term passive exposure to cigarette smoke. Probably there is a co-carcinogenic effect of smoking and industrial or environmental pollutants, e.g. radon gas from natural sources in the ground.

There is a dose–response relationship between the lung cancer death rate and the total amount of cigarettes smoked, such that the risk is increased 60–70-fold for a man smoking two packets a day for 20 years as compared with a non-smoker.

Conversely, the chance of developing lung cancer decreases with the cessation of smoking but may never return to the non-smoker's level. The recent increase in lung cancer rate in women is also associated with a rise in cigarette smoking.

While human lung cancer is not thought of as a genetic disease, a variety of molecular genetic studies have shown that lung cancer cells have acquired a number of genetic lesions, including activation of dominant oncogenes and inactivation of tumour suppressor or recessive oncogenes. Of these the most important are as follows:

- Dominant oncogenes: point mutations in the coding regions of the *ras* family of oncogenes (adenocarcinoma of lung), amplification, rearrangement, and/or loss of transcriptional control of the *myc* family of oncogenes (non-small cell cancers and small cell lung cancer), and overexpression of the telomerase gene.
- Recessive oncogenes (tumour suppressor genes), cytogenetic and allele-typing analyses have shown deletions (allele loss) involving several chromosome regions.

The large number of lesions shows that lung cancer, like many other epithelial malignancies, is a multistep process that is likely to involve both carcinogens and tumour promoters.

Nicotine may play a central role in lung cancer pathogenesis as carcinogenic derivatives of nicotine are formed in cigarette smoke.

35% of solitary pulmonary nodules, 1–6 cm in diameter, in adults aged 35 years and above, are malignant.

Clinical findings in lung cancer

Although 5–15% of patients are detected while asymptomatic, usually on a routine chest radiograph, the vast majority of patients present with some signs or symptoms.

Endobronchial growth of the primary tumour

This may result in cough, haemoptysis, wheeze and stridor, dyspnoea, and postobstructive pneumonitis (fever and productive cough).

Peripheral tumour growth

This could cause pain (pleural or chest wall involvement), cough, dyspnoea, and symptoms of lung abscess due to tumour cavitation.

Regional spread of tumour in the chest

Regional spread of tumour in the chest (by contiguous growth or metastasis to regional lymph nodes) may lead to tracheal obstruction, oesophageal compression with dysphagia, recurrent laryngeal nerve paralysis with hoarseness, phrenic nerve paralysis with elevation of the hemidiaphragm and dyspnoea, and sympathetic nerve paralysis with Horner's syndrome (ptosis, miosis, enophthalmos, and ipsilateral loss of sweating).

Pancoast's (or superior sulcus tumour) syndrome results from the local extension of a tumour growing in the apex of the lung with involvement of the 8th cervical and 1st and 2nd thoracic nerves. There is shoulder pain which characteristically radiates in the ulnar distribution of the arm, often with destruction of the first and second ribs seen on CXR.

Other problems of regional spread include superior vena cava syndrome from vascular obstruction, pericardial and cardiac extension with resultant tamponade, arrhythmia or cardiac failure, lymphatic obstruction with resultant pleural effusion, and lymphangitic spread through the lungs with hypoxaemia and dyspnoea.

Transbronchial spread

Transbronchial spread (especially bronchioloalveolar carcinoma) produces growth along multiple alveolar surfaces with resultant impairment of oxygen transfer, dyspnoea, hypoxia, and the production of copious sputum.

Paraneoplastic syndromes

These syndromes describe symptoms and signs resulting from extrapulmonary organ dysfunction unrelated to space-occupying metastases. They occur in 15–20% of lung cancer patients and are commonly due to tumour secretory products. Important paraneoplastic syndromes associated with lung cancer are listed in Fig. 31.4. Occasionally resection of the primary tumour may result in resolution of the syndrome.

Investigations

All patients with suspected lung cancer should have a full blood count, liver function tests, and measurement of electrolytes, calcium, and creatinine, in addition to a CXR. However, the diagnosis of lung cancer depends on histological diagnosis either from cytology or tissue.

Techniques for obtaining a tissue diagnosis are varied and include the following:
- Fibre-optic bronchoscopy: central or endobronchial disease.
- Percutaneous needle aspiration: peripheral lesions.
- Mediastinoscopy.
- Lymph node biopsy.
- Biopsy of other metastatic site, e.g. the skin.
- Open lung biopsy via thoracotomy: when simpler investigations are negative.

The diagnostic yield of cytological examination of different samples is shown in Fig. 31.5.

Imaging for lung cancer

The CXR is abnormal in most patients. Common findings are hilar masses (squamous and small cell), peripheral masses (adenocarcinoma), atelectasis, infiltrates, cavitation (squamous cell), and pleural effusions. These changes are not specific for lung cancer and comparison between old and current CXRs is very important.

Computed tomography (CT) scanning, magnetic resonance imaging (MRI), and ultrasound examination are additional useful investigations in patients with invasion of the lung parenchyma, pleura, or mediastinal disease.

Additional imaging may be required to investigate symptoms or signs that suggest the possibility of distant metastatic spread. These include X-rays of suspected bone metastases (or isotope bone scan), and a CT head scan or MRI of the brain for patients with central nervous system abnormalities.

Extent of disease and TNM staging

Small cell cancer is nearly always disseminated at presentation so the diagnosis of this histological type excludes surgical resection, except in very rare circumstances where there is a single, small, peripheral lesion. In all other cell types surgery is possible and the extent of disease is recorded by the TNM classification as shown in Fig. 31.6. The staging of disease using the TNM classification also helps to estimate the prognosis with treatment.

Assessment of patient's functional status before surgery

The patient's general status and respiratory status needs to be assessed before surgery can be offered.

This is usually assessed by the Karnofsky performance scale and by the following guidance regarding lung function testing (Fig. 31.7).

Treatment

Major treatment decisions are made on the basis of whether a tumour is classified histologically as a small cell carcinoma or as one of the non-small cell varieties

Important paraneoplastic syndromes associated with lung cancer		
Organ/system	**Syndrome**	**Lung cancer histology**
endocrine and metabolic	Cushing's	small cell
	SIADH	small cell
	hypercalcaemia	squamous cell
	gynaecomastia	large cell
connective tissue and bone	clubbing and HPOA	squamous cell, adenocarcinoma, and large cell
neuromuscular	peripheral neuropathy	small cell
	subacute cerebellar degeneration	small cell
	Eaton–Lambert (myasthenia)	small cell
	dermatomyositis	all
haematology	anaemia	all
	DIC	all
	eosinophilia	all
	thrombocytosis	all
cardiovascular	thrombophlebitis	adenocarcinoma
	marantic (non-infective) endocarditis	adenocarcinoma

Fig. 31.4 Important paraneoplastic syndromes associated with lung cancer. (SIADH, syndrome of inappropriate antidiuretic hormone secretion; HPOA, hypertrophic pulmonary osteoarthropathy; DIC, disseminated intravascular coagulation.)

The diagnostic yield of cytology and pleural biopsy in lung cancer		
Cytology/biopsy	**Diagnostic yield**	**Comments**
sputum cytology	40–60%	especially for central tumours
pleural fluid cytology	40–50%	in patients with malignant pleural effusions
closed pleural biopsy (Abrams' needle)	50–60%	with malignant effusion
pleural fluid cytology and closed pleural biopsy combined	75–85%	with malignant effusion

Fig. 31.5 The diagnostic yield of cytology and pleural biopsy in lung cancer.

TNM classification for lung cancer		
T/N/M	Stage	Characteristics
primary tumour (T)	T1	<3 cm diameter surrounded by lung or pleura
	T2	>3 cm diameter and/or collapse extending to hilum, invading pleura and more than 2 cm beyond the carina
	T3	any size extending to chest wall but not involving mediastinal structures (e.g. heart and great vessels); tumour within 2 cm of carina
	T4	any size invading mediastinum; malignant pleural effusion
lymph nodes (N)	N0	no involvement
	N1	ipsilateral hilar and peribronchial nodes
	N2	ipsilateral mediastinal and subcarinal nodes
	N3	contralateral mediastinal or hilar nodes; or any scalene or supraclavicular nodes
metastases (M)	M0	none known
	M1	distant metastases outside thorax

Fig. 31.6 TNM classification for lung cancer.

which include epidermoid, adenocarcinoma, large cell carcinoma, bronchioloalveolar carcinoma—a subtype of adenocarcinoma—and mixed versions of these). In general, small cell carcinomas have already spread at the time of presentation so that curative surgery cannot be performed, and they are managed primarily by chemotherapy with or without radiotherapy.

In contrast, non-small cell cancers that are found to be localized at the time of presentation should be considered for curative treatment with either surgery or radiotherapy (Fig. 31.8). Also, the response of non-small cell cancers to chemotherapy is usually not dramatic,

Assessment of patient for lung cancer surgery	
Score	Karnofsky performance level*
0–4	not self-caring (0, dead; 2, very ill; 4, disabled)
5–7	unable to work (5, often needs help; 7, self-caring)
8–10	normal activity (8, some symptoms; 10, normal)
Surgery	Lung function criteria
pneumonectomy possible	FEV_1 >2.0L (or 50% predicted) patients aged 70 years or less
lobectomy possible	FEV_1 >1.5L (or 40% predicted)
no lung resection possible	FEV_1 <1.2L or inability to walk 100 m on the level within 12 minutes hypoxia pO_2 <6.6 kPa when breathing air at rest, or any rise in arterial pCO_2

Fig. 31.7 Assessment of patient for lung cancer surgery. * Surgery is rarely curative in patients who are symptomatic from lung cancer.

Treatment strategies for lung cancer		
Histology	**Extent of disease**	**Treatment modality**
non-small cell lung cancer	stage 0–IIIa	surgery and/or postoperative radiotherapy (e.g. for node involvement)
	stage IIIb–IV	palliative radiotherapy for local complications or pain from bony metastases
small cell lung cancer	proven single peripheral lesion (rare)	curative surgery attempted
	limited stage	combination chemotherapy and radiotherapy
	disseminated at presentation (usual)	combination chemotherpy

Fig. 31.8 Treatment strategies for lung cancer.

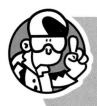

Treatment of lung cancer varies markedly for small cell versus non-small cell cancers

making chemotherapy less important in metastatic disease than it is in cases of small cell lung cancer.

Prognosis

Five-year survival rates in treated lung cancer patients are given in Fig. 31.9.

PNEUMONIA

Pneumonia is an infection of the pulmonary parenchyma. Various bacterial species, mycoplasmas, chlamydiae, rickettsiae, viruses, fungi, and parasites ca

Estimates of 5-year survival of treated patients with lung cancer		
	Stage	**5-year survival**
non-small cell lung cancer	0 (T1 N0 M0); carcinoma *in situ*	70–80%
	I (T1–2 N0 M0); no nodes or metastases	50%
	II (T1–2 N1 M0); ipsilateral local nodes only	30%
	IIIa (T1–3 N0–2 M0); more than T2 with ipsilateral mediastinal nodes	10–15%
	IIIb (any T, any N, M0); invading vital mediastinal structure, or non-resectable nodes but no extrathoracic spread	<5%
	IV (any T, any N, M1); extrathoracic distant metastases	<2%
small cell lung cancer	patients rarely live for 5 years after diagnosis— median survival with combined chemotherapy, e.g. with cisplatin-containing regimens is 40–70 weeks, compared with 6–20 weeks if untreated	

Fig. 31.9 Estimates of 5-year survival of treated patients with lung cancer.

cause pneumonia. Thus it is not a single disease but a group of specific infections, each with a different epidemiology, pathogenesis, clinical presentation, and clinical course. Identification of the aetiological micro-organism is of primary importance, since this is the key to appropriate antimicrobial therapy. However, because of the serious nature of the infection, antimicrobial therapy generally needs to be started immediately, often before laboratory confirmation of the causative agent.

Aetiology
Microbial pathogens enter the lung by one of several routes.

Aspiration from the oropharyngeal flora
This is the most common mechanism for the production of pneumonia. Healthy individuals transiently carry common pulmonary pathogens in the nasopharynx such as *Streptococcus pneumoniae*, *S. pyogenes*, *Mycoplasma pneumoniae*, *Haemophilus influenzae*, and *Moraxella catarrhalis*.

Airborne infection
Airborne infection is determined primarily by a particle diameter of less than 3–5 µm that contain one or perhaps two microorganisms. These droplets remain suspended in the atmosphere for long periods unless removed by ventilation or by filtration in the lungs of the individual breathing contaminated air. Inhaled particles of appropriate size may reach the alveoli and initiate infection.

Pneumonias typically acquired by droplet infection include TB, influenza, legionellosis, psittacosis, histoplasmosis, and Q fever.

Blood-borne infection
Blood-borne infection, usually with *Staphylococcus aureus*, disseminates to the lungs in patients (e.g. intravenous drug abusers) who have either right- or left-sided bacterial endocarditis and in patients with infections in intravenous catheter.

Epidemiology of pneumonia
The patient's living circumstances, occupation, travel history, pet or animal exposure history, and contacts with other ill individuals provide useful clues to the likely microbial cause for the pneumonia.

In community-acquired pneumonia requiring hospital admission the most frequent pathogens are *S. pneumoniae*, *H. influenzae*, *Chlamydia pneumoniae*, and *Legionella pneumophila*. *M. pneumoniae*, which usually causes mild illness, is common among outpatients with community-acquired pneumonia.

In hospital-acquired pneumonia, enteric, aerobic, Gram-negative bacilli and *Pseudomonas aeruginosa* are estimated to account for more than 50% of cases, while *S. aureus* is responsible for more than 10%.

Knowledge of the epidemiology of pneumonia is important because it guides antibiotic treatment used before the causative organism is identified.

Clinical features of pneumonia
Typical
The 'typical' symptoms of pneumonia are sudden onset of fever, cough productive of purulent sputum, and in some cases pleuritic chest pain. Signs of pulmonary consolidation (dullness, increased fremitus, bronchial breath sounds, and coarse crepitations) may be found on physical examination and coincide with abnormalities on the CXR.

This type of pneumonia is usually caused by the most common bacterial pathogen in community-acquired pneumonia, *S. pneumoniae*, but can also be due to other bacterial pathogens, such as *H. influenzae*.

Atypical
'Atypical' pneumonia usually causes a more gradual onset, a dry cough, and extrapulmonary symptoms (headache, muscle aching, fatigue, sore throat, nausea, vomiting, and diarrhoea). Abnormalities on the CXR may be seen despite few signs of pulmonary involvement other than crepitations on physical examination.

Atypical pneumonia is classically produced by *M. pneumoniae* but it can also be caused by *L. pneumophila*, *Chlamydia*, oral anaerobes, and

In hospital acquired pneumonia the organism and its treatment are often different from that of the community acquired infection.

Pneumocystis carinii, as well as some less frequently encountered pathogens.

Diagnosis of pneumonia
Chest X-ray
A CXR can confirm the presence of the pulmonary infiltrate and assess the extent of infection. Other features which may be present include pleural involvement, pulmonary cavitation, or hilar lymphadenopathy. Cavitation suggests the following infective causes for the pneumonia—oral anaerobic bacteria, enteric Gram-negative bacilli, *S. aureus*, *Pseudomonas*, *Legionella*, TB, and fungi.

It should be noted that a normal CXR does not exclude pneumonia especially early in the disease or in patients unable to mount an inflammatory response because of immunosuppression.

Sputum microscopy and culture
Sputum microscopy and culture is important in acute bacterial pneumonia. Unfortunately sputum is frequently contaminated by potentially pathogenic bacteria that colonize the upper respiratory tract without causing disease. Contamination therefore reduces the diagnostic specificity of lower respiratory tract specimens and so clinical judgement is required when interpreting the results.

Fibre-optic bronchoscopy
Fibre-optic bronchoscopy is rarely performed for pneumonia but has become the standard invasive procedure used to obtain lower respiratory tract secretions from seriously ill or immunocompromised patients. Samples are collected with a protected double-sheathed brush, by bronchoalveolar lavage or by transbronchial biopsy at the site of the pulmonary consolidation.

Treatment of pneumonia
The typical antimicrobial treatment of pneumonia is shown in Fig. 31.10.

RESPIRATORY FAILURE

Definition
Respiratory failure is defined as a dysfunction of gas exchange resulting in abnormalities of oxygenation or

Fig. 31.10 Drug choice for pneumonia.

Drug choice for pneumonia	
Community-acquired pneumonia for uncomplicated pneumonia	broad-spectrum penicillin, e.g. amoxycillin (or benzylpenicillin if previously healthy chest or erythromycin if penicillin allergic); add flucloxacillin if *Staphylococcus* suspected, e.g. with influenza or measles; add erythromycin if atypical pneumonia suspected
for severe pneumonia of unknown aetiology	erythromycin plus third generation cephalosporin (e.g. cefuroxime or cefotaxime) to cover common pathogens; add flucloxacillin if *Staphylococcus* suspected
for suspected atypical pneumonia	erythromycin (first choice)—severe *Legionella* infections may require addition of rifampicin or a 4-quinolone, e.g ciprofloxacin; tetracycline is an alternative for *Chlamydia* and *Mycoplasma* infections; atypical pneumonia requires treatment for at least 10–14 days
Hospital-acquired pneumonia	broad-spectrum cephalosporin (e.g. cefotaxime or ceftazidime) or an antipseudomonal penicillin, plus an aminoglycoside; add metronidazole if anaerobic infection suspected

carbon dioxide (CO_2) elimination severe enough to impair or threaten the function of vital organs.

Respiratory failure is said to be present in a patient breathing air at sea level when the pO_2 is less than 8.0 kPa as a result of lung disease. If hypoxia is combined with a normal or low pCO_2 (<6.7 kPa), this is type I respiratory failure, but if hypoxia is combined with a raised pCO_2, type II respiratory failure is present. Measurement of the ABGs is essential to the diagnosis of respiratory failure.

Type I respiratory failure

This is essentially hypoxaemia without CO_2 retention. Physiological causes include the following:

- A low inspired oxygen concentration (FIO_2), e.g. at high altitude.
- Mismatch of alveolar ventilation (V) to alveolar perfusion (Q).
- A shunt where blood passes form the pulmonary artery to the left heart without passing through ventilated alveoli.

In medical practice the common causes of type I respiratory failure include the following:

- Pneumonia.
- Asthma.
- COPD (predominant emphysema—'pink puffers').
- Pulmonary thromboembolism.
- Acute respiratory distress syndrome (ARDS) and non-cardiogenic pulmonary oedema.
- Cardiogenic shock.
- Tension pneumothorax.
- Pulmonary fibrosis.

Treatment of type I respiratory failure

The main therapeutic objective in acute hypoxaemic respiratory failure is to ensure adequate oxygenation of vital organs. Oxygen therapy is indicated when there is central cyanosis, tachycardia, systemic hypotension, and delirium. Consciousness can be lost suddenly without warning when the pO_2 falls below 4.0 kPa, even in previously healthy patients.

High concentrations of inspired oxygen (FIO_2 >50%) are safe in patients with type I respiratory failure, as there is no risk of CO_2 retention. However, pulmonary oxygen toxicity is a risk if the FIO_2 concentration remains over 60% for more than 48 hours continuously.

Other therapeutic objectives include the following:

- Specific therapy of the underlying cause, e.g. antimicrobial therapy for pneumonia, bronchodilators and steroids for asthma, or chest drain insertion for pneumothorax.
- General supportive care: adequate hydration, nutrition, and electrolyte balance, with measures to avoid stress gastritis, ulcers, deep venous thrombosis, and pulmonary embolism.

Type II respiratory failure

In a healthy subject a rise in arterial pCO_2 causes an increase in ventilation by central stimulation of the respiratory centres in the medulla resulting in an increase in breathing to lower the pCO_2. In type II respiratory failure this mechanism fails and signals that apart from lung disease there is also an abnormality of the ventilatory control mechanisms.

Clinical features of type II respiratory failure include central cyanosis (indicating hypoxaemia) but CO_2 retention can only be assessed accurately by the measurement of ABGs. There are however some clinical signs suggestive of CO_2 retention and these include the following:

- Tachycardia.
- Distention of the forearm veins.
- A flapping tremor of the outstretched hands.
- Clouding of consciousness.
- Papilloedema (rare).

These are unreliable signs because they can occur from other causes and their absence does not exclude significant CO_2 retention.

Common causes of type II respiratory failure include the following:

- COPD (predominant chronic bronchitis—'blue bloater').
- Respiratory muscle failure, e.g. bilateral diaphragmatic palsy.
- Kyphoscoliosis and other structural thoracic disorders.
- Muscular dystrophy.
- Guillain–Barré syndrome (acute demyelinating polyneuropathy).
- Poliomyelitis.
- Myasthenia.
- Opiate overdose.
- Head injury.
- Sleep apnoea.

Treatment of type II respiratory failure

As in type I, the main therapeutic objective is to ensure adequate oxygenation of vital organs by administering oxygen therapy. However, in the most common clinical setting—an acute exacerbation of COPD—patients may have chronic CO_2 retention. They are therefore dependent on hypoxic drive for ventilation, so that with oxygen therapy there is a real risk of inducing hypoventilation, worsening of the respiratory dysfunction, and progressive respiratory acidosis. Oxygen therapy must be carefully controlled so that sufficient oxygen is supplied, usually 24% via Ventimask, to prevent death from hypoxaemia but without precipitating severe respiratory acidosis. This needs repeated monitoring of ABGs.

Type II respiratory failure, as a consequence of causes other than COPD, are usually an indication for mechanical ventilation.

Other therapeutic objectives include the following:

- Specific therapy of the underlying cause, e.g. antimicrobial therapy for infective exacerbation of COPD or treatment of myasthenia.
- General supportive care is as for type I failure.
- Chemical (respiratory stimulants, e.g. doxapram), or mechanical ventilation should be considered if other measures fail.

Prognosis in acute respiratory failure

The course of the disease and its prognosis depend to a great extent on the underlying pathology. In patients with COPD who do not require mechanical ventilation the immediate prognosis is good. Patients developing ARDS associated with septicaemia have a very poor prognosis with mortality rates of about 90%. In general, patients requiring ventilation for respiratory failure have survival rates of about 60% to weaning off the ventilator, 40% to discharge from hospital, and about 30% 1-year survival.

MISCELLANEOUS RESPIRATORY CONDITIONS

Cystic fibrosis

Cystic fibrosis (CF) is an autosomal recessive disorder that presents as a multisystem disease, and occurs in 1 in 3,000 live births in Caucasians. Signs and symptoms typically occur in childhood but up to 5% of patients are diagnosed as adults. Improvements in therapy now

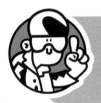

Beware! Patients with type II respiratory failure can stop breathing if given high dose oxygen.

mean that about a third of patients reach adulthood and nearly 10% live beyond 30 years old.

CF is characterized by chronic airway infection that ultimately leads to bronchiectasis, exocrine pancreatic insufficiency, intestinal dysfunction, abnormal sweat gland function, and urogenital dysfunction.

Diagnosis

The diagnosis of CF rests on a combination of clinical criteria and analyses of sweat chloride values. Typically in adults a chloride concentration of over 70 mmol/L discriminates between CF patients and patients with other lung diseases.

Treatment

The treatments for CF are to promote clearance of secretions (physiotherapy and bronchodilators), control infection in the lung (antibiotics), provide adequate nutrition (pancreatic enzyme and fat-soluble vitamin supplements), and prevent intestinal obstruction. Gene therapy with recombinant human DNAse may eventually become the treatment of choice.

Allergic bronchopulmonary aspergillosis

Allergic bronchopulmonary aspergillosis (ABPA) may resemble hypersensitivity pneumonitis and presents with systemic symptoms and recurrent pulmonary infiltrates, but with eosinophilia. It is the association with asthma and the typical peripheral eosinophilia (>1000/μL) that distinguishes it from hypersensitivity pneumonitis (or extrinsic allergic alveolitis).

ABPA is the most common example of the allergic bronchopulmonary mycoses and is sometimes confused with hypersensitivity pneumonitis because of the presence of precipitating antibodies to *Aspergillus fumigatus*. However, ABPA is an obstructive rather than a restrictive lung disease, and is associated with allergic (atopic) asthma. The bronchiectasis associated with ABPA is thought to result from a deposition of immune complexes in proximal airways. Adequate treatment usually requires the long-term use of systemic glucocorticoids.

Bronchiectasis

Bronchiectasis is an abnormal and permanent dilatation of the bronchi. It can be focal, involving airways supplying a limited region of the lung, or diffuse, involving airways in a more widespread distribution. Whatever the distribution the diagnosis is suggested by the clinical consequences of chronic or recurrent infection in the dilated airways and the associated copious purulent sputum that forms within these airways.

Aetiology

During childhood, bronchiectasis was often a complication of measles or pertussis but this is now rare as a result of effective immunization. Adenovirus and influenza are the main viral causes, and severe bacterial infections with necrotizing organisms, e.g. Staph. aureus, Klebsiella, TB, anaerobes, remain important causes of bronchiectasis.

Clinical features

Patients typically present with persistent or recurrent cough and purulent sputum production. Haemoptysis occurs in more than half of cases and can cause massive bleeding. Physical examination of the chest overlying an affected area may reveal any combination of crepitations and rhonchi, which reflect the damaged airways containing significant secretions. As with other chronic intrathoracic infections, clubbing may be present.

Patients with severe disease and chronic hypoxaemia, may develop cor pulmonale and right ventricular failure. Amyloidosis can result from chronic infection and inflammation, but it is now seldom seen in patients with bronchiectasis.

Treatment

Treatment strategies are similar to those described for CF except that pancreatic insufficiency is not usually present. Appropriate treatment should be started when a treatable cause is found, e.g. antituberculous drugs for TB or steroids for ABPA.

Interstitial lung diseases

Interstitial lung diseases (ILDs) represent a variety of conditions that involve the alveolar walls (septa), perialveolar tissue, and other adjacent structures. The ILDs are non-malignant and are not caused by any defined infectious agents. Although an acute phase of illness may occur, the onset is often insidious, and the disease is usually chronic in duration.

Aetiology

One useful approach to classification is to separate ILDs into two groups – known and unknown causes. Each of these groups can be divided into subgroups, according to the presence or absence of histological evidence of granulomas in interstitial or vascular areas.

Among the ILDs of known cause, the largest group comprises diseases due to exposure to occupational and environmental inhalants; e.g. inorganic dusts, organic dusts, and various irritative or noxious gases. These diseases can usually be recognized if the occupational history is pursued. The number of ILDs of unknown cause is very large but the major ones within this group are idiopathic pulmonary fibrosis, sarcoidosis, and the ILD associated with collagen vascular disorders.

Clinical features

In idiopathic pulmonary fibrosis, patients usually present with non-productive cough, progressive dyspnoea, fatigue, anorexia, weight loss, and arthralgias. The CXR often shows lower lung zone reticular or reticulonodular shadows, while pulmonary function tests show a restrictive pattern. This condition is also known as cryptogenic fibrosing alveolitis. Auscultation of the chest may be normal initially but as the disease advances, dry crepitations or fine crepitations on inspiration, are usually heard at the lung bases. There may be tachypnoea at rest, cyanosis, and clubbing. In later stages, cor pulmonale with right heart failure may develop.

Diagnostic investigation

This is by histological evaluation, microbial cultures, immunofluorescence, and electron microscopy studies. Samples are usually obtained by transbronchial biopsies, but if this does not yield sufficient tissue for diagnosis a thoracoscopic-guided or even an open lung biopsy should be considered.

A tissue diagnosis is vital before embarking on immunosuppressive therapy (with prednisolone and cyclophosphamide) as treatment has a high rate of possible complications.

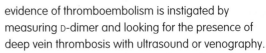

Pulmonary embolism

A triad of factors predispose to venous thrombosis, namely local trauma to the vessel wall, hypercoagulability and stasis (Virchow's triad).

Many patients who suffer pulmonary thromboembolism have an underlying inherited predisposition that remains clinically silent until an acquired stressor occurs, e.g. surgery (especially total hip replacement), obesity, or pregnancy. The most frequent inherited predisposition to hypercoagulability is resistance to the endogenous anticoagulant protein, activated protein C. The phenotype of activated protein C resistance is associated with a single point mutation termed factor V Leiden.

Other inherited hypercoagulable states include deficiencies in protein C, protein S, antithrombin III, and disorders of plasminogen.

Clinical features

Dyspnoea is the most frequent symptom and tachypnoea is the most frequent sign in pulmonary embolism (PE). Dyspnoea, syncope, hypotension, or cyanosis indicate a massive PE, while pleuritic pain, cough, or haemoptysis often suggest a small embolism located near the pleura. On examination, young or previously healthy individuals may simply appear anxious but otherwise seem well, even with a large PE.

Investigations

Investigations supporting the diagnosis of PE include the following:

- Electrocardiogram: tachycardia or the 'typical' $S_1 Q_3 T_3$ pattern.
- ABGs: hypoxaemia.
- CXR: usually normal but may show atelectasis or a small wedge shadow.
- A V/Q scan: unmatched V/Q defects.

If these investigations are negative but the clinical suspicion remains high, a search for corroborative evidence of thromboembolism is instigated by measuring D-dimer and looking for the presence of deep vein thrombosis with ultrasound or venography.

Pulmonary angiography is performed to make a definitive diagnosis in certain circumstances, e.g. pregnancy or acutely ill patients who may require embolectomy.

Treatment

The majority of patients are treated with intravenous heparin followed by oral warfarin for a period of 6 months; PE is a recurrent disease with an annual relapse rate of about 7%. When treatment is continued for only 6 weeks, the relapse rate is twice as high as with 6 months. Monitoring of maintenance warfarin treatment is performed 4–8 weekly in clinical practice, aiming to keep the international normalised ratio (INR) at about 3.0 (therapeutic range 2.0–3.5).

Patients who have recurrent thromboembolic events should be screened for the recognized hypercoagulable states mentioned above. They are also likely to need lifelong anticoagulation and should be considered for a caval filter if warfarin fails to prevent further emboli.

Occupational lung disease

Many acute and chronic lung diseases are directly related to occupational exposure to inorganic and organic dusts. A number of different clinical syndromes may result and these are shown in Fig. 31.11.

Sleep apnoea

Sleep apnoea is defined as an intermittent cessation of airflow at the nose and mouth during sleep. Periods of apnoea of 10 seconds duration are considered important but in most patients the apnoeas last from 20 seconds to as long as 3 minutes.

Sleep apnoea syndrome

This refers to a clinical disorder that arises from

Pulmonary embolism is life threatening and common. If in doubt heparinise and investigate fully.

Many drugs interact with warfarin to enhance or diminish its effect. Ask the patient to report any changes in treatment.

recurrent apnoeas during sleep. The clinical importance of sleep apnoea arises from the fact that it is a common cause of daytime sleepiness, occurring in about 2% of middle-aged women and 4% of middle-aged men.

Classification

Sleep apnoeas are classified into three types:

- Central sleep apnoea, where the neural drive to all the respiratory muscles is transiently abolished.
- Obstructive sleep apnoea, in which airflow ceases despite continuing respiratory drive because of occlusion of the oropharyngeal airway.
- Mixed apnoeas, which consist of a central apnoea followed by an obstructive component.

Treatment

Treatment of mild-to-moderate obstructive sleep apnoea is by modest weight reduction, avoidance of alcohol, improvement of nasal patency, and avoidance of sleeping in the supine posture. Moderate-to-severe cases are treated by uvulopalatopharyngoplasty and nasal continuous positive airways pressure during sleep.

Acute respiratory distress syndrome

Acute respiratory distress syndrome (ARDS; or adult respiratory distress syndrome) is a condition featuring acute hypoxaemic respiratory failure due to pulmonary oedema caused by increased permeability of the alveolar capillary barrier. Essential to the diagnosis are the following findings:

- A history of systemic or pulmonary insult, e.g. sepsis, shock, disseminated intravascular coagulation, high altitude, smoke inhalation.
- Respiratory distress: usually 12–48 hours after the initiating event.
- Bilateral pulmonary infiltrates: initially interstitial oedema but rapidly becomes alveolar with air bronchograms in over 80% of cases.
- Severe hypoxaemia refractory to oxygen treatment: due to shunting.

Common occupational lung diseases		
Disease	**Aetiology**	**Lung injury**
pneumoconiosis (chronic fibrotic lung disease)	coal dust silicosis asbestosis	diffuse nodular infiltrates on CXR
hypersensitivity pneumonitis	mouldy hay (farmer's lung) avian proteins (bird fancier's lung)	restrictive pulmonary dysfunction
obstructive airways disorders	grain dust wood dust tobacco pollen synthetic dyes formaldehyde	occupational asthma
toxic lung injury	irritant gases	pulmonary oedema bronchiolitis obliterans
lung cancer	asbestos	mesothelioma
	arsenic	all lung cancer types
	chromium	all lung cancer types
	hydrocarbons	all lung cancer types
pleural diseases	asbestos	may cause benign effusions and plaques
	talc	may cause benign effusions and plaques

Fig. 31.11 Common occupational lung diseases.

- Normal pulmonary capillary wedge pressure: this excludes cardiogenic pulmonary oedema.

Treatment

The treatment of ARDS includes the identification and treatment of any underlying cause, e.g. sepsis. Supportive therapy almost always includes intubation and mechanical ventilation. Positive end expiratory pressure improves hypoxaemia but does not affect the natural course of the disease.

Measures for avoiding a worsening of the pulmonary oedema are aimed at reducing the intravascular volume (with diuretics) and keeping the haematocrit high (by transfusions of packed red blood cells).

New treatments for ARDS currently being assessed include the following:

- Lung surfactant.
- Monoclonal antibodies to tumour necrosis factor.
- Human recombinant interleukin-1 receptor antagonists.
- Inhaled nitric oxide.

Prognosis

The prognosis is poor in ARDS with a mortality in excess of 50%, rising to 90% with associated sepsis. The major cause of death is non-pulmonary multiple organ failure. Patients who survive may be left with abnormal lung diffusing capacity.

Pneumothorax

A pneumothorax is the presence of gas in the pleural space. The following distinctions are made between the different types of pneumothorax:

- Spontaneous pneumothorax: occurs without trauma to the thorax.
- Primary spontaneous pneumothorax: occurs in the absence of lung disease.
- Secondary spontaneous pneumothorax: occurs in the presence of pre-existing lung disease.
- Traumatic pneumothorax: penetrating or non-penetrating chest injuries.
- Tension pneumothorax: the pressure in the pleural space is positive throughout the respiratory cycle.

Factors which predispose to pneumothorax include: spontaneous factors (tall, thin, healthy men), trauma, airways obstruction, cystic fibrosis, pulmonary abscess and Marfan's syndrome.

Primary spontaneous pneumothorax is usually due to the rupture of an apical pleural bleb that lays within or immediately under the visceral pleura. About 50% of patients with an initial primary spontaneous pneumothorax will have a recurrence.

Clinical features

Clinical features of pneumothorax include the following:

- Chest pain on the affected side.
- Shortness of breath.
- A mild tachycardia.
- Decreased vocal fremitus, hyperresonance and diminished breath sounds, may be detected if the pneumothorax is large.

A CXR will confirm the diagnosis by demonstrating a line of visceral pleura with absent lung markings beyond the line. The diagnosis may prove more difficult in secondary pneumothorax, especially if emphysematous bullae are present.

Treatment

The treatment for primary spontaneous pneumothorax is a simple aspiration. If the lung does not expand with aspiration, or if the patient has a recurrent pneumothorax, chest drain insertion with underwater seal drainage is indicated. Surgery by thoracoscopy or thoracotomy plus pleural abrasion is almost 100% successful in preventing further recurrences.

32. Gastrointestinal and Liver Disease

PEPTIC ULCER DISEASE

Peptic ulcer disease most commonly occurs in the duodenum, followed by the stomach, oesophagus, and jejunum in Zollinger–Ellison syndrome, or after a gastroenterostomy, or in a Meckel's diverticulum with ectopic gastric mucosa. It occurs in up to 15–20% of the population at some time, and is commoner in men. The incidence increases with age.

Although no cause is usually found, peptic ulceration is associated with gastric hypersecretion and impaired mucosal defences. *Helicobacter pylori* plays a central role. Exacerbating factors include stress (Curling's ulcer), smoking, alcohol, non-steroidal anti-inflammatory drugs (NSAIDs), and steroids. Ulceration is also associated with Zollinger–Ellison syndrome, multiple endocrine neoplasia (MEN) type I, and hyperparathyroidism.

Clinical features

The history is unreliable for separating duodenal ulcer (DU) from gastric ulcer (GU). Epigastric pain, often quite localized, is a frequent symptom. The pain may radiate to the back in posterior DU, and is episodic, often waking the patient at night, whereas the pain with GU is worse during the day. The pain is relieved with antacids or milk. The pain of DU is often relieved by food whereas with GU it is precipitated by food.

Other symptoms include nausea, and heartburn secondary to acid reflux. Anorexia, vomiting, and weight loss should lead to the suspicion of gastric carcinoma. If there is persistent and severe pain, complications such as perforation or penetration into other organs should be considered.

Examination reveals epigastric tenderness. A mass suggests carcinoma, and a succussion splash suggests pyloric obstruction.

Investigation

Gastroscopy or barium meal are the investigations of choice, although a trial of acid suppression may be given to younger patients as carcinoma is rarely present in those under 45 years old. All gastric ulcers should be biopsied to exclude malignancy but DUs are nearly always benign; biopsies should be taken for *H. pylori*.

Most gastric carcinomas are on the greater curve and in the antrum. They may have a rolled edge and a translucent halo around them.

Acid secretion status may be assessed if Zollinger–Ellison syndrome is suspected, before and after stimulation with pentagastrin.

Management

The patient should be advised to modify exacerbating factors such as smoking, diet, and alcohol. NSAIDs should be stopped if not absolutely necessary.

Antacids relieve the pain of ulcers but do not necessarily promote healing, and are best given when symptoms occur or are expected. Liquid preparations are more effective than tablets. They should preferably not be taken at the same time as other drugs as they may impair their absorption. They may also damage enteric coatings designed to prevent dissolution in the stomach. Prolonged high doses of calcium-containing antacids can cause hypercalcaemia and alkalosis, and can precipitate milk–alkali syndrome.

Aluminium hydroxide can lower serum phosphate levels, and magnesium carbonate can lead to diarrhoea and belching. Some antacids contain a high sodium content and should not be used in patients on salt-restricted diets.

H. pylori should be eradicated as this promotes long-term healing of duodenal and gastric ulcers. This is best achieved by acid inhibition combined with antibiotic treatment. A proton pump inhibitor (see below) and clarithromycin plus either amoxycillin or metronidazole given for 1 week produce *H. pylori* eradication in 90% of patients. Treatment failure may reflect poor compliance or antibiotic resistance, and antibiotic induced colitis is a possible risk.

H$_2$-receptor antagonists

These agents heal peptic ulcers by reducing gastric acid output as a result of H$_2$-receptor blockade. Examples include cimetidine 400 mg b.d. or ranitidine 150 mg b.d. Relapse rates are high on stopping treatment, and maintenance treatment may be required, especially in those with frequent severe recurrences and in the elderly. They are generally well tolerated but cimetidine is occasionally associated with gynaecomastia and acute psychosis. It also interacts with warfarin, phenytoin, and theophyllines.

Proton pump inhibitors
These inhibit gastric acid by blocking the hydrogen/potassium adenosine triphosphate enzyme system (the 'proton pump') of the gastric parietal cell. Examples include omeprazole 20–40 mg o.d., and lansoprazole 30 mg o.d. High doses may be used in Zollinger–Ellison syndrome.

Side effects include headaches, diarrhoea, rashes, pruritus, and dizziness.

Other drugs
Misoprostol is a synthetic prostaglandin analogue, and has antisecretory and protective properties, promoting peptic ulcer healing. It can prevent ulcers secondary to NSAIDs and is useful in patients in whom NSAIDs cannot be withdrawn. The usual dose is 800 μg daily in divided doses. The main side effect is diarrhoea.

Sucralfate may act by protecting the mucosa from acid–pepsin attack in peptic ulcers. It is a complex of aluminium hydroxide and sulphated sucrose but has minimal antacid properties.

Tripotassium dicitratobismuthate is a bismuth chelate effective in healing gastric and duodenal ulcers but not on its own in maintaining remission. It may be given in combination with two antibiotics to eradicate *H. pylori* but other regimens are preferable.

Surgery
Surgery is usually considered when medical treatment has failed, or for complications that include persistent haemorrhage, perforation, or pyloric stenosis. Operations include partial gastrectomy or now more commonly highly selective vagotomy and pyloroplasty. Haemorrhage may be controlled endoscopically by injection or diathermy, laser photocoagulation, or heat probe. Perforations are usually oversewn with an omental plug.

Complications of surgery include:
- Recurrent ulceration.
- Abdominal fullness.
- Bilious vomiting.

- Diarrhoea.
- Dumping syndrome. This is fainting and sweating after eating, possibly due to food of high osmotic potential being dumped into the jejunum and causing oligaemia because of rapid fluid shifts. 'Late dumping' is due to hypoglycaemia and occurs 1–3 hours after taking food.

Metabolic complications include:
- Weight loss.
- Malabsorption.
- Bacterial overgrowth (blind loop syndrome).
- Anaemia, usually due to iron deficiency following hypochlorhydria and stomach resection.

Complications
The three main complications secondary to peptic ulceration are bleeding, perforation, and pyloric stenosis. Perforation is commoner in DUs than GUs. Pyloric stenosis may also be prepyloric or in the duodenum. It occurs because of oedema surrounding the ulcer or from scar formation on healing. The patient often has projectile vomiting with food ingested up to 24 hours previously. There may be visible peristalsis and a succussion splash. Vomiting may lead to dehydration and a metabolic alkalosis.

Fluid and electrolyte replacement is needed, as is gastric aspiration with a nasogastric tube. Surgery is indicated if the patient does not settle with conservative management.

GASTROINTESTINAL HAEMORRHAGE

The differential diagnosis, history, and examination of patients with gastrointestinal (GI) bleeding is given on p. 33. Emergency resuscitative measures may be needed before a full assessment is made. All patients with a significant bleed should be admitted to hospital. The vast majority will stop bleeding spontaneously within 48 hours.

Management
Patients who have signs of shock suggested by tachycardia and low blood pressure or anaemia should be given blood immediately to expand the circulating volume and restore cardiac output and blood pressure. Blood should be sent for grouping and crossmatching.

Impending shock is indicated by, and requires intravenous fluids and transfusion:
- ○ **Pulse rate greater than 100 per minute.**
- ○ **Haemoglobin less than 10 g/dL.**
- ○ **Systolic blood pressure below 100 mmHg.**

The haemoglobin concentration will remain normal for several hours after a significant haemorrhage.

but if not immediately available colloid or crystalloids should be given. O Rhesus negative blood may be given in severe bleeding. Fluids should be administered via a large-bore cannula through a peripheral vein, or ideally through a central vein (jugular or subclavian) with central venous pressure (CVP) monitoring aiming to maintain the CVP at about 5–10cm saline.

The rate of transfusion should be monitored closely by the general clinical status, as should the pulse and blood pressure to ensure adequate replacement, and to avoid overtransfusion and consequent heart failure.

Blood should also be taken for clotting studies, full blood count (FBC), liver function tests (LFTs), and urea and electrolytes (U&Es). The patient is given oxygen if bleeding is severe. The urea may rise due to protein absorption from the gut but the creatinine is usually normal unless there is coexistent renal failure.

Bleeds from GUs carry twice the mortality of bleeds from DUs. Adverse prognostic factors in patient with GI haemorrhage are listed in Fig. 32.1.

If there are no signs of shock, and the patient is not anaemic, they may be managed 'conservatively', i.e. bed rest, nil by mouth, and close monitoring of the

pulse, blood pressure, and fluid balance. Blood should be grouped and saved, and normal saline should be given intravenously.

Once the patient is stable, endoscopy should be carried out within 24 hours. If varices are suspected, immediate endoscopy should be performed. The cause for the bleed will be apparent in over 80% of cases.

If there is active bleeding, a sclerosant can be injected, or bleeding vessels coagulated with a heat probe or with laser therapy. H_2-receptor antagonists or proton pump inhibitors are given to patients with ulcers for their long-term benefit, although there is little evidence of benefit in the acute situation.

Surgery is indicated if it is not possible to control the bleeding with medical management, especially for persistent or recurrent bleeding, although this is now becoming less common. It is more often carried out in the elderly and for those with GUs compared to DUs.

Management of bleeding oesophageal varices

Resuscitative procedures and endoscopy should be carried out as above. Acute variceal sclerotherapy and banding are the treatments of choice. This arrests bleeding in 80% of cases and reduces early rebleeding. Holding measures before endoscopy is carried out include vasoconstrictor therapy, which aims to restrict portal inflow by splanchnic arterial constriction. Two drugs are used:
- Octreotide is a long-acting analogue of the hypothalamic release-inhibiting hormone somatostatin, and will produce splanchnic vasoconstriction without significant systemic vascular effects.
- Vasopressin (antidiuretic hormone) will cause generalized vasoconstriction. It can precipitate myocardial infarction in patients with ischaemic heart disease.

Measures to prevent hepatic encephalopathy should be started, which include emptying the bowel with enemas

---

Adverse prognostic factors in patients with gastrointestinal haemorrhage

- age over 60 years
- recurrent haemorrhage
- initial presentation with shock
- more than 6 units of blood needed
- an active bleeding vessel seen on endoscopy
- bleeding from oesophageal varices, which can lead to liver failure and hepatic coma

Fig. 32.1 Adverse prognostic factors in patients with gastrointestinal haemorrhage.

or lactulose, and giving neomycin 1 g 6 hourly to reduce the number of bowel organisms. Vitamin K 10 mg i.v. is given, and platelets or fresh frozen plasma are given as needed.

If the bleeding continues, a Sengstaken–Blakemore tube can be passed through the oesophagus, with balloons to compress the gastric and oesophageal veins. Complications include aspiration pneumonia, oesophageal rupture, and mucosal ulceration, and produce a 5% mortality.

To prevent recurrent variceal bleeding, measures include long-term injection sclerotherapy leading to obliteration of the varices by fibrous tissues. This reduces rebleeding but does not necessarily improve mortality. Complications include oesophageal ulceration, mediastinitis, and strictures. Non-selective β-blockers, e.g. propanolol, decrease portal pressures and significantly reduce primary and secondary bleeding and mortality from large varices.

Surgical procedures include oesophageal transection with anastamosis, transthoracic transoesophageal ligation of varices, and gastric transection with reanastamosis.

About half of those bleeding from varices for the first time will die. The risk of recurrence is about 80% in the next 2 years. Adverse prognostic factors are jaundice, ascites, hypoalbuminaemia, and encephalopathy.

Lower gastrointestinal bleeding

The differential diagnosis of lower GI bleeding is listed in Fig. 32.2.

Differential diagnosis of lower gastrointestinal bleeding

- anal fissure
- haemorrhoids
- inflammatory bowel disease
- infective colitis
- gastrointestinal carcinoma: sigmoid, caecum, rectum
- ischaemic colitis
- diverticulitis
- intestinal polyps
- vascular abnormalities: angiodysplasia, arteriovenous malformations
- Meckel's diverticulum
- Peutz–Jeghers syndrome
- Osler–Weber–Rendu syndrome
- endometriosis

Fig. 32.2 Differential diagnosis of lower gastrointestinal bleeding

Resuscitation should be carried out as for upper GI bleeds, and further investigations are carried out when the patient is stable. Examination should include a rectal examination to exclude carcinoma, sigmoidoscopy, and colonoscopy. Barium enema may add to information, and angiography can be carried out if vascular abnormalities are suspected.

Lower GI bleeding may be occult and chronic, presenting with iron-deficiency anaemia, and general lethargy and fatigue. If the history does not suggest a particular site in the GI tract responsible for the blood loss, a sensible working plan is upper GI endoscopy followed by colonoscopy. If no diagnosis is apparent, a small bowel follow-through (enteroclysis) is next performed, followed by angiography if needed. Isotope-labelled red blood cells may localize the site of bleeding.

INFLAMMATORY BOWEL DISEASE

Inflammatory bowel disease usually implies ulcerative colitis and Crohn's disease. It is likely that these conditions represent a spectrum of disease resulting from a combination of genetic and environmental factors, although they typically differ in their natural history and response to treatment.

Aetiology

The primary cause of ulcerative colitis is unknown, although 10–15% of patients have a first-degree relative with ulcerative colitis or Crohn's disease. It may result from a genetically determined, inappropriately severe, and/or prolonged inflammatory response to a dietary or microbial product. Abnormalities of colonic epithelial cell metabolism have also been reported in ulcerative colitis, and there are associations with certain drugs such as NSAIDs and antibiotics, and with stress, although the significance is uncertain.

There may be a history of atopy, autoimmune disease, e.g. chronic active hepatitis and systemic lupus erythematosus, and the presence of circulating immune complexes and antibodies to colonocytes and neutrophil (pANCA) in ulcerative colitis.

Ulcerative colitis occurs almost exclusively among non-smokers whereas about two-thirds of patients who have Crohn's disease smoke cigarettes.

Ulcerative colitis

This is an idiopathic chronic relapsing inflammatory disease starting in the rectum and possibly spreading to involve all of the large intestine. It is commoner in the Western world with a prevalence of about 150 in 100 000, and an incidence of about 10 in 100 000 annually, and is maximal at 15–40 years of age. There is no major sex difference.

Clinical features

The disease may present with a single mild episode followed by remission for a prolonged period, or progressive symptoms over months with general ill health and chronic diarrhoea, or as an acute severe episode. In general, the severity of diarrhoea and systemic upset depends on the extent of the disease and depth of mucosal ulceration.

Active subtotal or total ulcerative colitis causes frequent bloody diarrhoea, often with fever, malaise, anorexia, weight loss, abdominal pain, anaemia, and tachycardia. With proctitis, characteristic symptoms are rectal bleeding and mucous discharge, but the stool is well formed and general health is maintained. The patient may present with a complication. Between relapses, the patient is usually symptomless.

Complications

Local

Toxic megacolon, perforation, or rarely massive haemorrhage can occur. There is an increased risk of colonic carcinoma in patients with subtotal or total ulcerative colitis. The cumulative incidence is 10–15% at 20 years.

Extraintestinal

Extraintestinal complications of ulcerative colitis include the following:

- Skin: erythema nodosum, pyoderma gangrenosum, vasculitis.
- Eyes: uveitis, episcleritis, conjunctivitis.
- Joints: large joint arthropathy, sacroilitis, ankylosing spondylitis.
- Liver: pericholangitis, sclerosing cholangitis, cirrhosis, chronic active hepatitis, cholangiocarcinoma.
- Vasculature: arterial and venous thrombosis.
- Renal stones and gallbladder stones: in Crohn's disease.

Diagnosis

Sigmoidoscopy and rectal biopsy show inflamed mucosa. If the disease is active there may be pus and blood, visible ulceration, and bleeding on contact with the sigmoidoscope. Other types of colitis should be excluded, and stool microscopy and culture is needed to exclude infection.

Histology shows inflammatory cells infiltrating the lamina propria with crypt abscesses. There is little involvement of the muscularis mucosa, and there is a reduction of goblet cells.

Barium enema shows loss of the normal haustral pattern and the bowel looks like a smooth tube ('hosepipe'). Ulcers and pseudopolyps may be seen, oedema of the colonic wall produces widening of the presacral space, and there may be narrowed areas secondary to strictures or carcinoma.

Management

General measures

A multidisciplinary approach is preferred with gastroenterologists, nursing staff, counsellors, and stoma therapists, in collaboration with primary health-care teams. Support groups are available. Some patients may improve with avoidance of cow's milk, and some with proctitis benefit from fibre supplements. Specific nutritional, haematinic, and electrolyte deficiencies may require correction. NSAIDs and antibiotics should be avoided.

Drugs

If the ulcerative colitis is not severe, the patient can usually be managed as an outpatient. Proctitis is treated with topical steroids and oral 5-aminosalicylic acid (5-ASA). Left-sided or extensive ulcerative colitis is treated with steroid enemas, oral 5-ASA, or oral prednisolone if necessary. Patients with an extensive, severe attack should be admitted. Infection should be excluded, and intravenous fluids and electroytes given as needed.

Extraintestinal manifestations of IBD are A PIE SAC: aphthous ulcers, pyoderma gangrenosum, iritis, erythema nodosum, sclerosing cholangitis, arthritis, and clubbing.

Transfusion may be required for extensive blood loss, and the patient should be given prophylactic subcutaneous heparin.

Antidiarrhoeal, antispasmodic, and anticholinergic drugs should be avoided as they can precipitate colonic dilatation. Patients are given intravenous hydrocortisone 400 mg per day, followed by high-dose prednisolone and a corticosteroid enema. About 70% of patients improve substantially within 7 days. If there is an inadequate response, urgent colectomy is required, or cyclosporin may be tried as adjunctive treatment. Unfortunately, there is a high relapse rate on stopping the cyclosporin, and surgery is required.

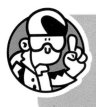

Indications for surgery in IBD are I CHOP: infection, carcinoma, haemorrhage, obstruction, and perforation.

To maintain patients in remission, oral 5-ASA is usually required unless relapse occurs less than once a year. For frequent relapses, oral azathioprine is of benefit.

Corticosteroids
Prednisolone is used for acute flare-ups, and their side effects can be reduced by restricting their use to less than 3 months. It may be given intravenously, orally, or topically, and as a suppository, liquid, foam, or enema.

Aminosalicylates
Examples include sulphasalazine 1–2 g t.d.s. This consists of 5-ASA, linked by an azo bond to sulphapyridine. The 5-ASA, the active component, is released in the colon by bacterial action. About 20% of patients cannot tolerate sulphasalazine because of adverse effects, mostly related to the sulphapyridine. These include headache and fever, blood dyscrasias, bone marrow suppression, rashes, and oligospermia, making newer compounds preferable in young men.

Mesalazine contains 5-ASA alone and may have less side effects.

The aminosalicylates help maintain remission, reducing annual relapse rates from 70% to 30%. They are also available as enemas and suppositories.

Immunosuppressive drugs
Azathioprine may be used in patients who relapse repeatedly on steroid withdrawal after an acute episode, or in whom aminosalicylates are ineffective for maintaining remission; it may take up to 4 months to effect a noticeable clinical benefit.

Serious adverse effects include bone marrow suppression and cholestatic jaundice, necessitating blood checks fortnightly for the first 3 months. Long-term safety data are still awaited.

Cyclosporin may be effective as an adjunct to steroids in refractory acute severe ulcerative colitis, but has serious side effects including hypertension, nephrotoxicity, epilepsy, and opportunistic infections. Close monitoring of the patient is needed.

Antibiotics
These may be used in severe attacks to prevent bacteraemia and endotoxic shock.

Surgery
Surgery is curative for colonic disease though not for extraintestinal complications. Options include panproctocolectomy with ileoanal pouch, permanent ileostomy, or rarely subtotal colectomy with ileorectal anastamosis. It may be considered electively for chronic intractable ulcerative colitis, colonic carcinoma, persistent mucosal dysplasia, or growth retardation in children.

Prognosis
About 70% of untreated patients relapse annually, and up to 30% eventually require surgery, although the overall mortality is close to that of the general population. The main risks to life are severe attacks of ulcerative colitis and colonic cancer. Patients with extensive ulcerative colitis of 10 years' duration or more are offered colonoscopy every 1 to 2 years to prevent colonic cancer by taking multiple biopsies to look for mucosal dysplasia, and to offer elective colectomy if appropriate, or to detect cancer at a curable stage.

CROHN'S DISEASE

Crohn's disease can affect any part of the GI tract from the mouth to the anus. It most frequently presents with ileocaecal disease followed by colonic, ileal alone, diffuse small intestinal, gastric, and oesophageal involvement. The overall prevalence in the Western world is about 1 in 1000 and is more common in Caucasians than Afro-Caribbeans.

Clinical presentation

The patient has diarrhoea and abdominal pain. There may be a fever, anaemia, and weight loss. The patient may be clubbed and there may be associated complications, e.g. joint, skin, or eye complications, as with ulcerative colitis.

The presentation depends on the site of disease, and on the tendency to perforate or fistulate rather than to fibrose and stricture, which is probably determined by genetic factors. Terminal ileal disease presents with right iliac fossa pain, often with an associated mass. This may present acutely, mimicking appendicitis, or chronically, mimicking irritable bowel syndrome.

Colonic Crohn's disease is distinguishable from ulcerative colitis by the presence of skip lesions (multiple lesions with normal bowel in between), rectal sparing, perianal skin tags, or fistulas with or without granulomata on biopsy, although the distinction is unclear in up to a third of patients.

Investigations

Diagnosis is made by endoscopy with or without barium studies. Barium enema shows skip lesions, a coarse cobblestone appearance of the mucosa, and, later, fibrosis produces narrowing of the intestine ('string sign') with proximal dilatation.

Serum C-reactive protein is raised in about 95% of cases with active disease.

Magnetic resonance imaging (MRI) is useful for evaluation of fistulas and abscesses.

Management

In most cases of active Crohn's disease, there are three therapeutic alternatives: surgery, corticosteroids or diet. These options should be discussed with the patient. Steroids have no proven maintenance effect and inappropriate long-term use produces unacceptable adverse effects.

Which IBD has Cobblestones on endoscopy? Crohn's disease.

Therapy with 5-ASA maintenance probably reduces the risk of recurrence.

Surgery

Postoperative fistulas used to be a common complication but are now rare, partly due to perioperative antibiotics, particularly metronidazole. Absolute indications for surgery include complete obstruction or peritonitis. After surgical resection, about half the patients remain symptom free for 5 years and half require further surgery within 10 years.

Perianal disease requires conservative management. Abscesses should be drained and fistulas treated with antibiotics, either metronidazole or ciprofloxacin. If there is coexistent active disease elsewhere, perianal disease may improve when the active disease is resected.

Dietary therapy

Enteral feeding should be considered for patients with extensive small bowel disease, or who have multiple or extensive small bowel resections, or for failure to respond to steroids. About two-thirds of patients achieve a satisfactory clinical and biochemical remission within about 3 weeks. The patient then gradually introduces components of the normal diet, although there is a 50% relapse rate 6 months after return to a normal diet.

Those with stricturing disease should avoid fruit and vegetable fibre, and may need vitamin C and folate supplements; also, vitamin B_{12} supplements will be necessary after extensive small bowel surgery. Patients can experiment to find a diet that suits them best.

Drugs
Steroids
Steroids may not modify the long-term course of the disease but are useful for acute episodes. High-dose prednisolone is usually given, and tailed off over several weeks. Within 4 weeks about a third of patients are in remission and a further third are considerably improved. Formulations of steroids are now available that deliver the drug to the distal ileum.

Azathioprine and other immunosuppressives

These may be used as an adjunct to steroids as with ulcerative colitis. They require close monitoring of the blood count. As well as maintaining remission, there is some evidence that they are helpful in healing fistulas.

Metronidazole and other antibiotics

A variety of bacteria and yeasts have been identified in Crohn's disease. Metronidazole is effective in colonic Crohn's disease, perianal disease, and in the prevention of recurrence following bowel resection. It should be given for 3 months. Longer maintenance doses carry a risk of peripheral neuropathy. Ciprofloxacin may also be of benefit.

Antidiarrhoeals and cholestyramine

Cholestyramine, an ion-exchange resin, is useful for chronic diarrhoea after ileal resection due to conjugated bile acids entering the colon. It should not be given at the same time as other medication as it impairs their absorption. Antidiarrhoeals such as loperamide are safe providing there is no evidence of obstruction.

Prognosis

A minority of patients have extensive disease or frequent recurrences, and account for most of the 10% who ultimately die of the disease. Around 10–20% of patients remain asymptomatic for 20 years after the first or second episode of symptomatic disease. Most patients need surgery within the first few years and further resections at intervals of 10–15 years but have a good quality of life for most of this time.

GASTROINTESTINAL TUMOURS

Oesophageal carcinoma

Squamous carcinomas occur in the mid-oesophagus. The incidence in the UK is 5–10 in 100000 but is higher in China and parts of Africa. It is commoner in men, heavy drinkers, and smokers. Predisposing factors include Plummer–Vinson syndrome (see p. 127), achalasia, coeliac disease, and tylosis (hyperkeratosis of the palms and soles).

Adenocarcinoma arises in columnar epithelium of the lower oesophagus, resulting from long standing reflux. Columnar metaplasia, called Barrett's oesophagus, increases the risk of adenocarcinoma by 40-fold.

Clinical features

The incidence peaks in the seventh decade. Dysphagia is common, progressing from difficulty in swallowing solids to difficulty with liquids. Odynophagia (pain on swallowing) may ensue. The lesions may ulcerate and cause strictures. Direct invasion of surrounding structures and regional lymph node involvement are common. Weight loss, anorexia, lymphadenopathy, and aspiration pneumonia may be found.

Investigations

Endoscopy with biopsy, and barium swallow are the main diagnostic investigations. Computed tomography (CT) scanning may show spread outside the oesophagus.

Management

Surgery is possible providing there is no evidence of metastases but it carries a high morbidity and mortality. Strictures may be dilated if causing dysphagia; laser photocoagulation via an endoscope is available in some centres. Overall survival is poor at around 2% at 5 years. Treatment is mainly symptomatic and palliative.

Gastric carcinoma

The incidence of gastric carcinoma is 15 in 100000, and it is commoner in men and the elderly. There is a link between gastric cancer and *H. pylori*, which may explain the higher prevalence in lower socio-economic groups. Suggested dietary links include alcohol, spicy foods, and nitrates, which are converted to nitrosamines by bacteria. It occurs more often in Japan due to the higher fish intake resulting in a high level of nitrosamines. It is commoner in smokers, in patients with achlorhydria, and in patients with blood group A.

Other predisposing conditions include pernicious anaemia, chronic gastritis with atrophy, areas of intestinal metaplasia, and partial gastrectomy.

Most cancers are adenocarcinomas and affect mainly the pylorus and antrum. They are polypoid or ulcerating lesions with rolled edges.

Clinical features

In the early stages, the symptoms are similar to GU with epigastric pain but the patient may present later with anorexia, nausea and vomiting, weight loss, and iron-deficiency anaemia. Metastases occur to the liver, bones, brain, and lungs.

A palpable epigastric mass and upper abdominal tenderness may be present, and there may be a palpable lymph node in the left supraclavicular fossa (Virchow's node). Other signs include dermatomyositis and acanthosis nigricans.

Investigation
Blood tests include a FBC to look for signs of chronic blood loss, and LFTs for possible metastases. Diagnosis is made on gastroscopy with multiple biopsies.

Treatment
The 5-year survival is about 10% but the 5-year survival with gastrectomy (if found early) is up to 50%.

Colonic tumours
Colonic polyps are common and often found incidentally during investigation of coincidental GI symptoms such as pain, altered bowel habit, or bleeding haemorrhoids. They may be sessile or pedunculated, vary from a few millimetres to up to 10 cm in diameter, and they may be solitary or multiple.

Peutz–Jeghers syndrome consists of mucocutaneous pigmentation and polyps anywhere along the GI tract, most commonly in the small bowel. It has a Mendelian dominant inheritance.

Adenomatous polyps may bleed and lead to iron-deficiency anaemia. Sessile villous adenomas of the rectum may present with profuse diarrhoea and hypokalaemia. Once the polyp is removed endoscopically, continuous colonoscopic surveillance every 3–5 years is recommended due to the high probability of recurrence.

Familial adenomatous polyposis is Mendelian dominant. Patients have multiple polyps throughout the GI tract. In high-risk patients, colectomy with ileorectal anastamosis may be performed, with continued surveillance of the rectal stump.

Colonic adenocarcinoma is the second commonest tumour in the UK with a lifetime incidence of 1 in 50. It is commoner in the elderly and less common in Africa and Asia. It may be related to low fibre and high animal fat diets. Predisposing conditions include ulcerative colitis and familial adenomatous polyposis. Genetic factors also play a role, with a 2–3-fold increased risk of developing colon cancer with one first-degree affected family member. Two-thirds of tumours occur with ulceration, and spread by direct infiltration, invading the lymph nodes and blood vessels leading to metastases.

Clinical features
Left-sided tumours present with altered bowel habit and abdominal pain. They may be asymptomatic, or present with an iron-deficiency anaemia or with obstruction. Rectosigmoid tumours commonly bleed. Examination should always include a rectal examination.

Investigation
FBC for anaemia, and U&Es for electrolyte abnormalities with diarrhoea. Colonoscopy and barium enema will identify most tumours. Ultrasound is useful for staging and to detect liver metastases.

Treatment
The overall 5-year survival is about 30% but is over 90% if resected early. Adjuvant chemotherapy and radiotherapy increase survival in more advanced stages.

Endocrine tumours of the gut
Although these are all very rare they are sometimes discussed in examinations.

They arise from APUD (amine precursor: uptake and decarboxylation) cells, which secrete a number of hormones, e.g. gastrin, glucagon, and vasoactive intestinal peptide (VIP). They may occur with other endocrine tumours as part of MEN syndromes.

Zollinger–Ellison syndrome
This is usually due to a gastrin-secreting pancreatic adenoma, which stimulates excessive acid production leading to multiple recurrent ulcers in the stomach and duodenum. About half are malignant and 10% are multiple.

Patients commonly get diarrhoea due to the low pH in the upper intestine, and steatorrhoea due to the inactivation of lipase by the low pH. The diagnosis is made by a raised fasting serum gastrin level; the gastric acid output is also raised. Treatment is by removal of the primary tumour (provided there is no evidence of metastases) and omeprazole or octreotide.

Insulinomas
These are tumours of the pancreatic islet ß-cells; 5% are malignant and 5% are multiple. The patient presents

with recurrent or fasting hypoglycaemia, which may manifest in bizarre behaviour, epilepsy, dementia, or confusion. The diagnosis is confirmed by the demonstration of hypoglycaemia in association with inappropriate and excessive insulin secretion. Treatment is by surgical excision of the tumour. If surgery is not feasible, diazoxide or octreotide are useful.

Vipomas

These tumours release VIP, which produces intestinal secretions leading to watery diarrhoea, hypokalaemia, and sometimes achlorhydria. Diagnosis is by high serum levels of VIP. The tumour should be resected if possible. Octreotide is useful for controlling symptoms.

Glucagonomas

These are tumours of the α-cells of the pancreas, which release glucagon. Symptoms include diabetes, diarrhoea, a necrolytic migratory erythematous rash, weight loss, anaemia, and glossitis.

Carcinoid tumours

These tumours originate from the argentaffin cells of the intestine. They may appear in the appendix, terminal ileum, rectum, or other site in the GI tract. They have malignant potential; 80% of large tumours produce metastases. Presentations include appendicitis (10% of tumours arise in the appendix), GI obstruction, and ,in 5% of cases, the carcinoid syndrome.

Carcinoid syndrome

This only occurs when liver metastases are present. Clinical features include flushing (which may be prolonged and lead to telangiectases), abdominal pain, diarrhoea, bronchospasm, and oedema associated with pulmonary stenosis or tricuspid regurgitation. Symptoms are due to the release of pharmacologically active mediators, e.g. 5-hydroxytryptamine (5-HT), prostaglandins, and kinins.

Diagnosis is by measurement of 5-hydroxyindoleacetic acid (5-HIAA) in 24-hour urine collection, which is a metabolite (5-HT).

Abdominal CT scan or laparotomy may be needed to localise the tumour.

Treatment: Food and drink which precipitate flushing should be avoided, e.g. alcohol, coffee. Surgery is best for localised tumours and may be curative. Octreotide

alleviates flushing and diarrhoea. Other useful drugs include cyprohepatiine (an antihistamine with 5-HT and calcium channel blocking properties), and methysergide (which also blocks 5-HT). Other procedures include enucleation of liver metastases, hepatic artery ligation, embolisation, and 5-fluorouracil injection.

Prognosis: the median survival is 5–10 years after diagnosis.

MALABSORPTION

Causes of malabsorption are given in Fig. 32.3.

Clinical features

Symptoms include anorexia and weight loss, abdominal distension and borborygmi, pale, greasy stools with an offensive odour, tiredness, and parasthesiae. There may be signs of wasting, abdominal distension, petechiae (vitamin K malabsorption), anaemia, bone pain (hypocalcaemia), oedema and ascites (hypoproteinaemia), clubbing, tetany, and peripheral neuropathy (vitamin B deficiency). There may also be signs of the underlying disease, e.g. jaundice or lymphadenopathy with lymphomas.

Investigations

The following investigations are important in the patient with malabsorption:

- General blood tests: FBC may show a microcytic, macrocytic, or mixed picture. Albumin and calcium may be low. Electrolytes (e.g. sodium, potassium, and magnesium) may be low. LFTs are abnormal if liver pathology is responsible for the malabsorption, and prothrombin time may be increased.
- Specific blood tests: serum folate, vitamin B_{12}, and serum iron may help to confirm malabsorption.
- Faecal fat estimations: high fat content in stools.
- Glucose tolerance test: this is 'flat'.
- Radiology: plain X-ray may reveal fluid levels, pancreatic calcification or gallstones. Small bowel enemas are useful for Crohn's disease, lymphoma or diverticula. Jejunal biopsy is indicated in coeliac disease.
- Pancreatic function tests: if pancreatic disease is suspected. Endoscopic retrograde cholangiopancreatography (ERCP) will give further information.

Fig. 32.3 Causes of malabsorption.

Causes of malabsorption	
Cause	**Examples**
mucosal disease	gluten-sensitive enteropathy tropical sprue intestinal lymphangiectasia Whipple's disease
structural abnormalities	gastric surgery intestinal resections blind loops diverticula, fistulae small bowel malignancy arterial insufficiency systemic sclerosis
infections	acute enteritis postinfective malabsorption traveller's diarrhoea tuberculosis parasites
impaired digestion	biliary and liver disease pancreatic disease Zollinger–Ellison syndrome
biochemical disorders	alactasia abetalipoproteinaemia hypogammaglobulinaemia
iatrogenic	drugs surgery radiotherapy
disorders outside the gastrointestinal tract	endocrine disorders, e.g. thyroid disease, Addison's disease, hypoparathyroidism collagen disorders malignant disease widespread skin diseases

• Breath hydrogen tests: indicated in bacterial overgrowth.

Specific diseases

Coeliac disease

Coeliac disease is a gluten-sensitive enteropathy. In this disease there is an abnormal jejunal mucosa leading to malabsorption. The condition improves with a gluten-free diet but relapses when gluten is reintroduced.

Gluten is present in wheat, barley, rye, and oats.

Coeliac disease is commoner in Europeans, with an incidence of about 1 in 2000 in the UK. There is an increased incidence within families, and it is associated with HLA-B8 and DR3. It is also associated with a blistering subepidermal eruption of the skin (dermatitis herpetiformis). The aetiology is thought to be due to α-gliadin, a peptide present in gluten, which is injurious to the small bowel mucosa. Immunogenic mechanisms and possibly environmental factors (e.g. viral infections) may also play a role.

Clinical features

The disease can present at any age. The peak incidence in adults is in the third and fourth decades, and it is more common in women. Symptoms may be non-specific, e.g. lethargy and malaise. There is usually a history of diarrhoea or steatorrhoea, with abdominal discomfort, and there may be weight loss. Other features include mouth ulcers, anaemia, and less commonly tetany, osteomalacia, neuropathies, and myopathies.

There is an increased incidence of autoimmune disease, e.g. thyroid disease and insulin-dependent diabetes. Coeliac disease may be complicated by GI lymphoma and gastric or oesophageal carcinoma.

Investigations

The following investigations are important in the patient with coeliac disease:

- Jejunal biopsy: villous atrophy with chronic inflammatory cells in the lamina propria.
- FBC: may show anaemia (folate, vitamin B_{12}, or iron deficiency).
- Antireticulin antibodies and anit-endomysial antibodies: usually present.
- Serum albumin: hypoalbuminaemia.
- Prothrombin time: may be prolonged due to vitamin K deficiency.

Management

The condition improves on a gluten-free diet. Deficient vitamins are replaced. If symptoms persist, it may be that the patient is not complying with the diet.

Bacterial overgrowth

Although bacterial overgrowth may occur spontaneously, especially in the elderly. It is normally associated with a structural abnormality of the small intestine, e.g. in diverticula or postoperative blind loops. Aspiration of jejunal contents reveals *Escherichia coli* or *Bacteroides* in concentrations greater than 10^6/mL as part of a mixed flora. The bacteria can deconjugate bile salts, which can be detected in aspirates; this deficiency of conjugated bile salts leads to steatorrhoea. The bacteria also metabolize vitamin B_{12} leading to its deficiency.

Management

Underlying small bowel lesions should be corrected if possible. The condition may respond to intermittent courses of metronidazole 400 mg 8 hourly or oxytetracycline 250 mg 6 hourly.

Tropical sprue

In this condition there is severe malabsorption usually accompanied by diarrhoea and malnutrition. It occurs in most of Asia and the Caribbean. The aetiology is unknown but it is thought to be infective. The onset can be insidious or acute with anorexia, weight loss, and abdominal distension, as well as diarrhoea. There may be features of vitamin deficiency, especially vitamin B_{12}. Jejunal histology shows partial villous atrophy.

Management

Severe cases may need intravenous fluids and electrolytes, and replacement of nutritional and vitamin deficiencies. Patients often improve when they leave an endemic area. Patients may be helped with tetracycline 250 mg 6 hourly and folic acid.

Whipple's disease

This is a rare cause of malabsorption, usually affecting men over 50 years old. As well as steatorrhoea, there is fever, weight loss, arthralgia, lymphadenopathy, and sometimes involvement of the heart, lung, and brain. Histologically, cells of the lamina propria are replaced by macrophages which contain periodic acid–Schiff (PAS) positive glycoprotein granules. The organism responsible is *Tropheryma whippelii*. Treatment is with antibiotics, e.g. tetracycline or chloramphenicol.

DISEASES OF THE GALLBLADDER

Gallstones

The incidence of gallstones rises with age, and is more common in women on the oral contraceptive pill.

Bile contains cholesterol, bile pigments, and phospholipids, and it is the relative concentrations of these that determines the kind of stone that is formed. Pigment stones are small and radiolucent, and they are occasionally associated with haemolytic anaemia due to increased formation of bile pigment from haemoglobin.

Cholesterol stones are large, often solitary, and are radiolucent. Mixed stones contain calcium salts, pigment and cholesterol; 10% are radiopaque. (Compare with renal stones, of which about 90% are radiopaque.)

Gallstones may be asymptomatic but may cause acute or chronic cholecystitis, biliary colic, or obstructive jaundice. Other presentations include cholangitis (infection of the bile ducts causing right upper quadrant pain, jaundice, and fever with rigors), pancreatitis, empyema, and gallstone ileus where the gallstone perforates the gallbladder, ulcerates into the duodenum and passes on to obstruct the terminal ileum.

Investigations

If pigment stones are suspected or found operatively, a haemolysis screen should be obtained. Plain abdominal X-ray and ultrasound should detect most stones. A cholecystogram or intravenous cholangiography may performed in cases of uncertainty. Operative cholangiography will reveal stones in the bile ducts, which might otherwise be missed.

Gallstones are most common in people with the 'six Fs':

- Fair.
- Fat.
- Fertile.
- Female.
- Forty
- (Low) Fibre diet.

Management

If the patient is symptomatic, treatment is by cholecystectomy. Sphincterotomy via ERCP may release stones in the common bile duct. Other options include the medical dissolution of small, cholesterol-rich radiolucent stones (with ursodeoxycholic acid given for up to 2 years) or shockwave lithotripsy.

Acute cholecystitis

This disease is most common in overweight, middle-aged women, but may occur at any age. It usually follows the impaction of a stone in the cystic duct and leads to fever, rigors, epigastric or right upper quadrant pain, vomiting, local peritonism, or a gallbladder mass. If the stone moves to the common bile duct, jaundice may occur. Murphy's sign may be positive; this is pain on inspiration when two fingers are placed over the right upper quadrant, due to an inflamed gallbladder impinging on the examiner's fingers.

Differential diagnosis

The differential diagnosis of acute cholecystitis includes the following:

- Appendicitis in a highly-situated appendix.
- Right basal pneumonia.
- Perforated peptic ulcer.
- Pancreatitis.
- Myocardial infarction.

Investigations

The white cell count is elevated. A chest X-ray (CXR), electrocardiogram (ECG), serum amylase and cardiac enzymes should be taken to help exclude differential diagnoses. Ultrasound will show a thickened gallbladder wall and stones.

Management

Management is usually initially conservative, unless complications ensue, e.g. perforation of the gallbladder. The patient should be on bed rest, nil by mouth with intravenous fluids, and analgesia and antibiotics, e.g. cefuroxime or cefotaxime, should be given. Cholecystectomy is either performed after 48 hours, or the inflammation is allowed to settle and the gallbladder is removed after 2–3 months.

Chronic cholecystitis

Recurrent episodes of cholecystitis are usually associated with gallstones, leading to intermittent colic and chronic inflammation. There is abdominal discomfort, bloating, nausea, flatulence, and intolerance of fats.

The differential diagnosis includes myocardial ischaemia, hiatus hernia and oesophagitis, peptic ulcer disease, irritable bowel syndrome, chronic relapsing pancreatitis, and tumours of the GI tract. Treatment is by cholecystectomy.

DISEASES OF THE PANCREAS

Carcinoma of the pancreas

The incidence of pancreatic carcinoma is increasing. Risk factors include smoking and possibly diabetes. About three-quarters of tumours occur in the head, the rest occurring in the body or tail. Secondary diabetes is uncommon. Pancreatitis may occur due to obstruction of the pancreatic duct.

Clinical features

There is dyspepsia or epigastric pain radiating to the back, anorexia and weight loss, fever, and obstructive jaundice with an enlarged gallbladder. There may be hepatomegaly from biliary obstruction or metastases. Thrombophlebitis migrans occurs in 10% of patients.

Investigations

Ultrasound and CT scan may show the tumour, ERCP may confirm the diagnosis, and needle biopsy can be performed under CT control.

Management

A minority of patients may be suitable for operative treatment although survival is not usually greater than 1 year, even after surgery. Patients with ampullary carcinoma often present early with jaundice, and surgical removal may therefore be more successful.

Without treatment, survival is usually only a few weeks after diagnosis.

Acute pancreatitis

Aetiology
Most cases are secondary to gallstones or alcohol. It may be also be idiopathic.

Clinical features
There may be a history of cholecystitis or other complications of gallstones. Alcohol intake should be ascertained. The patient complains of severe abdominal pain radiating to the back or shoulder, which may be relieved by sitting forward. There may be associated vomiting.

On examination there is abdominal tenderness with guarding and rebound tenderness. There may be a tachycardia, fever, jaundice, hypotension, and sweating. There may be bruising around the umbilicus (Cullen's sign) or in the flanks (Grey–Turner's sign).

Differential diagnosis
This includes any cause of an acute abdomen, e.g. cholecystitis, mesenteric ischaemia, and intestinal perforation. Myocardial infarction and dissecting aortic aneurysm should also be excluded.

Investigations
The following investigations are important in the patient with acute pancreatitis:

- Serum amylase: markedly raised (over 1000 IU/mL). Amylase is also raised with cholecystitis and perforated peptic ulcer, but usually to a lesser extent.
- Abdominal X-ray: gallstones, pancreatic calcification indicating previous inflammation, an absent psoas shadow due to retroperitoneal fluid, and a distended loop of jejunum ('sentinel loop').
- Serum calcium: may be low.
- White cell count: usually raised.
- ECG: to exclude myocardial infarction.
- Arterial blood gases: metabolic acidosis.
- CXR: widened mediastinum in aortic dissection; gas under the diaphragm in perforated peptic ulcer.

Management
Management is usually conservative. Intravenous fluids should be given to maintain the circulating volume, and

The causes of pancreatitis can be recalled from the mnemonic GET SMASH'D: gallstones, ethanol, trauma, steroids, mumps, autoimmune diseases, scorpion stings, hypertriglyceridaemia, and drugs, e.g. azathioprine or diuretics.

a central venous catheter may be helpful for assessing the volume of fluid required. If the patient is shocked, plasma expanders will be required.

Pain relief is with intravenous or intramuscular opiates, e.g. pethidine 50–150 mg 4 hourly or pentazocine 30–60 mg 4 hourly, with an antiemetic such as prochlorperazine 12.5 mg 8 hourly. A nasogastric tube should be inserted. Blood tests, especially U&Es, glucose, and calcium should be monitored.

Surgery should be considered for suspected haemorrhagic necrosis of the pancreas. Some give H_2-receptor antagonists, prophylactic antibiotics, or peritoneal lavage, although these measures are of unproven value.

Prognosis
Mortality is 5–10% but recurrence is uncommon in patients who recover. Death may be from shock, renal failure, sepsis, or respiratory failure. Other complication include hypocalcaemia due to the formation of calcium soaps, transient hyperglycaemia, pancreatic abscess requiring drainage, and pseudocyst (i.e. fluid in the lesser sac presenting as a palpable mass), persistently raised serum amylase or liver function tests, and fever. Patients should be investigated to exclude gallstones, and alcohol should be avoided.

Chronic pancreatitis
The main cause of chronic pancreatitis is chronic excessive alcohol intake. Other causes include gallstones, cystic fibrosis, and haemochromatosis. The patient is generally ill with weight loss and has recurrent abdominal pain radiating to the back. Steatorrhoea is secondary to malabsorption from pancreatic insufficiency. Diabetes may occur due to

involvement of pancreatic islet ß-cells, and there may be intermittent or persistent obstructive jaundice.

Investigations
These are similar to those for acute pancreatitis although serum amylase is not helpful in the diagnosis as it is usually only slightly raised. In addition the following investigations should be performed:
- Plasma glucose: raised in diabetes.
- CT scan: may show dilated ducts.
- ERCP: outlines the anatomy of the ducts and shows calculi.

Investigations of consequences or complications of pancreatitis should also be carried out, e.g. tests of malabsorption, jaundice, and pancreatic exocrine function.

Management
Alcohol should be avoided, and the patient should be advised to follow a low-fat diet because of malabsorption. Fat-soluble vitamins, calcium, and pancreatic enzymes are given. Insulin is required if the patient develops diabetes, and gallstones should be removed.

For recurrent attacks causing unremitting pain, pancreatectomy should be considered. Patients often have chronic persistent pain and can become addicted to opiates.

ACUTE VIRAL HEPATITIS

Hepatitis A
Epidemiology
Hepatitis A virus (HAV) is a member of the picornavirus family. The incubation period varies from 3–6 weeks. Transmission is by the faecal–oral route. Clinical disease with jaundice is uncommon in infants and young children, and the infection may go unnoticed. It may be acquired by eating partially cooked shellfish from estuaries contaminated by sewage.

Spread amongst drug smugglers by faecal contamination of condom-borne drugs has also been reported.

Serology
At the onset of symptoms, immunoglobulin (Ig)M anti-HAV antibody is present in serum. High titres persist for 3–12 months, so a positive test in a patient with acute hepatitis indicates recent acute infection. Previous infection, and therefore immunity, can be diagnosed by the presence of IgG anti-HAV without IgM anti-HAV.

Outcome
Relapses and cholestatic jaundice may occur but hepatitis A does not progress to chronic hepatitis.

Prevention and control
Prophylaxis can be obtained by immune serum immunoglobulin or active immunization. The latter induces higher levels of anti-HAV.

Hepatitis B
Epidemiology
The complete infectious virion (Dane particle) consists of the following:
- Hepatitis B surface antigen (HBsAg): the outer lipoprotein 'surface' envelope.
- Hepatitis B core antigen (HBcAg): the internal core, which surrounds the viral genome of DNA.
- Hepatitis B e antigen (HBeAg): a subunit of HBcAg; it can be detected in serum and is a useful marker of circulating virions and infectivity.

Transmission is parenteral through cutaneous and mucosal routes, across breaks in the skin or mucous membranes, and the mean incubation period is 75 days. In developed countries hepatitis B occurs sporadically.

Risk factors are male homosexuality, low socio-economic status, intravenous drug abuse, ethnic group, sexual promiscuity, residence in institutions, mental handicap, and employment in health professions. In endemic areas such as China and southern Africa, the disease is often acquired in childhood, and can occur by inoculation of infectious blood during the birth process. Infection is characteristically anicteric, asymptomatic, and chronic.

Serology
Following exposure to hepatitis B virus (HBV), HBsAg can be detected throughout the prodromal phase and is not usually cleared from the serum until convalescence. Other early markers include anti-HBc and HBeAg. A positive IgM anti-HBc test typically distinguishes acute from chronic hepatitis B. The presence of HBeAg implies high infectivity but it is often no longer detectable by the time the patient consults the physician.

The loss of HBeAg is a good prognostic sign, indicating that the patient will clear HBsAg and will not develop chronic infection. The disappearance of HBeAg is usually followed by the appearance of serum anti-HBe. Anti-HBs is the last marker to appear in serum.

Outcome

Acute infection may lead to fulminant hepatic failure. The disease may progress to chronic hepatitis, particularly in males and older people. It occurs in less than 5–10% of people with clinically apparent hepatitis B. Cirrhosis and hepatocellular carcinoma are complications of chronic hepatitis.

Prevention and control

Infection can be prevented by active immunization.

Hepatitis C
Epidemiology

Hepatitis C (HCV) is an RNA virus, and can be divided into many major types and subtypes. Transmission is most common after transfusion of whole blood products, and the mean incubation period is 9 weeks. There is a high prevalence in haemophiliacs, thalassaemics, haemodialysed patients, transplant recipients, and intravenous drug abusers.

Serology

Anti-HCV develops 1–3 months after the onset of clinical illness, and in some patients will not be detected for up to 1 year afterwards. Identification of the viral RNA in serum is possible using the polymerase chain reaction. HCV antigens cannot be detected in serum.

Outcome

The acute disease is often asymptomatic and leads to chronic infection in over 50% of patients. In about 20% of patients, cirrhosis may develop insidiously within 10 years, and patients may develop a clinical picture resembling autoimmune hepatitis. Systemic manifestations include cryoglobulinaemia, porphyria cutanea tarda, and membranous glomerulonephritis. Hepatocellular carcinoma is recognized with chronic infection.

Prevention and control

Blood bank screening for anti-HCV, and genetically engineered factor VIII preparations for haemophiliacs limit the occurrence of hepatitis C.

Hepatitis D
Epidemiology

Hepatitis D (delta) virus (HDV) is an RNA virus. The virion particle is encapsulated by the coat protein of HBV, i.e. HBsAg. Thus infection by HDV only occurs in patients affected by hepatitis B. Transmission is similar to HBV and the incubation period is 35 days. In developed countries, infection occurs mainly in drug addicts, haemophiliacs, and institutionalized persons.

Serology

IgM anti-HD, IgG anti-HD, and HDAg can be detected.

Outcome

The disease is not usually progressive but outbreaks of fulminant hepatitis caused by HBV plus HDV are described. Chronic infection can occur.

Prevention and control

The prevention of HBV infection will also prevent HDV infection as HDV cannot replicate in the absence of HBsAg.

Hepatitis E
Epidemiology

This RNA virus is transmitted via the faecal–oral route with a peak of epidemic infection 6–7 weeks after primary exposure and low secondary attack rate.

Serology

Serological tests are still in development.

Outcome

This is usually self limiting and progression to chronic hepatitis does not occur. There is a high mortality (20%

Prevention and control

This is dependent on high standards of public sanitatic and sewage elimination.

Clinical features

The clinical features of the various forms of acute viral hepatitis are similar. In the pre-icteric phase, the main symptoms include malaise, fatigue, listlessness, and lack of energy. Anorexia, nausea, and vomiting occur, which may be induced by fatty food. There is often a distaste for cigarettes. There may be right upper quadrant pain, change in bowel habit, myalgia, fever, and headaches.

In 10% of patients, acute hepatitis B may be accompanied by a serum sickness-like syndrome, which is characterized by low-grade fever, urticarial rash, and arthralgia.

The prodromal symptoms become less severe as jaundice appears. The urine darkens and the stools are pale. During the first week, the jaundice may deepen, and anorexia and fatigue may worsen in this period. There may be accompanying weight loss.

During recovery, symptoms gradually resolve although malaise and fatigue may persist and mild relapses can occur in 1–5% of patients. Exercise tolerance is generally depressed for some weeks; depression may be a prominent symptom.

Physical signs are usually minimal. Common findings are jaundice, hepatic tenderness, hepatomegaly, splenomegaly, and occasionally lymphadenopathy. Skin rashes may be noted.

Fulminant hepatitis leads to hepatic encephalopathy with severe jaundice, ascites, and oedema, and is usually accompanied by haemorrhage caused by coagulopathies. The disturbance of consciousness reflects a combination of hepatic coma, hypoglycaemia, and cerebral oedema.

Investigations

The following investigations are important in the patient with acute viral hepatitis:

- Liver enzymes, alanine aminotransferase (ALT), and aspartate aminotransferase: these are markedly elevated. Bilirubin concentration is also increased. During recovery, liver enzymes return to normal. A persistently raised ALT 6 months after the acute onset of hepatitis usually indicates progression of the disease.
- Prothrombin time: may be prolonged if fulminant hepatic failure occurs.
- Serum albumin concentrations: may fall slightly during the course of hepatitis, and serum globulin may rise.
- Hypoglycaemia: may occur with fulminant hepatic failure.
- Serum α-fetoprotein values: increased transiently in patients with acute viral hepatitis.

Management

Most patients can be cared for at home although hospital admissions may be required for diagnosis, social reasons, or if complications occur. Patients should be barrier nursed in hospital. All unnecessary drugs should be stopped. Paracetamol is the preferred analgesic, and is not hepatotoxic in low doses. Cholestyramine may alleviate itching.

For uncomplicated acute viral hepatitis, no specific treatment is required. Rest is recommended and alcohol should be avoided.

CHRONIC LIVER DISEASE

Chronic hepatitis

Clinically, chronic hepatitis is defined as any hepatitis lasting 6 months.

Chronic hepatitis may follow viral hepatitis, or develop with alcohol or drug use, e.g. isoniazid and methyldopa. Clinical features may include general malaise and lethargy, anorexia, hepatosplenomegaly, and signs of chronic liver disease. There may be remissions and exacerbations, and either complete recovery or progression to cirrhosis.

Management of chronic liver disease

The principal problems in severe chronic liver disease are the degree of hepatocellular failure and the complications of portal hypertension.

Management of variceal bleeds

This is described on p.255.

Ascites

Ascites is the presence of free fluid within the peritoneal cavity. Factors leading to the formation of ascites include salt and water retention as a result of cirrhosis, hypoalbuminaemia resulting in decreased plasma colloid pressure, portal hypertension, and increased hepatic lymph production.

Clinically, there may be abdominal distension, shifting dullness, and a fluid thrill, if the ascites is tense. Associated features include hernias, divarifaction of the recti, abdominal wall venous distension, ankle oedema, and distension of the neck veins.

Investigations include diagnostic paracentesis. The ascites is clear and yellow unless it is infected, when it appears turbid. If the tap is non-traumatic, blood signifies intra-abdominal malignancy. The protein content is usually less than 15 g per litre. Higher values indicate infection, hepatic venous obstruction, or malignancy. Fluid should be sent for cytology to look for malignant cells and for culture.

The patient should be on bed rest with restricted salt and fluids. The first choice of diuretic is spironolactone 100–200 mg per day. This can cause painful gynaecomastia in men, and amiloride can be substituted. If there is a poor response to spironolactone, frusemide is added. Fluid balance, weight, and U&Es should be monitored daily. Ascites can also be treated with therapeutic paracentesis and albumin infusion.

Overdiuresis may result in dehydration, uraemia, and hyponatraemia, and may precipitate hepatic encephalopathy, oliguria, and hepatorenal syndrome.

Hepatic encephalopathy

Encephalopathy can either be reversible and episodic, or lead to coma and death (Fig. 32.4). Liver failure results in diminished hepatic metabolism of substances derived from the gut, which can cause neurotoxicity. Clinical features include impaired conscious level, personality disturbances, inversion of the normal sleep pattern, slurred speech, constructional apraxia, flapping tremor (asterixis), hepatic fetor, brisk tendon reflexes, increased muscle tone and rigidity, and hyperventilation in deep coma.

Management

Initial treatment aims to correct or remove the precipitating cause. These may include electrolyte abnormalities, sepsis, hypovolaemia, hypoxia, bleeding, and constipation. Diuretics, sedatives, and opiates should be stopped, and intracranial pathology should be excluded, especially in alcoholic patients. CT scanning of the brain is useful to exclude subdural haematomas.

Measures should then be instituted to remove nitrogenous material, and bacteria from the bowel. The patient is put on a low-protein, high-calorie diet. In alcoholics, intravenous thiamine is given to treat possible Wernicke's encephalopathy.

Once over the acute phase, routine measures include lactulose to ensure two soft bowel motions per day. Protein intake is restricted, and the patient is educated to avoid precipitating causes, including alcohol. In difficult cases of chronic encephalopathy, a trial of

Grading of conscious level in hepatic encephalopathy	
Grade	**Features**
1	confusion, altered behaviour, psychometric abnormalities
2	drowsy, altered behaviour
3	stupor, obeys single commands, very confused
4	coma responding to painful stimuli
5	coma unresponsive to painful stimuli

Fig. 32.4 Grading of conscious level in hepatic encephalopathy.

bromocriptine is required. Recurrent acute-on-chronic encephalopathy is an indication for liver transplantation.

Haemochromatosis

Haemochromatosis is due to excess iron in the tissues.

Classification

Haemochromatosis may be classified as hereditary ('primary') or secondary.

Hereditary haemochromatosis is autosomal recessive. Secondary haemochromatosis may result from excessive iron administration, e.g. blood transfusion or iron tablets.

Clinical features

Affected organs are the liver, endocrine system, heart, and joints. Most patients are asymptomatic or have non-specific symptoms such as arthralgia and lethargy until the effect of iron overload becomes apparent in the fifth or sixth decade. Joints are involved by chondrocalcinosis.

In the early stages, pain and swelling of the second and third metacarpophalangeal joints is characteristic. There is slate-grey skin, due to melanin, and iron deposition. Symptoms include asthenia, abdominal pain, impotence, arthralgia, and amenorrhoea. Signs include hepatomegaly, splenomegaly, jaundice, and gynaecomastia. The disease may lead on to cirrhosis.

The prevalence varies from 1 in 200 to 1 in 2000, and men are 5–10 times more affected than women, indicating that environmental and genetic factors modify disease expression. Women are usually affected at a later age partly due to loss of iron during pregnancy or menstruation. Alcohol may exacerbate the problem by influencing iron metabolism and absorption.

Pathology

Total body iron is increased in haemochromatosis from 4 g up to as much as 60 g. There is cellular damage and fibrosis, leading to a rusty colour of the liver, pancreas, spleen, and abdominal lymph nodes. The liver is usually enlarged and may be cirrhotic. Iron is found in all liver cell types and in cardiac myocytes, the adrenals, pituitary, pancreas, and testes. Chondrocalcinosis in the joints is associated with synovial haemosiderin and loss of intra-articular space.

Investigations

- Serum iron is elevated and saturation of plasma transferrin is high. Serum iron is reduced in inflammatory conditions and is subject to diurnal variation.
- Serum ferritin is usually high.
- Definitive diagnosis of haemochromatosis depends on histology of liver biopsies.
- CT scanning and MRI can be used to detect increased tissue iron but are not routine.

Course and prognosis

Complications include diabetes mellitus, cirrhosis, heart disease with arryhthmias, and liver cancer.

Life expectancy and hepatic and cardiac function in primary haemochromatosis are improved by iron depletion. The 5-year survival rate increases from 18% to 66%. Removal of iron does not prevent the development of cancer in patients with established cirrhosis.

Venesection does not improve endocrine failure or joint disease.

Treatment

Patients should be venesected regularly, e.g. 500 mL weekly, until they develop a mild microcytic anaemia. Care is needed in patients with severe hepatic disease since vigorous bleeding may be complicated by hypoproteinaemia. Folate supplementation may be needed to optimize erythropoiesis. Seriously ill patients with overt cardiac haemochromatosis may require high-dose parenteral chelation therapy with desferrioxamine to reverse life-threatening disease.

Patients with established haemochromatosis should be investigated for cardiac involvement and pituitary as well as target organ endocrine failure, and replacement therapy should be instituted when necessary. Patients should be reviewed to monitor diabetic control, to care for joint disease, and to search for the development of complications, e.g. hepatocellular carcinoma.

Physical examination and screening tests to search for disordered iron metabolism should be carried out in family members to identify presymptomatic individuals so that iron can be removed before cirrhosis and other complications occur. Genetic studies may be of help.

Primary biliary cirrhosis

Primary biliary cirrhosis (PBC) is a disease of unknown aetiology primarily affecting the middle-sized intrahepatic bile ducts as a non-suppurative, destructive cholangitis leading to bile duct damage, cholestasis, fibrosis, cirrhosis, and death from liver failure. It is more common in Europe than Africa and Asia with a prevalence of 3–35/100 000 and an incidence of 6–15/million/year.

Clinical features

The disease is nine times more common in women. It usually presents in middle age with lethargy and pruritus. Pigmentation and xanthomata may be present, jaundice may develop, and portal hypertension may lead to ascites or oesophageal varices. There may be stigmata of chronic liver disease. About 80% have hepatomegaly at presentation, and 50% have splenomegaly. The patient may be asymptomatic at presentation, or present with liver failure.

The average life expectancy is 10 years from diagnosis. If the serum bilirubin is greater than 180 μmol/L, the life expectancy is 18 months.

PBC is associated with autoimmune conditions, e.g. Sjögren's syndrome, thyroid disease, Addison's disease, Raynaud's syndrome, systemic sclerosis, and coeliac disease. It is also associated with malabsorption, extrahepatic malignancies, particularly of the breast, and hepatocellular carcinoma.

Investigations

LFTs show an obstructive pattern with elevated serum alkaline phosphatase and gamma-glutamyl transpeptidase (GGT). As the disease progresses, serum bilirubin rises.

With regard to immunology, HLA-B8 and C4B2 are associated with a threefold increase in the risk of PBC. Serum immunoglobulins are raised, especially immunoglobulinM. Antimitochondrial antibody is positive in about 90%.

Ultrasound of the liver is important to exclude obstruction. It can also show evidence of portal hypertension and splenomegaly.

Histology of the liver will confirm the diagnosis. Initially there is asymmetrical destruction of middle-sized bile ducts and surrounding lymphocytic infiltrate. Granulomas may be present. Increasing fibrosis, and eventually cirrhosis, develops.

Differential diagnosis
This includes autoimmune hepatitis, sarcoidosis, and drug reactions, e.g. phenothiazines.

Treatment
Immunosuppressive agents may have a small effect. Bile salts, e.g. ursodeoxycholic acid, may help with cholestasis. Antifibrotic agents, e.g. colchicine, may be of help. Liver transplantation is indicated for intractable symptoms or end-stage disease.

Itching can be treated with cholestyramine. Alternatives include enzyme inducers, e.g. phenobarbitone, and opiate antagonists, e.g. naloxone or propofol. Patients with jaundice should receive supplementation with fat-soluble vitamins A, D, and K. Diarrhoea is treated with a low-fat diet and pancreatic supplements.

Hepatolenticular degeneration (Wilson's disease)
This is an autosomal recessive disorder of copper metabolism leading to deposition of copper in the following:
- Liver: cirrhosis with its ensuing complications.
- Basal ganglia: tremor and choreoathetosis.
- Cerebrum: dementia and fits.
- Eyes: Kayser–Fleischer rings (a brown pigmentation of the periphery of the iris).
- Renal tubules: renal tubular acidosis.
- Bones: osteoporosis and osteoarthritis.
- Red blood cells: haemolytic anaemia.

Clinical features are usually due to hepatic or CNS involvement.

Investigations
There is a high concentration of copper in the blood, and low caeruloplasmin, the copper binding protein.

Management
The dietary intake of copper should be reduced, and penicillamine is given to aid the elimination of copper ions. Regular blood counts are mandatory due to potential agranulocytosis and thrombocytopenia with treatment. Other side effects include oedema, proteinuria, haematuria, rashes, loss of taste, and muscle weakness. Relatives should be screened. The prognosis is generally good.

Alcoholic liver disease
Men who drink over 80 g of alcohol per day, or women who drink over 40 g per day have a significant risk of developing cirrhosis. However, cirrhosis is not inevitable. Only 10–20% of chronic alcoholics develop cirrhosis even though they drink the same amount of alcohol over the same period as other alcoholics. Risk factors for developing cirrhosis include genetics, gender (women develop alcoholic hepatitis and cirrhosis younger, and after less intake, than men), nutrition (alcohol is better tolerated under optimal dietary conditions), and a synergistic effect with hepatotropic viruses.

Pathology
Initially there are fatty changes within the liver. With alcoholic hepatitis, there is liver cell necrosis and an inflammatory reaction. Cells contain alcoholic hyaline or Mallory's bodies. Later there is deposition of collagen around the central veins, which may spread to the portal tracts.

Cirrhosis may result, which is initially micronodular. Extensive fibrosis contributes to the development of portal hypertension. With continued cell necrosis and regeneration, the cirrhosis may progress to a macronodular pattern.

Clinical features
The patient may initially be asymptomatic. With alcoholic hepatitis, there may be fatigue, anorexia, nausea, and weight loss. There may be signs of chronic liver disease (Chapter 10). Ascites may develop and complicating hypoglycaemia can precipitate coma.

Hepatic decompensation leads to encephalopathy and liver failure, and can be precipitated by the factors listed in Fig. 32.5.

With advanced cirrhosis, there may be signs of malnutrition, ascites, encephalopathy, and a tendency to bleed. Signs include bilateral parotid enlargement, palmar erythema, Dupuytren's contractures, and multiple spider naevi. Men develop gynaecomastia and testicular atrophy. Portal hypertension develops, leading to splenomegaly and distended abdominal wall veins.

There may be signs of alcohol damage in other organs, e.g. peripheral neuropathy, cardiomyopathy, proximal myopathy, or pancreatitis.

Investigations

The mean corpuscular volume (MCV) and GGT are sensitive indices of alcohol ingestion. Important variables for predicting outcome include the prothrombin time, serum albumin, serum bilirubin, and haemoglobin.

Ultrasound will demonstrate fatty liver, and histology of liver biopsy will show the pathological changes discussed above.

Management

Patients should abstain from alcohol. General measures for the management of chronic liver disease should be instigated. Patients may need nutritional support including vitamins B and C.

Prognosis

Fatty liver alone carries a good prognosis if the patient abstains from alcohol. If the patient is encephalopathic and malnourished, the mortality is up to 50%. Ascites, peripheral oedema, persistent jaundice, uraemia, and the presence of collateral circulation are unfavourable prognostic signs.

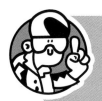

If you see a triad of high MCV, high GGT and low urea, think about excessive alcohol intake.

MISCELLANEOUS GASTROINTESTINAL DISORDERS

Gastro-oesophageal reflux disease

Reflux of gastric or duodenal contents into the oesophagus causes heartburn and pain often radiating to the back which is worse on stooping or lying down, and with hot drinks. There may be bleeding from the oesophagus resulting in anaemia. There may be oesophageal ulceration and stricture formation. Barrett's ulcer is a premalignant chronic peptic ulceration of the lower oesophagus, and may lead to dysphagia, vomiting, and haematemesis.

Predisposing factors include conditions that raise intra-abdominal pressure, e.g. tight clothes and obesity, a lax lower oesophageal sphincter, e.g. with smoking and pregnancy, and drugs, e.g. tricyclic antidepressants and anticholinergic agents.

Management

Patients should avoid tight clothes, stop smoking, avoid aggravating foods, and lose weight if overweight. Patients should be advised to prop themselves up in bed with pillows and put a block under the end of the bed to avoid slipping down. Drug treatment is initially with antacids or alginates, which coat the oesophagus. Metoclopramide will increase the tone of the lower oesophageal sphincter and relieves nausea. H_2-receptor antagonists are prescribed for severe symptoms. Proton pump inhibitors are the treatment of choice for erosive oesophagitis. Anaemia should be investigated and managed appropriately.

Irritable bowel syndrome

Irritable bowel syndrome is the commonest diagnosis made in GI clinics, although there is no accepted definition. It occurs mainly in young women. There is intermittent colicky abdominal pain which is relieved

---

Factors that can precipitate hepatic decompensation

- constipation
- vomiting and diarrhoea
- GI bleeding
- intercurrent infection
- alcohol
- morphine
- surgery
- electrolyte imbalance

Fig. 32.5 Factors that can precipitate hepatic decompensation.

by bowel action, diarrhoea or frequent passage of small amounts of stool, and bloating. The diarrhoea may alternate with periods of constipation. Some people have a sense of incomplete evacuation or 'rectal dissatisfaction'. Symptoms may be precipitated by certain foods, drugs, e.g. antibiotics or stress.

Investigation
The diagnosis is one of exclusion. It is important not to miss more serious disease, e.g. inflammatory bowel disease or malignancy. It is prudent to check the FBC and erythrocyte sedimentation rate, faecal occult blood, and perform a sigmoidoscopy. Older patients, or patients in whom colonic carcinoma is suspected, warrant a barium enema.

Treatment
Symptoms may improve with a high-fibre diet, with bran or with other agents which increase stool bulk. Specific aggravating foods should be avoided. In some patients there may be important psychological aggravating factors which respond to reassurance. Antimotility drugs such as loperamide may relieve diarrhoea, and antispasmodic drugs, e.g. mebeverine 135 mg t.d.s., may relieve pain. Opioids with a central action such as codeine are best avoided because of the risk of dependence.

Pseudomembranous colitis
Pseudomembranous colitis is caused by colonization of the colon with *Clostridium difficile*, which produces toxins. It usually follows antibiotic therapy and should be suspected in patients in hospital who develop diarrhoea after a period of antibiotics. It is usually of acute onset but may run a chronic course. The most frequently implicated antibiotic is clindamycin but few antibiotics are free of this side effect. Clinical features include diarrhoea, fever and abdominal cramps.

Diagnosis
Diagnosis is by identification of the toxin in stool specimens. Sigmoidoscopy reveals an erythematous, ulcerated mucosa, which is covered by a membrane. The appearances are not however essential for the diagnosis.

Management
Suspected antibiotics should be stopped and patients should be isolated. Oral vancomycin or metronidazole are used as specific treatments.

Diverticular disease
A diverticulum is an outpouching of the wall of the gut. Diverticula can occur anywhere in the gut but are most common in the colon, especially the sigmoid colon. Diverticulosis implies the presence of diverticula, and diverticulitis implies that there is inflammation within a diverticulum. They are due to high intracolonic pressure with weakness of the colonic wall. The mucosa therefore herniates through the muscle layers of the gut. The incidence increases with age and affects up to a third of the population although most people are asymptomatic. It is more common in women then men.

Clinical features
There may be colicky left-sided abdominal pain and tenderness, nausea, and flatulence. The pain may be relieved with defecation and there may be a change in bowel habit with constipation or diarrhoea. With diverticulitis, pain is more severe, and the patient is pyrexial. Diverticula may perforate and lead to localized or generalized peritonitis or fistula formation. Fistulae may communicate between the colon and bladder (vesicocolic fistula) leading to pneumaturia and recurrent urinary tract infection. They may also form between the colon and vagina or small bowel. Rectal bleeding may occur and is usually sudden and painless. Subacute obstruction may occur due to stricture formation.

Management
In acute diverticulitis, treatment is with bed rest, analgesia, and antibiotics. The patient may have to be kept nil by mouth and given intravenous fluids. Abscesses may need to be drained, and peritonitis following perforation or obstruction may necessitate resection and colostomy. Patients with profuse rectal bleeding may require transfusion and colonic resection. Treatment of fistulae is surgical.

For diverticulosis, a high-fibre diet is recommended, and bran supplements and bulk-forming agents can be prescribed. Antispasmodics may provide symptomatic relief when colic is a problem. Drugs which slow intestinal motility, e.g. codeine and loperamide, could exacerbate symptoms and are contraindicated.

GLOMERULAR DISEASE

Glomerular disease is often found to be confusing because there is a poor correlation between the clinical findings and the histology. Systemic disorders that can involve the glomerulus are listed in Fig. 33.1.

Clinical features

Clinical features of glomerular disease include the following:

- Proteinuria (see also Chapter 13): up to 150 mg of proteinuria daily is normal but this may increase in pregnancy, febrile states, and following exercise. It may be preglomerular, as in the overproduction of small-sized proteins which pass freely across the glomerular basement membrane, e.g. Bence Jones protein in myeloma. It may be postglomerular with tubular damage. Gross proteinuria, which leads to hypoalbuminaemia and oedema, is called *nephrotic syndrome.*
- Haematuria.
- Raised blood urea or creatinine.
- *Nephritic syndrome*: this is a combination of proteinuria, haematuria and impaired renal function, often in association with oliguria and hypertension.

The causes of secondary nephrotic syndrome, i.e. not of direct renal origin, are DAVID: diabetes mellitus, amyloidosis, vasculitis, infections, and drugs.

Most patients present with nephrotic syndrome, asymptomatic proteinuria, or haematuria. Presentation with oliguria or a nephritic syndrome is less common.

History

The history should include asking about haematuria and proteinuria (e.g. is there frothy urine?). There may also be a history of previous nephritis. Ask about associated systemic diseases, e.g. arthritis, diabetes, hypertension or evidence of malignancy. A full drug history should be taken including exposure to toxins.

Hearing impairment is present in Alport's syndrome, and there may be a family history of renal disease. Ask about recent upper respiratory tract infections and valvular heart disease.

Consequences of glomerular dysfunction

The consequences of glomerular dysfunction include the following:

- Iron deficiency secondary to haematuria in a patient with limited iron reserves.
- Protein loss. The absolute level of plasma albumin necessary to induce oedema varies from patient to patient.
- Hypovolaemia resulting in postural hypotension or prerenal failure.
- Altered drug metabolism, usually secondary to hypoalbuminaemia, leading to reduced binding and increased circulating levels of free drug.

Systemic disorders that can involve the glomerulus
• diabetes • amyloidosis • systemic lupus erythematosus • rheumatoid arthritis • ankylosing spondylitis • neoplasia • myeloma • vasculitic syndromes • liver disease • sarcoidosis • partial lipodystrophy

Fig. 33.1 Systemic disorders that can involve the glomerulus.

- Hyperlipoproteinaemia and hypercholesterolaemia.
- Hypercoagulability.
- Cardiovascular disease, including increased risk of venous and arterial thrombosis.
- Changes in serum immunoglobulins: IgG often falls and IgM is often raised in many patients with severe proteinuria. In IgA nephropathy up to 50% of patients have abnormally high serum IgA levels.
- Hormonal changes, including low circulating levels of 25-hydroxycalciferol and 1,25-dihydroxy-cholecalciferol. This results in decreased bone mobilization and gut absorption of calcium, and hence hypocalcaemia.
- Increased risk of infection.
- Pancreatitis precipitated by high serum triglyceride levels.

Investigations

The following investigations are important in the patient with glomerular disease:

- Plasma albumin and creatinine, creatinine clearance, and 24-hour urinary protein excretion serve as a baseline, and can be used to monitor progress and response to treatment.
- Urine microscopy for red blood cell casts indicating glomerular disease.
- Blood glucose: to exclude diabetes mellitus (DM).
- Anti-DNA and antinuclear antibodies in systemic lupus erythematosus (SLE).
- Antiglomerular basement membrane (anti-GBM) antibodies for the diagnosis of anti-GBM disease.
- Hepatitis B surface antigen to exclude hepatitis B.
- Tests for rheumatoid arthritis, e.g. Rose–Waaler and Latex tests.
- Serum immunoelectrophoresis to exclude myeloma.
- Antineutrophil cytoplasmic antibodies are often present in microscopic polyarteritis and Wegener's granulomatosis.
- Cryoglobulins.
- Serological tests for syphilis.
- Serum complement levels: C3 may be low in postinfectious glomerulonephropathy, mesangiocapillary glomerulonephropathy, and SLE; C4 may be depleted in SLE and mesangiocapillary glomerulonephropathy.
- Chest X-ray: this may show pulmonary oedema, malignancy, pulmonary haemorrhage, and cavitation in Wegener's granulomatosis.

Histological classification, treatment, and prognosis

The terms 'focal' and 'diffuse' refer to the kidney as a whole, i.e. some or all of the glomeruli are involved. 'Segmental' and 'global' refer to individual glomeruli, i.e part or all of each glomerulus is involved. As there is clinical overlap, the diagnosis is confirmed only after renal biopsy. Biopsies should not be taken if there is only one functioning kidney, bilateral small kidneys, or if there is a bleeding disorder.

General principles of management

In glomerulonephritis with a specific aetiology, specific action can be taken, e.g. withdrawal of an offending drug, or treatment of a malignancy or infection. Adequate protein and calorie intake is most important. Potent acting loop diuretics may be needed to produce natiuresis and reduce oedema. It may be necessary to give an infusion of salt-poor albumin to maintain plasma volume at the same time.

Patients tend to have hyperlipidaemia and are at high cardiovascular risk. If there is any evidence of coronary artery disease, treatment with a statin should be started. Hypertension should be controlled and nephrotoxic agents should be stopped. If renal function does not improve, treatment of chronic renal failure should be introduced.

Minimal change nephropathy

This is most common in boys under 5 years of age, and accounts for 90% of children in the UK who present with nephrotic syndrome. Renal biopsy is therefore not always indicated. Light microscopy is normal but electron microscopy reveals retraction and fusion of the epithelial foot processes at the glomerular basement membrane. There are no deposits of immunoglobulin or complement on immunofluorescence. There is usually severe and selective proteinuria, which remits with corticosteroid therapy. In patients with frequently relapsing disease, a course of cyclophosphamide for a maximum of 8 weeks can be considered.

Focal and segmental glomerulosclerosis

Histology shows a proliferation of sclerotic lesions but electron microscopy and immunofluorescence findings are variable. Nephrotic syndrome is the usual presentation and progressive renal impairrment occurs in 80–90% of patients. It is associated with SLE, polyarteritis nodosa (PAN), subacute bacterial endocarditis, Henoch–Schönlein purpura, and Wegener's granulomatosis.

In patients not responsive to steroids, the 5-year renal survival is about 50%.

Diffuse mesangial proliferation

This is associated with IgA deposition (Berger's disease) seen on immunofluorescence, and cellular proliferation within the glomerular mesangium. It usually presents with intermittent haematuria in the second and third decades of life. There may be an associated upper respiratory tract or gut infection.

It is also associated with SLE, cirrhosis, hepatitis B infection and Henoch–Schönlein purpura. About a third of patients will eventually require dialysis or transplantation.

Membranous nephropathy

This is most common in adults with a peak age at onset of 40–50 years. It may be idiopathic with strong human lymphocyte antigen associations, or may occur in association with drugs such as gold and penicillamine, neoplasms, or infections such as hepatitis B. Patients usually present with proteinuria or nephrotic syndrome.

Histologically there is thickening of the glomerular wall, with subepithelial deposits of antigen–antibody complexes visible on electron microscopy. Immunofluorescence shows deposition of IgG and C3. About a third of patients improve spontaneously, a third have persistent proteinuria, and a third progress to renal failure. Women and children have a better prognosis than men. When renal function is declining quickly, corticosteroids and azathiaprine may be effective.

Mesangiocapillary glomerulonephritis

This presents with haematuria, proteinuria, nephrotic syndrome, or renal impairment. There appears to be a layer of tissue beneath the glomerular basement membrane giving it a double contour on light microscopy. In type I, there may be subendothelial extension of mesangial matrix and cells containing immune deposits and C3, and in type II or dense deposit disease, there may be electron dense material incorporated into the membrane.

Overall, type I lesions have a 50% 5-year survival, and type II is generally regarded as having a worse outcome.

Diffuse proliferative glomerulonephritis

This often occurs in association with acute infections, classically with streptococcus. It often heals completely after an acute nephritic illness. Light microscopy shows hypercellular glomerular tufts with proliferation of mesangial cells which have a neutrophilic and mononuclear cell infiltrate. Complexes containing IgG can be seen on immunofluorescence along the glomerular basement membrane and in the mesangium.

Crescentic glomerulonephritis

This is usually rapidly progressive, and presents with haematuria, oliguria, and hypertension. It results from the proliferation of epithelial cells. It may occur in SLE, anti-GBM disease, and vasculitides, but often occurs in the absence of underlying disease. The prognosis is usually poor but it is potentially curable if treatment is instituted sufficiently early.

Antiglomerular basement membrane disease

There is the even and linear deposition of IgG along the glomerular basement membrane, with a variable inflammatory response. At its most destructive, this produces a neutrophilic cell infiltrate, heavy fibrin deposition, and extensive epithelial crescent formation.

Goodpasture's syndrome is anti-GBM disease associated with pulmonary haemorrhage. Note, however, that patients with SLE, Henoch–Schönlein purpura, Wegener's granulomatosis, and microscopic polyarteritis can also have pulmonary haemorrhage. Goodpasture's syndrome is strongly associated with cigarette smoking.

Treatment with plasma exchange and immunosuppressive drugs remove and suppress the antibody, together with the reversal of its renal and pulmonary effects.

Wegener's granulomatosis and microscopic polyarteritis

The incidence of these uncommon conditions appears to be increasing. They are strongly associated with circulating antibody directed at cytoplasmic components of normal neutrophils. Early recognition is important as treatment may prevent progression.

Combination of prednisolone and immunosuppressive therapy produces a survival of 80% at 5 years.

ACUTE RENAL FAILURE

Acute renal failure (ARF) is a rapid decline in glomerular filtration rate (GFR) sufficient to cause uraemia. Oliguria (below 15 mL per hour) is often a feature, although 'non-oliguric' renal failure can also occur, particularly in patients with severe burns, nephrotoxic damage, or patients with oliguric renal failure that has been converted to non-oliguric renal failure by aggressive management with fluids, diuretics, and other agents.

Aetiology
It is useful to classify ARF into prerenal, renal, and postrenal causes (Fig. 33.2). However, the aetiology is often multifactorial. For example, in postsurgical ARF, fluid depletion, systemic infection, and nephrotoxic drugs may all play a role. ARF may also complicate chronic renal failure.

Clinical features
The clinical features depend on whether there is pre-existing chronic renal impairment, and whether the cause is pre-, intrinsic-, or post-renal failure. A full history should be taken focusing on previous renal disease, a history of hypertension or analgesic abuse, symptoms of prostatism, recent diarrhoea, vomiting or blood loss, and recent operations.

Symptoms of renal failure include:
- Thirst.
- Polyuria.
- Nocturia.
- Anorexia.
- Nausea and vomiting.
- Fatigue.
- Itching.
- Confusion.
- Oliguria.
- Dehydration.
- Signs of volume overload, e.g. pulmonary oedema, and ankle or sacral oedema with nephrotic syndrome.
- Signs of volume depletion, e.g. postural hypotension, a rapid small volume pulse, reduced tissue turgor.

The examination should focus on both the cause and consequences of the renal failure. The patient may have a yellow-brown pallor of uraemia, and brown lines at the ends of the finger nails. If acidotic, there is

Causes of acute renal failure	
prerenal failure (ischaemic)	extracellular volume loss: GI loss (e.g. severe diarrhoea or vomiting), urinary loss (polyuria with salt-losing kidneys), burns intravascular volume loss or redistribution: sepsis, haemorrhage (e.g. postpartum or at operation), hypoalbuminaemia decreased cardiac output: heart failure (e.g. postmyocardial infarction), cardiac tamponade, cardiac surgery miscellaneous: hypercalcaemia, hepatorenal syndrome, rhabdomyolysis
renal failure (intrinsic)	postischaemic acute tubular necrosis: shock, trauma, sepsis, hypoxia nephrotoxic acute tubular necrosis: antibiotics, analgesics, contrast media, heavy metals, solvents, proteins glomerulonephritis: acute diffuse proliferative nephritis acute pyelonephritis acute interstitial nephritis: antibiotics, analgesics, leptospirosis, *Legionella*, viral infections vasculitis: polyarteritis intratubular obstruction: myeloma (Bence–Jones protein), urate coagulopathies: acute cortical necrosis, haemolytic uraemic syndrome, thrombotic thrombocytopoenic purpura, postpartum renal failure miscellaneous: malignant hypertension
postrenal failure	renal tract obstruction: stones, tumour (prostatic or pelvic), prostatic hypertrophy, surgical mishap (e.g. accidental ligation of ureters), periureteric fibrosis, bladder dysfunction major vessel occlusion: renal artery thrombosis, renal vein thrombosis

Fig. 33.2 Causes of acute renal failure. (GI, gastrointestinal.)

deep sighing (Kussmaul's) respiration. There may be palpable kidneys with polycystic kidney disease or hydronephrosis. There will be a palpable bladder with outflow obstruction.

Pericarditis occurs in advanced uraemia, and twitching, hiccoughs, and uraemic frost also occur late. Check the blood pressure (are there other signs of malignant hypertension, and/or is there a postural drop suggesting volume depletion?) and look for bruising.

Perform a rectal examination for prostatic hypertrophy or carcinoma, and a vaginal examination for pelvic masses.

Investigations

Urea, creatinine, and electrolytes should be assessed. This will confirm renal impairment and serve as a useful baseline for monitoring the patient's progress. If the patient is acidotic, serum bicarbonate will be low. It is crucial to check the potassium as hyperkalaemia can be life threatening, and immediate measures to lower the potassium need to be taken.

Urine should be sent for microscopy, culture, and sensitivity. In patients with acute tubular necrosis there will be casts, whereas these are absent in prerenal failure.

Patients with established acute tubular necrosis cannot concentrate the urine or conserve sodium. Consequently urinary sodium is usually over 20 mmol/L; the urine is dilute (osmolality below 310 mmol/L) with a urine/plasma osmolality ratio below 1.1:1; and urinary urea is below 150 mmol/L with a urine/plasma urea ratio below 3:1.

Conversely, in prerenal failure, urinary sodium is below 20 mmol/L; the urine is concentrated (osmolality over 450 mmol/L) with a urine/plasma osmolality ratio over 1.5:1; and urinary urea is over 330 mmol/L with a urine/plasma urea ratio over 8:1.

In addition, the following investigations are important in the patient with ARF:

Full blood count: a normochromic normocytic anaemia suggests pre-existing chronic renal impairment.

Clotting screen for coagulopathies.

Urine for Bence–Jones protein; serum immunoglobulins and electrophoresis.

Blood cultures to look for infection.

Electrocardiogram (ECG) for the precipitating cause, e.g. myocardial infarction, or complications such as pericarditis or hyperkalaemia.

- Abdominal X-ray: look for renal size; normal kidneys are 13 ± 2 cm; small kidneys suggest pre-existing renal disease; the kidneys may be large in polycystic disease; stones in the renal tract may be visible.
- Abdominal ultrasound will demonstrate kidney size, stones, and dilatation of the pelvicalyceal system in outflow obstruction.
- Isotope renography will demonstrate kidney function.

Management

Immediate thoughts should be to correct hypovolaemia, exclude obstruction, and assess the presence of previous intrinsic renal disease. Fluids should be replaced and electrolytes should be corrected quickly. Monitoring with a central venous pressure line is essential for proper assessment of fluid balance. Appropriate antibiotics should be given for septicaemia or other infections. Bilateral nephrostomy tubes will relieve obstruction. Surgery can then be performed later.

If there is established acute tubular acidosis, intravenous fluids may still be needed. Vasoactive agents, e.g. dopamine and dobutamine, may be necessary to achieve a blood pressure which is appropriate for the patient's age and history. Correction of hypoxia and acidosis may also improve cardiac and renal function.

If oliguria persists after adequate circulation is established, or if the patient has established renal failure and is volume overloaded, intravenous frusemide should be given, either as slow boluses or as an intravenous infusion. Strict fluid balance should be kept with daily weights and regular assessment of fluid, electrolyte, and nutritional requirements. In general, patients should be given 500 ml of fluid per 24 hours as well as the volume of urine output from the previous 24 hours. In patients with fluid retention a weight loss of 0–1 kg per day should be aimed for.

Note, however, that fluid overload may occur in patients without any change in weight, as negative nutritional balance may cause a loss of 1–2 kg per day. Careful examination is necessary to detect fluid accumulation, which should be counteracted by further sodium and water restriction. Patients should be on a low-protein, high-carbohydrate diet. In many cases, the patient's appetite is poor and calorie supplements may be required.

279

Treatment of hyperkalaemia

This may be life threatening and so the reduction of potassium should be the top priority if it is over 7 mmol/L, particularly if ECG changes are present. These ECG changes can be reversed temporarily by boluses of calcium chloride of 20–40 mmol/L. The patient should also be on a cardiac monitor.

Potassium should be redistributed intracellularly by the correction of acidosis with sodium bicarbonate 100–150 mmol/L and the administration of glucose 50–100 mg. Insulin may be necessary to control hyperglycaemia. It is usually necessary to give these drugs in small volumes in order to avoid fluid overload. Polystyrene sulphonate resin 15 g 6 hourly orally or as an enema (30 g) will maintain a low potassium.

Do not give calcium chloride i.v. through the same canula as sodium bicarbonate—it forms chalk!

Indications for dialysis in renal failure

Indications for dialysis in renal failure are as follows:
- Persistent hyperkalaemia, e.g. serum potassium above 6.5 mmol/L.
- Severe acidosis, e.g. bicarbonate below 15 mmol/L.
- Symptomatic uraemia, e.g. confusion and hiccoughs.
- Pericarditis.
- Pulmonary oedema or progressive fluid retention.

Prognosis

The prognosis of patients with ARF depends on the cause. Patients with non-oliguric ARF have a lower mortality. A particularly high mortality is found in older patients and those who have severe burns, severe pancreatitis, hepatorenal syndrome, intra-abdominal sepsis, pre-existing cardiovascular disease, and patients with serious complications, such as pulmonary infection. Those patients who recover generally return to health and independent living, and this justifies an aggressive approach to treatment.

CHRONIC RENAL FAILURE

Chronic renal failure is a reduction in GFR to below around 15 mL per minute. Features that suggest chronic rather than acute renal failure include a long history of urinary symptoms and chronic ill health, anaemia, osteodystrophy, and small kidneys.

Causes

Finding the cause of renal failure is important because some are reversible and treatment can delay or prevent progression to end-stage renal failure (ESRF). In addition the prognosis can be better determined, risks of rejection with renal transplantation can be assessed, and diagnosis of familial disease may benefit other members of the family by early diagnosis, treatment, and genetic counselling. Common causes include the following:
- Glomerulonephritis: the commonest single cause of ESRF accounting for more than a third of cases.
- Infection: mainly due to obstruction or vesicoureteric reflux.
- Obstruction: most cases are due to prostatic hypertrophy and stones.
- Renovascular causes: renovascular atheroma and consequent ischaemia is becoming increasingly recognized reflecting the ageing population. Risk factors include age, a history of cardiac, cerebral or peripheral vascular disease, smoking, hypertension and diabetes.
- Drugs: analgesic nephropathy should be considered in patients with chronic painful conditions, but may also be taken for 'social' reasons. Non-steroidal anti-inflammatory drugs (NSAIDs) can cause ESRF.
- Interstitial nephritis: this may be idiopathic but also secondary to NSAIDs and chronic diuretic therapy with frusemide.
- DM: both insulin-dependent and non-insulin-dependent diabetes can lead to ESRF.
- Hypertension: the incidence of ESRF seems to be decreasing due to better identification and treatment of hypertension. It is more common in the black population.
- Inherited disease: the two most common conditions are polycystic kidney disease and Alport's disease.
- Idiopathic causes.
- Less common causes are amyloidosis, myeloma, SLE, PAN, gout, hypercalcaemia, and retroperitoneal fibrosis.

Clinical features

These are outlined in the features of ARF.

Specific questions in the history should include symptoms of prostatism, previous urinary tract infections, a drug history (especially of analgesics), and family history (polycystic kidneys?).

There may be signs of anaemia and brown lines on the finger nails. The skin is classically 'lemon yellow' and there may be bruising. There may be a pericardial rub or signs of neuropathy, and hyperventilation secondary to acidosis may be present. The blood pressure may be elevated. Examine for signs of obstruction, e.g. a palpable bladder, and perform a rectal examination for prostatic hypertrophy or pelvic masses. The kidneys are large in polycystic disease.

Investigations

The following are important investigations in the patient with chronic renal failure:

- Urine: microscopy for casts and culture to exclude infection. Urinary electrolytes and osmolality should be determined. 24-hour urinary protein and creatinine clearance should be measured.
- Urea and electrolytes will help determine the degree of renal dysfunction and acidosis. Serum calcium may be low secondary to hyperphosphataemia or acquired vitamin D resistance. The acidosis protects the patient from tetany by increasing the ionized portion of the reduced calcium. Serum phosphate is high and plasma uric acid is often raised although clinical gout is uncommon.
  A random blood glucose should be requested to exclude diabetes. Other investigations include those to elucidate an underlying cause for the renal failure such as a myeloma screen.
  Plain abdominal film will define kidney size, and ultrasound will exclude obstruction. X-rays of the chest and hands may show evidence of secondary hyperparathyroidism.

- Renal biopsy should be considered once prerenal and postrenal disease have been excluded, especially if renal size is normal suggesting more acute disease.

Management

The aims of treatment are to prevent further deterioration in renal function, and to prevent or treat the complications of renal failure. Renal function should be monitored with reciprocal plots of serum creatinine (Fig. 33.3). Whenever an abrupt decline or acceleration in the slope is noted, its cause must be determined and rectified.

Possible causes include uncontrolled hypertension, infection, hypovolaemia or fluid overload, urinary tract obstruction, drugs, and pregnancy. Always question whether the drugs that the patient is on are necessary, in particular NSAIDs, and angiotensin-converting enzyme (ACE) inhibitors in patients with renovascular disease. Other drugs to avoid include tetracycline, polymyxin, nitrofurantoin, aminoglycosides, and potassium-sparing diuretics, e.g. amiloride and spironolactone.

Prevention of decline in renal function

Hypertension should be tightly controlled (to about 130/85 mmHg).

Restriction of dietary phosphate intake may delay the decline in renal function, although it is difficult to

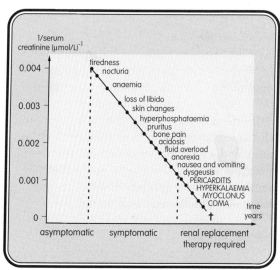

Fig. 33.3 Inverse creatinine plot with typical progressive onset of the non-specific symptoms and signs of chronic renal failure.

More than 50% of glomeruli may be lost before the U&Es become abnormal

achieve as it is often accompanied by a concomitant decrease in calcium intake, which can accelerate the development of renal osteodystrophy.

A low-protein diet may also reduce the decline in renal function and can reduce the symptoms of uraemia. Protein intake is reduced from a normal 85 g per day to 40 g per day. If protein intake is lowered further, essential amino acids should be added and the overall calorie intake should be high enough to suppress the breakdown of body protein using carbohydrate supplements if necessary. Total serum protein, albumin, transferrin, vitamin B_{12}, and red blood cell folate levels should be estimated at regular intervals.

Potassium restriction may be necessary to prevent hyperkalaemia, and sodium restriction to prevent fluid retention.

ACE inhibitors slow down the decline in renal function associated with diabetic nephropathy.

Prevention of complications

Hypertension
Regular measurements of blood pressure are necessary as the onset of hypertension is insidious. Control of hypertension can slow the deterioration of renal function and prevent cardiovascular complications. High doses of frusemide are often required and, in resistant cases, minoxidil is a potent antihypertensive agent. All classes of antihypertensives may be used but ACE inhibitors are contraindicated in renal artery stenosis.

Renal osteodystrophy
Renal osteodystrophy is due to a combination of disturbed vitamin D metabolism and secondary hyperparathyroidism. Serum alkaline phosphatase is raised. Management is by the normalization of serum phosphate by diet and oral phosphate-binding agents such as calcium carbonate. Serum calcium should be maintained in the normal range with synthetic vitamin D analogues. Frequent monitoring of serum calcium is required for the early detection of hypercalcaemia, which will further decrease renal function.

Systemic acidosis
Systemic acidosis accompanies declining renal function and may contribute to increased potassium levels. Sodium bicarbonate supplements will help to maintain serum bicarbonate levels within the normal range.

Anaemia
In renal failure there is a normochromic normocytic anaemia. Evidence of blood loss should be sought if there is an inappropriately low haemoglobin. Vitamin B_{12} and folate deficiency should be corrected with diet and supplements if needed. Recombinant human erythropoietin will increase the haemoglobin and improve symptoms attributable to anaemia, but it can cause hypertension and convulsions.

Nausea and vomiting
This often responds to protein restriction or antiemetics, e.g. metaclopramide. Dialysis should be considered if these measures are unsuccessful.

Pruritus
This can lead to excoriation of the skin, bleeding and secondary infection. The correction of serum calcium and phosphate may help, and antipruritic agents such as chlorpheniramine may also be of value.

Peripheral neuropathy
Dialysis should produce an improvement.

Hyperuricaemia
Treatment with allopurinol may be required.

End-stage renal failure
End-stage renal failure (ESRF) is identified on biochemical and clinical grounds as that point when, despite conservative measures, the patient will die without the institution of renal replacement by dialysis or transplantation. Specific indications for dialysis in ESRF include symptomatic uraemia, hyperkalaemia, metabolic acidosis, peripheral neuropathy, pericarditis central nervous system disorders, and poor control of ESRF by conservative treatment. Problems with dialysis include infection, hypotension, haemorrhage, and the maintenance of fluid and electrolyte balance.

Renal transplantation is becoming increasingly common. Patients are on immunosuppressive drugs, e.g. cyclosporin, prednisolone, and azathioprine, which have their own problems such as susceptibility to opportunistic infections, skin malignancies, and cyclosporin-induced nephrotoxicity.

Other complications of transplantation include rejection, obstruction at the ureteric anastamosis, and persisting hypertension.

URINARY TRACT INFECTION

Urinary tract infections (UTIs) are one of the most common infections encountered in general practice. Women are more prone to UTIs than men, except during the first few months of life, and in old age. Approximately 25–35% of all women have symptoms of UTI at some stage in their lives.

UTI is a general term referring to the presence of micro-organisms in the urine. Significant bacteriuria is defined as urine that yields more than 100 000 organisms per mL on culture. The causes of UTI are given in Fig. 33.4.

The causes of sterile pyuria (a common exam question) are:
- Tuberculosis of the urinary tract.
- Analgesic nephropathy.
- Neoplasms.
- Catheterization.
- Fevers in children.
- Intra-abdominal inflammation, e.g. appendicitis.
- Surgery involving the urinary tract.

Lower urinary tract infections

Lower UTIs may take the following forms:

- Cystitis: a symptomatic infection of the bladder in the presence of significant bacteriuria.
- Asymptomatic bacteriuria: the patient has no symptoms, but urine culture yields a growth of over 100 000 per mL.
- Acute urethral syndromes: symptomatically similar to cystitis but the urine culture may be sterile.

Upper urinary tract infections

Upper UTIs may take the following forms:

- Acute pyelonephritis: an inflammatory process within the renal parenchyma, most commonly caused by bacterial infection.
- Chronic pyelonephritis: this is usually the result of long-standing bacterial infection, which usually occurs in childhood. Urinary tract obstruction and vesicoureteric reflux are associated with eventual parenchymal scarring, which is characteristic of chronic pyelonephritic kidneys.

Infection usually occurs by ascent of the invading organism from the urethra into the bladder. Colonization of the ureters may then occur, and from there to the kidneys. This is facilitated by vesicoureteric reflux. The haematogenous route of infection is less common but may occur secondarily to bacteraemia, septicaemia, or endocarditis.

The commonest pathogen is *Escherichia coli*. Other organisms include *Proteus*, *Klebsiella*, staphylococci, and streptococci. *Pseudomonas* may be present after catheterization. In patients with long-term catheters mixed infections can be a significant problem.

Clinical features

Symptoms of lower UTI are suprapubic pain, frequency, nocturia, dysuria, and strangury. Upper UTIs such as acute pyelonephritis or renal abscesses present with fever, rigors, loin pain, vomiting, and weight loss.

Investigations

Obvious predisposing factors such as pregnancy or diabetes should be considered. Indications for further investigations include relapsing infections, childhood onset, male sex, urological symptoms, persistent haematuria, unusual organisms (such as *Pseudomonas*), and frequent recurrence of infections.

Initial investigations should involve an ultrasound scan, which will determine renal size, cysts, obstruction, and

---

Precipitating causes of urinary tract infection

- stones
- obstruction
- polycystic kidneys
- papillary necrosis
- diabetes mellitus
- analgesic nephropathy
- sickle cell disease
- sexual intercourse
- pregnancy
- bladder catheterization

Fig. 33.4 Precipitating causes of urinary tract infection.

residual urine; abdominal X-rays involving the kidneys, ureters, and bladder will detect radiopaque stones.

An intravenous urogram (IVU) often complements the above investigations, and gives a better demonstration of parenchymal scars and calyceal clubbing. A micturating cystogram is used to detect vesicoureteric reflux, and bladder and urethral abnormalities, especially in children. Scarring may also be demonstrated on isotope and computed tomography (CT) scanning.

Management

Treatment is usually started after urine has been sent for culture and antibiotic sensitivities, but before results are available. Antibiotics may then be changed if necessary according to the results. High fluid intake should be encouraged. More than 80% of lower UTIs respond to a 48-hour course of an antibiotic such as trimethoprim or amoxycillin. If the urinary tract is structurally abnormal, a 5–10 day course of therapy is indicated. Follow-up microscopy and culture should be carried out to ensure eradication of organisms and pyuria.

Patients with acute pyelonephritis usually require admission to hospital for intravenous fluids and antibiotics. Paracetamol will reduce the temperature but stronger analgesia may be required.

Patients with frequent reinfection require a high fluid intake, and frequent and complete voiding should be encouraged. Long-term, low-dose prophylaxis using antibiotics such as trimethoprim 100 mg or nitrofurantoin 50 mg per day may be of benefit, but the need for continued treatment should be reassessed after 6 months.

If infection is related to sexual intercourse, the patient should void after intercourse and may benefit from a single dose of an antibiotic.

FLUID AND ELECTROLYTE BALANCE

In a 70 kg man, the total fluid volume is 42 L, i.e. 60% of the body weight. The intracellular fluid volume is 28 L or two-thirds of the total body fluid, and the extracellular fluid volume is 14 L or a third of the total body fluid. The intravascular component is 3 litres (plasma contributing to 5 L of blood).

The average total fluid intake in 24 hours is 2500 mL (1500 mL drunk, 800 mL in food, and 200 mL via the metabolism of food). The output matches this via urine, insensible loss, and stool.

Sodium ingestion is about 80 mmol in 24 hours and potassium is also 80 mmol in 24 hours.

Salt and water balance

Water depletion results from reduced intake or increased losses. Examples of the former include an inability to get water (e.g. unconsciousness or extreme weakness), inability to swallow (e.g. causes of dysphagia), and nausea. Increased losses usually occur via the skin (e.g. fever, thyrotoxicosis), lungs (e.g. hyperventilation), and urine (e.g. diabetes insipidus).

Water and sodium depletion tend to occur together. Causes of mixed depletion of water and sodium include loss from the following:

- Gastrointestinal tract, e.g. vomiting, watery diarrhoea, fistulous drainage, and paralytic ileus.
- Urinary tract, e.g. overuse of diuretics, osmotic diuresis (in DM), chronic renal failure, renal tubular damage (such as the relief of obstruction), and Addison's disease.
- Skin, e.g. excessive sweating, exfoliative dermatitis, and burns.
- Others, e.g. ascites and inferior vena caval thrombosis.

Clinically, hyponatraemia (Fig. 33.5) leads to confusion and fits. Hypernatraemia (Fig. 33.6) leads to thirst, confusion, and coma.

Water deficiency may show as hypotension. The pulse will be thready and fast, the skin is dry and turgor is reduced, and there is peripheral vasoconstriction. The urea, haemoglobin, packed cell volume, and plasma protein tend to rise. Water excess (Chapter 12) leads to hypertension, cardiac failure, oedema, headache, anorexia, nausea, muscle weakness, and later on confusion, fits, and coma. Investigations show haemodilution (reduced packed cell volume).

Management of hyponatraemia

Treat the underlying cause. If the patient is not dehydrated fluid intake should be restricted to 500–1000 mL in 24 hours; diuretics should also be considered. If the patient is dehydrated, an infusion of 0.9% saline can be given.

Causes of hyponatraemia	
Cause	**Examples**
sodium and water retention	secondary hyperaldosteronism, e.g. cardiac failure hypoproteinaemia, e.g. nephrotic syndrome reduced GFR, e.g. renal failure
sodium and water depletion	losses from GI tract, renal and skin (see above)
normal total body sodium (excessive ADH effect)	CNS disease, e.g. encephalitis drugs, e.g. chlorpropamide, carbemazepine glucocorticoid deficiency inappropriate ADH secretion
artefact	blood taken from arm with i.v. fluids marked hyperlipidaemia or hypoproteinaemia

Fig. 33.5 Causes of hyponatraemia. (ADH, antidiuretic hormone; CNS, central nervous system; GFR, glomerular filtration rate; GI, gastrointestinal; i.v., intravenous.)

Causes of hypernatraemia	
low total body sodium	extrarenal, e.g. sweating, diarrhoea renal—osmotic diuresis
normal total body sodium	high temperatures diabetes insipidus

high total
body sodium
	steroid excess, e.g. Cushing's, Conn's
	iatrogenic, e.g. hypertonic sodium
	    infusions
	self-induced, e.g. ingestion of
	    sodium chloride tablets

Fig. 33.6 Causes of hypernatraemia.

Hyperkalaemia causes large T waves on the ECG, hypokalaemia causes small ones—large pot, lots of tea; small pot, no tea.

Too rapid an increase in sodium may lead to central pontine myelinolysis, or severe shrinking of the brain cells, which can lead to death.

Management of hypernatraemia

Treat the underlying cause. Water is given orally or as intravenous 5% dextrose guided by the urine output and plasma sodium. In severe hypernatraemia, 0.9% saline should be used initially to avoid too rapid a drop in sodium concentration (to avoid cerebral oedema).

Hypokalaemia

The causes of hypokalaemia are given in Fig. 33.7. The clinical features of hypokalaemia are muscle weakness, apathy, anorexia, confusion, ileus, increased cardiac excitability, digitalis toxicity, thirst, polyuria, renal lesions (e.g. Fanconi's syndrome), interstitial inflammation, and

fibrosis in severe prolonged depletion. The ECG changes are described in Chapter 29.

Management

The underlying cause should be identified and treated. If hypokalaemia is mild, oral potassium supplements are given. These are rarely required for patients on thiazides. If the patient is severely hypokalaemic, the cautious infusion of intravenous potassium should be considered (but not more than 20 mmol per hour).

Hyperkalaemia

The causes of hyperkalaemia are given in Fig. 33.8. The management of hyperkalaemia is described on p.280.

Hypercalcaemia

The causes of hypercalcaemia are given in Fig. 29.21.

Hypocalcaemia

The causes of hypocalcaemia are given in Fig. 33.9.

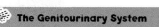
Causes of hypokalaemia	
Cause	**Examples**
losses	gastrointestinal: chronic laxative abuse, diarrhoea and vomiting, villous papilloma of the colon renal: diuretics (e.g. thiazides and frusemide), hyperaldosteronism, glucocorticoid excess (including treatment with steroids, and ACTH-secreting tumours), renal tubular acidosis, Bartter's syndrome inadequate replacement: postoperative, diuretic phase of acute renal failure
redistribution of potassium	alkalosis insulin overdose familial periodic paralysis
ACTH-secreting tumour	
secretion of atrial natriuretic peptide	paroxysmal SVT

Fig. 33.7 Causes of hypokalaemia (ACTH, adrenocorticotrophic hormone; SVT, supraventricular tachycardia.)

Causes of hyperkalaemia	
Cause	**Examples**
excessive oral intake	potassium supplements
diminished renal excretion	renal failure potassium sparing diuretic in combination with renal failure, e.g. amiloride, spironolactone
redistribution of potassium	haemolysis, e.g. incompatible blood transfusion, DIC acidosis tissue necrosis, e.g. burns
artefact	delay in separation of plasma or serum, improper storage conditions

Fig. 33.8 Causes of hyperkalaemia (DIC, disseminated intravascular coagulation).

Causes of hypocalcaemia	
Cause	**Examples**
hypoproteinaemia	nephrotic syndrome
renal disease	chronic renal failure
inadequate intake of calcium or vitamin D	malabsorption
hypoparathyroidism	—
target organ resistance	pseudohypoparathyroidism
neonatal hypocalcaemia	—
others	acute pancreatitis, cystinosis, cytotoxic drugs

Fig. 33.9 Causes of hypocalcaemic

Management

Treat the underlying cause. If mild, give oral calcium supplements. If severe, give 10 mL 10% intravenous calcium gluconate over 3 minutes and repeat as necessary.

MISCELLANEOUS GENITOURINARY CONDITIONS

Adult polycystic kidney disease

This is an autosomal dominantly inherited disease, the gene lying on chromosome 16. Patients are usually between the ages of 30 and 50. Cysts develop in the kidney and lead to progressive renal failure. About 30% of patients also have cysts in the liver.

Clinical features

Haematuria or abdominal pain are presenting features in about a third of patients. The patient may have signs or symptoms of chronic renal failure. There is an association with subarachnoid haemorrhage. Examination reveals large irregular palpable kidneys, and the patient is often hypertensive. There may be bruits from intracranial vascular anomalies.

Investigations

Ultrasound shows multiple cysts. IVU shows large kidneys and 'spider calyces'.

Management

Blood pressure should be controlled and infections treated. Renal failure is progressive and may necessitate dialysis or renal transplantation. Screening first degree relatives and genetic counselling is recommended.

Hepatorenal syndrome

This mainly occurs in patients with obstructive jaundice. Renal failure may be precipitated by surgery to relieve the jaundice, overvigorous diuretic therapy, diarrhoea, or paracentesis for ascites, although there may be no precipitating factor found. Histology of the kidney is usually normal early on but may advance to produce an acute tubular necrosis.

The cause of the renal failure is not fully understood but may be due to the toxic effects of bilirubin on the kidney, or peripheral vasodilatation mediated through nitric oxide leading to hypotension.

This then activates the renin–angiotensin system and other humoral mechanisms to cause constriction of renal vessels.

Opiates should be avoided preoperatively and euvolaemia should be ensured with intravenous fluids. Urine output and serum electrolytes should be monitored. If renal failure occurs, the prognosis is usually poor.

The differential diagnosis includes leptospirosis, which may cause hepatic and renal failure. The organism can be grown from urine and blood, and is penicillin sensitive.

Haemolytic uraemic syndrome

Haemolytic uraemic syndrome is a disorder usually affecting infants under 3 years old. The aetiology is unknown but the syndrome often follows an infective illness such as gastroenteritis or upper respiratory tract infection. The infection may trigger endothelial damage and cause clotting disturbances characteristic of the condition. There is intravascular haemolysis with red blood cell fragmentation. Fibrin deposition is seen in renal arterioles. Thrombocytopaenia also occurs and the condition is similar to thrombotic thrombocytopaenic purpura in adults. See Chapter 37 for more details.

Treatment is with heparin, prostacyclin, fresh frozen plasma, plasma exchange, and dialysis for renal failure. Most children recover spontaneously.

Urinary tract malignancies
Renal cell carcinoma

Renal cell carcinoma is the commonest renal tumour in adults and is twice as common in men. The peak age of onset is between 50 and 60 years of age. It may be solitary, multiple, or occasionally bilateral. Clinically, patients present with haematuria, loin pain, and an abdominal mass. Other features may include pyrexia, polycythaemia, anaemia, hypercalcaemia, and left-sided varicocele associated with left renal vein obstruction. A tendency to grow into the inferior vena cava (IVC) is a typical characteristic. About a quarter of patients present with metastases.

Investigations include urinalysis for red cells, chest X-ray for metastases, ultrasound, IVU, and CT or magnetic resonance imaging of the abdomen. Angiography will reveal the circulation of the tumour.

Treatment is by nephrectomy. Metastases may regress after the primary tumour is removed.

Radiotherapy has no proven value. Progesterone may be of help in controlling metastatic disease. The overall 5-year survival is about 40% but is better if the tumour is confined to the renal parenchyma and worse if there are metastases or lymph node involvement.

Nephroblastoma

This is seen in infants. It presents as an abdominal mass or occasionally with haematuria. Treatment is with nephrectomy, radiotherapy, and chemotherapy, and is often curative.

Transitional cell carcinoma

This occurs mainly in the over 40s and most commonly affects the bladder. It is four times more common in men than women. Predisposing factors include cigarette smoking, exposure to industrial carcinogens, exposure to drugs (e.g. phenacetin and cyclophosphamide), and chronic inflammation (e.g. schistosomiasis).

Patients usually present with painless haematuria although pain may occur. There may be symptoms similar to UTI. Investigations include urine cytology, IVU, cystoscopy, abdominal CT scanning, and retrograde urography.

Treatment options include local resection with follow-up cystoscopy, cystectomy, radiotherapy and local or systemic chemotherapy.

Prostatic carcinoma

Prostatic carcinoma is the third most common malignancy in men. The incidence increases with age and may be very indolent. Patients are often asymptomatic, but may present with symptoms of prostatism, e.g. hesitancy, frequency, and postmicturition dribbling, or with symptoms arising from metastatic spread, especially to bone. There is a hard irregular prostate on rectal examination.

Investigation includes prostate-specific antigen (PSA) transrectal ultrasound, and prostatic biopsy, which shows an adenocarcinoma. Evidence of metastases should also be sought.

Treatment for local disease may be by transurethral resection of the prostate, radical prostatectomy, or radiotherapy. Metastases can be treated with orchidectomy, luteinizing hormone-releasing hormone analogues, and antiandrogens, e.g. cyproterone acetate.

34. Central Nervous System

CEREBROVASCULAR DISEASE

Stroke

A stroke is a focal neurological deficit due to a vascular lesion that lasts for more than 24 hours. About 80% are due to infarction secondary to thrombosis or embolism, and 20% are due to intracerebral haemorrhage. The overall incidence is about 150 in 100 000 but rises with age so that the incidence at 75 years is 1000 in 100 000.

Risk factors for stroke are summarized in Fig. 34.1. The main cause of thrombotic strokes are thromboembolism from arteries and emboli from the heart. Uncommon causes of thrombosis are vasculitis, polycythaemia rubra vera, and meningovascular syphilis. Thrombus *in situ* may also occur following hypotension. Cerebral haemorrhage is usually due to rupture of microaneurysms in perforating arteries or intracerebral vessels.

Less common causes of haemorrhagic stroke include haemorrhage, tumour, abscess, or secondary to blood dyscrasias.

The sudden onset of any symptom usually suggests either a vascular or neurological aetiology.

Clinical features

Signs and symptoms usually appear rapidly whereas a gradual progression over days suggests a tumour. Clinical features relate to the distribution of the affected artery, although in practice this may not be clear-cut due to collateral circulation and the development of cerebral oedema. The commonest presentation is hemiplegia due to infarction of the internal capsule.

Types of infarction

Cerebral hemisphere infarcts

Cerebral hemisphere infarcts may be classified by vascular territory:

- Anterior cerebral artery infarcts: proximal to the medial striate branch, they cause contralateral hemiplegia; distal to the medial striate branch, they cause contralateral paralysis with sparing of the arm and face.
- Middle cerebral artery infarcts: causes contralateral hemiplegia often sparing the leg, and hemianopia. Aphasia is present if the dominant hemisphere is affected.
- Posterior cerebral artery infarcts: causes contralateral hemianopia.

Motor signs are upper motor neurone.

Lacunar strokes

Lacunar strokes are due to small areas of infarction usually occurring around the basal ganglia, thalamus, and pons. Clinical features include pure motor or sensory signs, a mixed motor and sensory picture, ataxia, and dysarthria. They may also be asymptomatic, and found at post-mortem.

Risk factors for stroke	
major risk factors	hypertension atrial fibrillation previous transient ischaemic attacks diabetes mellitus ischaemic heart disease peripheral vascular disease oral contraceptive pill
other risk factors	smoking obesity excessive alcohol intake polycythaemia arteritis bleeding disorders hyperlipidaemia* low cholesterol†

Fig. 34.1 Risk factors for stroke. *Hyperlipidaemia is associated with cerebral infarction. †Low cholesterol may be associated with cerebral haemorrhage.

Brainstem infarcts

Clinical features include hemi- or quadriplegia, sensory loss, diplopia, facial weakness and numbness, nystagmus, dysphasia, and coma due to damage to the reticular formation.

The locked-in syndrome results from upper brain-stem infarction. The patient is conscious but unable to respond.

The commonest brainstem vascular syndrome is lateral medullary syndrome (Wallenberg's syndrome), which is due to thromboembolism of the posterior inferior cerebellar artery. The patient presents with sudden vertigo and vomiting. Ipsilateral signs include 9th and 10th nerve lesions, Horner's syndrome, spinothalamic sensory loss in the face, diplopia, and cerebellar signs in the limbs. Contralateral signs include spinothalamic sensory loss in the body.

Investigations

The following investigations should be performed in patients who have suffered a stroke:

- Full blood count (FBC): polycythaemia or thrombocytopenia.
- Clotting screen: bleeding disorders.
- Erythrocyte sedimentation rate (ESR): giant cell arteritis.
- Blood glucose: hyper- or hypoglycaemia may lead to impaired consciousness.
- Chest X-ray (CXR): primary tumour; left atrium enlarged with mitral stenosis.
- Syphilis serology.
- Computed tomography (CT) scan: this will distinguish between haemorrhagic and ischaemic infarction if done within 2 weeks; also aids diagnosis of other conditions in cases of uncertainty, such as tumour or subdural haematoma; should always be performed in cerebellar stroke as haematoma requires urgent evacuation.
- Cartoid duplex scan: stenoses.

Management

Prevention

Risk factors such as hypertension, smoking, diabetes mellitus (DM), high cholesterol, and atrial fibrillation should be identified and managed appropriately. Following stroke, the blood pressure may be high for some days, and a decision on antihypertensive drugs is not usually made for about 2 weeks.

Cholesterol should be lowered to reduce coronary risk because myocardial infarction is the major cause of death during the period following the acute stage of stroke or transient ischaemic attacks (TIAs). Anticoagulation should be considered for patients with atrial fibrillation and thromboembolic stroke.

If there is a severe internal carotid artery stenosis (of more than 70%) and the patient has had TIAs within the last 6 months, endarterectomy should be considered.

Treatment

If the patient is unconscious or severely impaired, a decision on the most appropriate degree of intervention needs to be taken in liaison with relatives, and the patient if possible. Factors to consider include prognosis, quality of life, and the patient's wishes. Raised intracranial pressure should be suspected if the blood pressure rises, the pulse falls, and there is papilloedema. An urgent CT scan should be considered.

Hydration should be maintained, and this should be done parenterally if there is no gag reflex.

The patient should be turned regularly to prevent pressure sores. If incontinent, urinary catheterization should be considered. Physiotherapy will prevent contractures and hasten mobility.

Speech therapy and occupational therapy are important later on.

Aspirin 75–300 mg daily for people with thrombotic stroke reduces the rate of further strokes and vascular deaths. Complications, e.g. pneumonia, depression, and constipation, should be managed appropriately.

Prognosis

Features associated with a poor prognosis include impaired consciousness, severe hemiplegia, incontinence, a defect in conjugate gaze, and increasing age. About 20–25% of patients with thromboembolic infarction and 75% of patients with intracerebral haemorrhage die at 1 month. Recurrent strokes are common. About a third of survivors make a complete recovery and a third are left with severe disability.

Transient ischaemic attacks

These are focal neurological deficits due to vascular events that settle within 24 hours with a complete clinical recovery. They are usually due to emboli from the carotid or vertebrobasilar arteries, but emboli may also arise from the heart or other vessels. The annual incidence is about 50 per 100 000.

Other possible causes are arteritis, e.g. giant cell arteritis, polyarteritis nodosa (PAN), systemic lupus erythematosus (SLE), syphilis, arterial trauma, and haematological causes, e.g. polycythaemia rubra vera and sickle cell disease.

Clinical features

There is a sudden focal neurological deficit, which gradually resolves over minutes or hours, leading to complete recovery within 24 hours. In the internal carotid artery territory, platelet emboli obstruct blood flow leading to loss of function in part of the brain. The platelet aggregates then break up, restoring blood flow and hence function. This may lead to dysphasia and dysarthria, contralateral hemiparesis, hemisensory loss, homonymous hemianopia, and ipsilateral amaurosis fugax. The latter is due to emboli passing through the retinal arteries leading to a sensation of a curtain passing across the vision.

TIAs in the vertebrobasilar system may again result from emboli, or from a pinching of the vertebral arteries by osteophytes arising from the cervical vertebrae. Symptoms include diplopia, vertigo, nausea and vomiting, ataxia, hemiparesis or hemisensory loss, tetraparesis, deafness, cortical blindness, occasionally loss of consciousness, and transient global amnesia.

Sources of emboli should be sought. Risk factors are the same as for stroke, and should be identified and managed appropriately.

Differential diagnosis

This includes all conditions that may cause transient neurological symptoms. Epilepsy is usually distinguished by features such as jerking, and migraine is usually associated with headache, which is rare in TIAs. Hypoglycaemia, multiple sclerosis (MS) and intracranial lesions should be excluded.

Investigations

These should identify risk factors, find the cause of the TIA, and exclude other causes of symptoms, as for stroke. Carotid doppler studies or angiography may identify stenoses (Fig. 34.2).

Treatment

Risk factors should be controlled, particularly hypertension. Cholesterol should be lowered to reduce coronary risk. Aspirin 75–300 mg daily reduces the risk of subsequent non-fatal stroke, myocardial infarction, and vascular deaths. More recent evidence suggests that dipyridamole MR 200 mg daily has a protective effect for subsequent neurological events, which are additional to the protective effect of aspirin.

Anticoagulation should be considered if TIAs continue despite antiplatelet treatment, or if there is a known cardiac source of embolism. Carotid endarterectomy is indicated for recurrent TIAs in the appropriate distribution if the responsible carotid stenosis is over 70% of the luminal diameter.

Prognosis

Patients with TIAs in the carotid distribution fare worse than those in the vertebrobasilar territory. The risk of stroke and myocardial infarction are significantly increased, at about 5% per year each.

Extracerebral haemorrhage
Subarachnoid haemorrhage

Subarachnoid haemorrhage (SAH) is due to bleeding into the subarachnoid space. The annual incidence is 15 in 100 000. Most cases are due to rupture of a congenital berry aneurysm in the circle of Willis and its adjacent branches (Fig. 20.2); 15% are multiple.

Berry aneurysms are associated with coarctation of the aorta, polycystic kidneys, and Ehlers–Danlos syndrome. About 5–10% of SAHs are due to arteriovenous malformations but in 15% of patients no cause is found.

Bleeds may occasionally be due to ruptures, mycotic aneurysm from endocarditis, and bleeding diatheses.

Clinical features

The classic history is of a feeling like a sudden blow to the back of the neck. This is usually followed by faintness, nausea, vomiting, and sometimes loss of consciousness.

On examination, there is photophobia and neck stiffness, and a positive Kernig's sign. If bleeding continues, the level of consciousness deteriorates. There may be signs of raised intracranial pressure, or pressure effects on surrounding structures, e.g. cranial nerve palsies. There may be a bruit over the skull due to an arteriovenous malformation.

291

Investigations

A CT scan usually shows blood in the subarachnoid space, and it can also identify arteriovenous malformations. A lumbar puncture shows raised pressure, uniform blood staining in consecutive samples, and xanthochromia (yellow colour) which persists for several days. Angiography will show the aneurysm, and is carried out if surgery is considered.

Management

Immediate treatment is bed rest, analgesia, and supportive measures. About a third of patients rebleed, most commonly about a fortnight after the initial event.

Angiography should therefore be performed before then if the aneurysm is to be clipped. Blood pressure should be monitored and lowered if severely raised.

Nimodipine 60 mg 4 hourly is used to prevent vascular spasm following SAH, and reduces mortality. It is related to nifedipine but the smooth muscle relaxant effect preferentially acts on cerebral arteries. It should be started within 4 days and continued for 21 days.

Prognosis

Nearly half of patients with SAH are dead or moribund before reaching hospital. A further 30% will rebleed in the next few days.

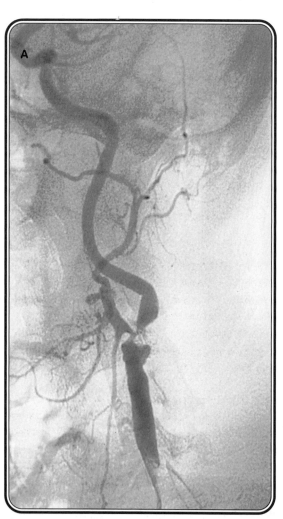
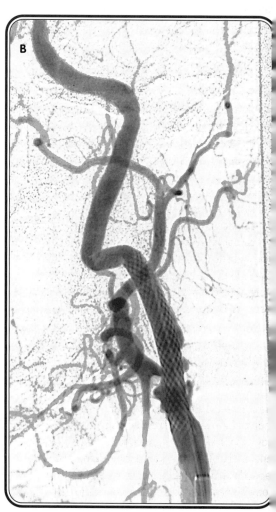

Fig. 34.2 (A) Carotid angiogram showing a severe atheromatous plaque leading to stenosis of the internal carotid artery. (B) The same vessel is shown after angioplasty and stent insertion.

Patients who have severe neurological deficits have a poor prognosis. Of patients who survive 1 year, about a third will have made a full recovery.

Subdural haematoma

These are due to bleeding from bridging veins between the cortex and venous sinuses. An initial small haemorrhage gradually enlarges by absorbing fluid osmotically from the cerebrospinal fluid (CSF). It is more common in the elderly, epileptics, and alcoholics. Although it is often secondary to trauma, the initial event may not be recalled.

Symptoms develop insidiously. They include headache, confusion, a fluctuating level of consciousness, and sometimes a personality change. There may be focal neurological signs (which may develop many days after the initial insult), signs of raised intracranial pressure, or secondary epilepsy.

A CT scan should show the haematoma, which may be bilateral. Treatment is by removal of the haematoma, which often leads to a full recovery if performed early.

Haematomas may resolve spontaneously, and in the very elderly they can be monitored with serial CT scans.

Extradural haematoma

This results from tearing of the middle meningeal artery or its branches following head injury. The classic picture of a sudden brief loss of consciousness followed by a lucid interval. The patient's conscious level then deteriorates and the ipsilateral pupil dilates, followed by bilateral fixed dilated pupils and death. Treatment is by evacuation of the clot through Burr holes.

MANAGEMENT OF CONDITIONS CAUSING HEADACHE

The differential diagnosis of headache is given in chapter 15. Headache is a common symptom, which may either be of trivial significance or the expression of serious disease. The clinical approach to headache depends on a detailed analysis of symptoms and a thorough general and neurological examination.

Acute headache

The most common cause of acute severe headache is acute meningeal irritation as a result of SAH or meningitis. Headache also occurs with encephalitis, hydrocephalus, and after head injury. CT scanning is usually the first investigation used to exclude a mass lesion, haematoma, or hydrocephalus. Lumbar puncture may be necessary to examine the CSF for SAH and meningitis. Occasionally acute migraine can produce a meningitic picture.

Recurrent and chronic headache
Tension headache

Tension headaches are extremely common and classically present as intermittent attacks of diffuse tightness, pressure or heaviness over the vertex, or in the neck or occiput. It may occasionally be unilateral. The headache may be relieved by analgesics but is not accompanied by vomiting or visual disturbance. When the headaches are constant and occur daily, analgesics are ineffective, and excessive medication may itself induce headache. Tension headaches are commonest in middle-aged women.

Enquiries should be made for the common and often concealed fear of a brain tumour or stroke.

Migraine

Migraine affects about 10% of the population, and is slightly commoner in women than men (ratio of 1.5:1). About 75% of people have their first attack before the age of 20 years.

Clinical features

The frequency of headaches varies from one to two each week to a few attacks scattered over a lifetime. The prodrome may consist of yawning, euphoria, or depression, and sometimes a craving for, or a distaste of, food in the 24 hours before the headache.

This is followed by an aura 30–60 minutes before the headache. It is usually visual, consisting of teichopsiae (flashes of light), scotomata, and fortification spectra (zigzag castellations). There may be micropsia and metamorphosia. Circumoral tingling and parasthesiae in the hands may also occur. In hemiplegic migraine, a hemiparesis, sometimes with dysphasia, occurs.

The headache is commonly unilateral. It usually starts in the day and is classically throbbing or pulsating. Associated features include nausea and vomiting, diarrhoea, chills, faintness, and fluid retention. There may be photophobia and sonophobia. The headache is usually worse with movement, and lasts for 24–48 hours.

Occasionally, especially in older people, the aura may occur without the headache—'migraine sine cephalgia'.

Pathology
The mechanism of migraine attacks are not well understood but a reduction in cerebral blood flow leads to the aura. This is followed by an increased blood flow associated with vasodilatation leading to headache. The process involves neurohumoral triggers including 5-hydroxytryptamine (5-HT) and noradrenaline.

The cerebral mechanism is responsive to mood, emotions, tiredness, relaxation, hormonal changes, and peripheral stimuli, e.g. bright lights and noise. There is often a seasonal and/or diurnal pattern.

Management
Precipitating factors should be identified and avoided, such as certain foods including cocoa, cheese, citrus fruits, and alcohol. Acute attacks should be treated with simple analgesia, e.g. aspirin, paracetamol, or codeine, combined with an antiemetic, e.g. domperidone or metochlopramide.

Ergotamine is used in patients who do not respond to analgesics. It relieves migraine headache by constricting cranial arteries but the aura is not affected and vomiting can be made worse. Common side effects include nausea, vomiting, abdominal pain, and muscular cramps. It should not be used for hemiplegic migraine, in patients with peripheral vascular disease, or in coronary heart disease. The frequency of administration should be limited to no more than twice a month to avoid habituation.

Sumatriptan and other 5-HT antagonists are of value for treatment of acute attacks, although experience is still relatively limited. They should not be given to patients with ischaemic heart disease or previous myocardial infarction, coronary vasospasm, or uncontrolled hypertension.

Prophylaxis
Prophylactic drugs are indicated in patients who have two or more attacks each month, and includes pizotifen, β-blockers, and tricyclic antidepressants. The need for continuing therapy should be reviewed every 6 months.

β-Blockers, such as propanolol, are effective but their use is limited by contraindications and interaction with ergotamine.

Pizotifen is an antihistamine and serotonin antagonist related to the tricyclic antidepressants. It may cause weight gain and drowsiness, which can be avoided by starting with low doses at night and gradually increasing the dose.

Tricyclic antidepressants, such as amitriptyline, can be effective in low doses, even in patients who are not depressed.

Cyproheptadine can be tried in refractory cases. It is an antihistamine with serotonin antagonist and Ca^{2+} channel-blocking properties.

In patients with severe recurrent migraine refractory to all the above treatment, methysergide may be tried under hospital supervision. Dangerous side effects include retroperitoneal fibrosis and fibrosis of the heart valves and pleura. If side effects start to occur, treatment should be stopped immediately.

Cluster headache
Cluster headaches are 10 times more common in men than women. Attacks usually start in adulthood. Headaches are of agonizing severity around one eye, and often occur at night. Attacks last for 30–120 minutes and usually occur every day for 4 weeks to 3 months. There is then usually a total remission until the next cluster ensues a year or two later.

The pain may radiate to the face, jaw, neck, and shoulder, and the eyes may water and become red. The nostrils may also run or feel blocked. Meiosis occurs in 20% of attacks, and in about 5% a permanent partial Horner's syndrome occurs. Attacks can be precipitated by vasodilators, e.g. alcohol, nitrites, and Ca^{2+} channel blockers.

Treatment is with ergotamine given in anticipation of the attacks or with pizotifen or verapamil for the duration of the cluster. Oxygen affords prompt relief in some patients. Sumatriptan will stop attacks in 5–10 minutes in 70% of patients.

Brain tumours and other space-occupying lesions
These present with headaches in about 50% of patients but are uncommon causes of headache overall. The following symptoms may be present:
- Raised intracranial pressure: headache, vomiting, and papilloedema.

- Generalized or focal epilepsy.
- Progressive focal signs: hemiparesis, hemianopia, and dysphasia.
- Mental changes: depression, apathy, dementia, and hallucinosis.

Headaches often occur in the mornings and are worse with coughing, exertion, or a change in posture. Focal signs are suggestive of tumours. Investigations should include CT scanning to show primary or secondary tumour.

Cranial (giant cell) arteritis

This disease usually occurs in patients over 60 years old. The classical features include engorged, reddened, tender, non-pulsatile temporal arteries (Fig. 34.3) but this is not invariably present. The headache is severe and often worse at night, and may be accompanied by sweats, fever, malaise, and pain in the jaw during eating ('masseter claudication'). It may be associated with

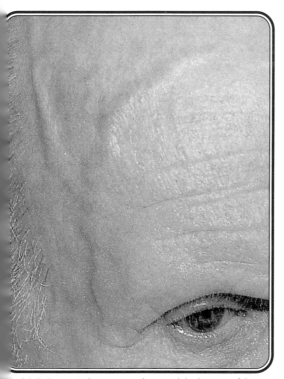

Fig. 34.3 Temporal arteritis with typical thickening of the right temporal artery. This patient presented with temporal pain and sudden visual impairment in the right eye but responded to prompt treatment with systemic steroid. (Courtesy of Dr. C.D. Forbes and Dr. W.F. Jackson, Color Atlas and Text of Clinical Medicine, Mosby, 1993.)

polymyalgia rheumatica. Involvement of the vertebral arteries may lead to TIAs or stroke, and disease of the ophthalmic arteries may lead to retinal ischaemia or infarction, which is irreversible.

Investigation
The ESR is markedly raised at around 100 mm per hour. A biopsy of the temporal artery should be taken within 24 hours of starting steroid therapy. 'Skip lesions' may lead to false negatives, and so a long biopsy specimen should be obtained. Inflammatory cells infiltrate the tunica, and the internal elastic lamina is commonly destroyed or disrupted and intraluminal thrombosis may be found.

Treatment
Treatment is with high doses of prednisolone (60 mg daily). This relieves the headache within 24 hours and averts the risk of blindness, which occurs in up to 50% of patients if untreated. The prednisolone is gradually reduced to a maintenance level, and the dose is monitored by symptoms and serial ESRs. Treatment may have to be continued for many years.

Glaucoma
Localized pain in the eye and forehead may be a recurrent source of headache, and glaucoma should be considered in hypermetropic, middle-aged or elderly patients. In acute attacks, there may be vomiting, blurred vision, cloudiness of the cornea, and discoloration of the iris with a dilated pupil and circumorbital injection. Tonometry will confirm the elevated intraocular pressure.

Standard treatments include miotics, acetazolamide, and iridectomy, which should be supervised by an ophthalmologist.

Paget's disease of the skull
This is a common condition presenting with diffuse headaches, somnolence, deafness, and enlargement of the skull. Headaches result from local bony changes with vascular hyperaemia. Hydrocephalus may later be an additional factor of importance.

Trigeminal neuralgia
This condition of unknown cause is seen most commonly in the elderly and is more common in women. In young patients, MS should be suspected. It is unilateral in 96% of patients, and consists of

paroxysms of stabbing pain in the distribution of the trigeminal nerve. The face may screw up with pain, hence the alternative name of tic douloureux.

The pain may be brought on by touching a specific trigger zone such as the side of the nose, and is thus provoked by factors such as eating, shaving, or talking. If left untreated the condition usually progresses with shorter periods of remission.

Treatment is with carbamazepine, phenytoin, or occasionally clonazepam or baclofen. Surgical procedures such as sectioning of the sensory root or thermocoagulation of the ganglion is reserved for failure of medical therapy.

Other neuralgias include glossopharyngeal neuralgia and auriculotemporal neuralgia, which are precipitated by swallowing. Postherpetic neuralgia occurs in patients with previous herpes zoster.

Atypical facial pain

This refers to episodes of prolonged facial pain for which no cause can be found. It is commoner in women, and is often bilateral. It is associated with depression and may respond to tricyclic antidepressants.

Benign intracranial hypertension

This is also known as pseudotumour cerebri. The aetiology is often unknown but it may be related to steroids in some patients. A few cases are secondary to thrombosis of the dural venous sinuses. The condition occurs mainly in overweight young women, and there may be a history of menstrual irregularities or recent pregnancy. Symptoms include headache and vomiting. There is marked papilloedema which, if long standing, can lead to optic atrophy and infarction of the optic nerve causing blindness.

A CT scan shows no mass lesion, and the ventricles are of normal or small size. Thiazides or frusemide may reduce the intracranial pressure, and repeated lumbar puncture may induce a remission. In resistant cases, or if visual acuity deteriorates, a ventriculoperitoneal CSF shunt may be necessary.

PARKINSONISM

Parkinsonism comprises the syndrome of tremor, rigidity, and bradykinesia; Parkinson's disease is only one type of parkinsonism.

First described by James Parkinson in 1817 it is now known to be due to a relative deficiency of the neurotransmitter dopamine, resulting in a neurohumoral imbalance. Pathologically, there is progressive degeneration of the basal ganglia predominantly affecting the substantia nigra, and the appearance of eosinophilic inclusion bodies (Lewy bodies). The cause of the degeneration is unknown.

People with Parkinson's disease are less likely to be smokers. The incidence increases with age, and affects 1 in 200 people over 70 years old. It affects men and women equally and there does not appear to be a genetic predisposition.

Clinical features

Early on the patient may complain of fatigue, muscular discomfort, or restlessness. Fine movements may be difficult.

Tremor

Initially this is intermittent and may only appear when the patient is tired. It commonly affects one hand, spreading to the leg on the same side, and later to the other limbs. The frequency of the tremor is 3–6 beats per second and is most marked at rest (whereas a cerebellar tremor is more marked on intention). There is a 'pill rolling' movement of the thumb over the fingers.

Rigidity

There is resistance to passive movement, which may be smooth throughout its range ('lead pipe' rigidity). When combined with tremor, resistance to passive movement is jerky and termed 'cogwheel' rigidity.

Bradykinesia

Bradykinesia means difficulty in initiating movements and varying posture. It may be difficult rising from a chair. Writing becomes small (micrographia), spidery and cramped. The face is expressionless and mask-like (Fig. 34.4), and the voice is monotonous and unmodulated. There is a shuffling, 'festinant' gait, and the patient stoops (Fig. 34.5). The arms do not swing and the frequency of spontaneous blinking reduces.

Other features

Due to a disorder of the normal pattern of swallowing saliva gathers and drips from the half-open mouth.

To examine for bradykinesia, ask the patient to unbutton and button his or her shirt.

Constipation and urinary difficulties are common. Rigidity may be accompanied by pain in the muscles. Late on in the disease, dementia may occur. Depression is common.

Other causes of parkinsonism

Other causes of parkinsonism include the following:
- Drugs, e.g. neuroleptics.
- Atherosclerosis: look for symptoms and signs of atherosclerosis in other regions, e.g. TIAs or intermittent claudication.

- Postencephalitis: following outbreaks of encephalitis lethargica (as in 1917–25).
- Progressive supranuclear palsy: a symptom complex comprising a parkinsonism-like illness, dementia, and a failure of upward gaze.
- Shy–Drager syndrome: parkinsonism, orthostatic hypotension, and atonic bladder.
- Poisoning with heavy metals or carbon monoxide.
- Wilson's disease (hepatolenticular degeneration).
- 'Punch drunk' syndrome: brain damage in boxers.

Management

The disease is treated symptomatically. Physiotherapy can improve the gait and help build confidence. Physical aids such as high chairs and rails may help with daily activities.

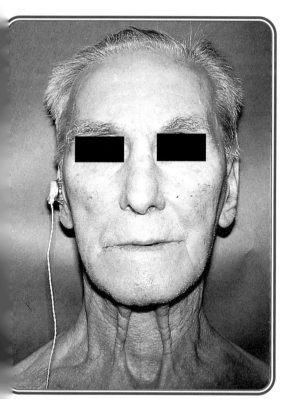

Fig. 34.4 Parkinson's disease is characteristically associated with a mask-like face which is devoid of motion. The patient often drools and has monotonous speech. (Courtesy of Dr. C.D. Forbes and Dr. W.F. Jackson, Color Atlas and Text of Clinical Medicine, Mosby, 1993.)

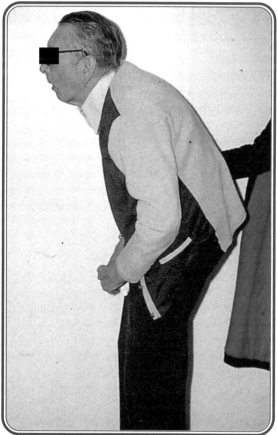

Fig. 34.5 Typical posture in Parkinson's disease. (Courtesy of Dr Kamal, St. George's Hospital, Lincoln.)

Drugs

The aim of drug therapy is to correct the neurohumoral imbalance. This may greatly improve the quality of life but does not prevent progression of the disease. Ten to twenty percent of patients are unresponsive to treatment.

Drugs may cause confusion in the elderly, and it is important to start treatment with low doses, and use small increments.

Dopaminergic drugs

Levodopa

Levodopa (L-dopa) is used with a dopa decarboxylase inhibitor and is the treatment of choice for idiopathic Parkinson's disease. It is less helpful for elderly patients or those with long standing disease who may not tolerate the high doses required to overcome their deficit. It is also less valuable in patients with postencephalitic disease, who are particularly susceptible to side effects.

Parkinsonism caused by generalized degenerative brain disease does not normally respond to levodopa. It should not be used for neuroleptic-induced parkinsonism.

Levodopa is the amino acid precursor of dopamine, and acts mainly by replenishing depleted striatal dopamine. It helps bradykinesia and rigidity more than tremor. It is generally administered with a extracerebral dopa decarboxylase inhibitor, e.g. benserazide or carbidopa. These prevent the peripheral breakdown of levodopa to dopamine, but unlike levodopa do not cross the blood–brain barrier. Effective brain concentrations of dopamine can thus be achieved with lower doses of levodopa.

The reduced peripheral formation of dopamine decreases peripheral side effects, e.g. nausea, vomiting, and cardiovascular effects. There is less delay in the onset of therapeutic effect and a smoother clinical response. There is however an increased incidence of abnormal involuntary movements.

Side effects of levodopa include nausea and vomiting which may be limited by domperidone. Late side effects include the sudden unpredictable swings of the 'on-off' syndrome', dyskinesia, and 'end-of-dose' deterioration. In the last, the duration of benefit after each dose becomes progressively shorter. This may be improved with modified-release preparations.

Selegiline

This is a monoamine oxidase B inhibitor used in severe parkinsonism in conjunction with levodopa to reduce end-of-dose deterioration. Early treatment with selegiline may delay the need for levodopa therapy but does not delay disease progression.

Bromocriptine

This is one of the ergot derivatives, which act by direct stimulation of surviving dopamine receptors. It should be reserved for patients in whom levodopa alone is no longer adequate or who despite careful titration cannot tolerate it. Occasionally it may cause neuropsychiatric side effects and retroperitoneal fibrosis.

Ropinirole

Ropinirole is a dopamine D_2 receptor agonist which improves the symptoms and signs in Parkinson's disease. Its side effects are similar to those of dopamine.

Amantadine

This improves mild bradykinetic disabilities as well as tremor and rigidity. Few patients derive much benefit and tolerance develops to its effects.

Apomorphine

Apomorphine is a potent stimulator of dopamine receptors, which is sometimes helpful in stabilizing patients experiencing unpredictable 'off' periods with levodopa treatment.

Antimuscarinic drugs

Examples of antimuscarinic drugs used in the treatmer of Parkinson's disease include orphenadrine and benzhexol. They are less effective than levodopa in idiopathic Parkinson's disease although they may be used to supplement its action.

Antimuscarinic drugs may be used first in patients with mild disease, especially when tremor is the predominant symptom. They are also of value in postencephalitic parkinsonism. They correct the relativ central cholinergic excess thought to occur in parkinsonism as a result of dopamine deficiency. They also reduce the symptoms of drug-induced parkinsonism seen with antipsychotic drugs.

Side effects include blurred vision, dry mouth, tachycardia, urinary retention, and constipation.

MULTIPLE SCLEROSIS

Multiple sclerosis (MS), also called disseminated sclerosis, is an inflammatory, demyelinating disorder. It is the most common cause of neurological disability in young adults in the UK. The prevalence of MS varies worldwide and is much higher in temperate zones. The overall prevalence in the UK is 100 in 100 000, rising to as high as 300 in 100 000 in the Shetland and Orkney Islands.

There is a female preponderance with a male:female ratio of 1:1.5. The mean age of onset is 30 years but there is a bimodal distribution with a major peak at 21–25 years and a lesser peak at 41–45 years.

Aetiology

The cause of MS is unknown. Evidence suggests that in a genetically susceptible individual an environmental agent is responsible. The causative agent is likely to be a virus and it is possible that a range of viruses may be involved. First-degree relatives have an increased chance of developing MS.

Pathology

The hallmark of MS is the presence of multiple lesions disseminated in site and time. These are characterized by demyelination with relative preservation of the axons, gliosis, and varying degrees of inflammation. Sites of predilection include the optic nerve, spinal cord, periventricular areas, and the brainstem. Each small lesion is orientated around a venule, which, in the acute stages, shows perivascular cuffing with lymphocytes and plasma cells.

Axonal loss is seen in established lesions and may result in an expansion of the extracellular space. Chronic lesions show marked astrocytic gliosis. There are also a number of immunological abnormalities.

Clinical features

The diagnosis depends on the demonstration of physical signs that can only be explained by lesions in at least two sites in the central nervous system (CNS). There is a wide spectrum of disease activity, and the course of the disease is extremely variable. The onset is monosymptomatic in 85% of patients, while in the remainder there is clear evidence of involvement at a number of sites. Common presentations include optic neuritis, symptoms referable to the brainstem and

Cerebellar lesions lead to VANISH'D: vertigo, ataxia, nystagmus, intention tremor, slurred speech, hypotonic reflexes, and dysdiadochokinesia.

cerebellum (including diplopia and ataxia), sensory disturbance of the limbs, and leg weakness.

Optic neuritis

The patient develops increasingly blurred vision in one eye, which may progress to complete uniocular blindness during a period of a few hours or 2–3 days. Central vision is usually more severely affected. The affected eye may be painful, and colour vision is almost always affected. The optic nerve head appears normal unless the plaque is very anterior, when the disc may be swollen. Vision usually improves after 3–4 weeks and often returns to normal within 2 months. Transient blurring of vision lasting minutes, associated with exercise or raised body temperature (Uthoff's phenomenon), may occur.

Diplopia

This is a common symptom caused by a brainstem plaque involving fibres of the 3rd, 4th, or 6th cranial nerves, or by a lesion in the medial longitudinal bundle causing an internuclear ophthalmoplegia.

Motor weakness

Motor weakness is more common in the arms than in the legs, reflecting involvement of the thoracic spinal cord.

Sensory symptoms

These include paraesthesia and dysaesthesia, proprioceptive disorders resulting in sensory ataxia and incoordination, and diminished vibration sense. Flexion of the neck may lead to an electric shock sensation in the back and limbs (Lhermitte's sign), and is associated with a lesion in the cervical cord.

Cerebellar signs

Cerebellar signs include nystagmus, dyssynergia (fragmentation of voluntary movements resulting in intention tremor), dysdiadochokinesia, incoordination of the heel–shin test, titubation (continuous rhythmical tremor of the head and trunk), and dysarthria.

Other manifestations

Other manifestations include the following:

- Cognitive impairment: especially of memory, sustained concentration, and abstract conceptual reasoning.
- Psychiatric abnormalities: most commonly depression; about 10% of patients suffer psychotic symptoms; euphoria may be present in severely disabled patients.
- Pain: this occurs in up to 50% of patients; trigeminal neuralgia is 300 times more common in patients with MS than in the general population.
- Paroxysmal symptoms: these include tonic seizures, and rapid flickering contraction in the facial muscles (myokymia).
- Bladder disturbance: this occurs in 50–75% of patients and is the presenting symptom in 10%; frequency, urgency, and incontinence are the most common symptoms; sexual dysfunction is common.
- Uncommon manifestations: 'useless hand' syndrome (an upper limb ataxia), lower motor neurone signs, swallowing and respiratory problems, and extrapyramidal movement disorders.

Diagnosis and differential diagnosis

The diagnosis of MS is based on clinical findings, and the exclusion of conditions producing a similar clinical picture.

Initially, individual plaques may cause diagnostic difficulty and must be distinguished from compressive, inflammatory, and mass or vascular lesions. Inflammatory conditions include isolated angiitis of the CNS, SLE, primary Sjögren's syndrome, Behçet's disease, and PAN.

The differential diagnosis also includes infectious diseases, e.g. Lyme disease and brucellosis, multiple emboli, and granulomatous disorders, e.g. sarcoidosis and Wegener's granulomatosis.

Investigations

The following investigations are important in the patient with MS:

- Examination of CSF shows a pleocytosis, raised protein, and immunoglobulin (Ig) G. Oligoclonal IgG is seen in 90% of patients with clinically definite MS

but is not specific for MS as it is also seen in a wide range of inflammatory and infectious disorders.
- Delay in the visually evoked response follows optic neuropathy, which may be subclinical. It is useful in providing evidence of a second lesion in patients whose neurological deficits are only attributable to a single lesion.
- Magnetic resonance imaging (MRI) is very useful and can show plaques in the vast majority of patients with clinically definite disease.

Prognosis

The progression of MS is very variable. There are four distinctive clinical presentations:

- Intermittent relapses followed by remissions. With each ensuing attack, the remissions are less complete, so that within 10–20 years the patient is physically disabled.
- Rapid deterioration with numerous relapses and only partial remissions in the first year or two of illness.
- Infrequent attacks with long periods of remission.
- Continuous deterioration without remission.

Once the particular pattern has been established, the disease tends to develop along its declared path. After 5 years, 70% of patients are still employed. After 20 years, only 35% are employed, and 20% are dead from complications.

Management

No cure for MS has been found. Adrenocorticotrophic hormone or corticosteroids have an established role in acute relapses but do not alter the course of the disease. Intravenous pulses of steroids may be effective in acute disease, but there is no justification for subjecting patients to the hazards of long-term corticosteroid therapy.

β-Interferon may be used for patients with relapsing–remitting MS who are able to walk unaided. It is indicated for reducing the frequency and degree of severity of clinical relapses. There is no evidence of an effect on the progression of the disease, the duration of exacerbations, or on disability. Not all patients respond, and an accelerated deterioration has been observed in some. It should not be used in those with a history of severe depressive illness, inadequately controlled epilepsy, or decompensated hepatic impairment. Side effects include irritation at the injection site, and influenza-like symptoms, although these decrease with time.

Symptomatic treatment is of great importance. Physiotherapy and occupational therapy maintain maximum function. Spasticity may respond to baclofen, dantrolene, or vigabatrin. The intention tremor resulting from the involvement of the cerebellum may respond to isoniazid and pyridoxine, or to β-blockers. Trigeminal neuralgia and paroxysmal symptoms may respond to carbamazepine, and chronic dysaesthetic pain may respond to tricyclic antidepressants.

The management of patients with bladder disturbance has been revolutionized by the introduction of clean intermittent self-catheterization. Anticholinergic agents, particularly oxybutynin, may alleviate urinary frequency. In men with erectile dysfunction, intracorporeal papaverine may be helpful.

MENINGITIS

Meningitis is inflammation of the membranous coverings of the brain and spinal cord. It may be caused by the following:

• Infection: bacteria, viruses, and fungi.
  Malignant cells.
• Blood following SAH.
• Air, drugs or contrast media during encephalography.

The term 'meningitis' is usually reserved for infection of the meninges by organisms.

Pathophysiology

In acute bacterial meningitis, a dense exudate forms over the base of the brain and extends towards the convexity along the sulci. It may affect emerging cranial nerves giving rise to ocular palsies. Sulcal pockets of the exudate may become encysted or it may occlude the foramina of Magendie and Luschka with consequent hydrocephalus.

In tuberculous meningitis, the meninges over the base of the brain are most severely affected. A tough gelatinous exudate often involves the cranial nerves and the blood vessels. The subsequent arteritis may lead to occlusion of the vessel and infarction of the tissues which it supplies. In the case of miliary dissemination, choroidal tubercles can often be found in the optic fundus.

Viral meningitis consists mainly of a lymphocytic inflammatory reaction in the CSF without the formation of pus or adhesions.

Predisposing factors

Outbreaks of meningitis tend to occur with overcrowding, poverty, and malnutrition. Infection may spread in institutions such as prisons or universities. Secondary meningitis can occur after head injury, sinusitis, mastoiditis, or extension of infection from the ears and nasopharynx. Immunocompromised patients such as those with acquired immunodeficiency syndrome (AIDS), carcinoma, or those on cytotoxic drugs, and following splenectomy are at increased risk. People with congenital meningeal defects or CSF shunts are also prone to infection.

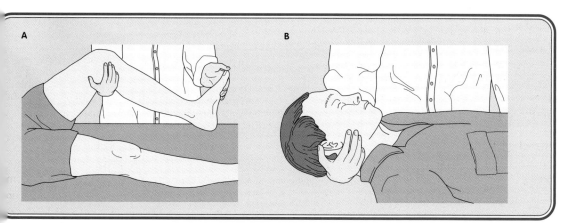

Fig. 34.6 (A) Eliciting Kernig's sign. (B) Testing for neck stiffness.

Clinical features

The features of meningitis are headache, neck stiffness, and clouding of consciousness. Bacterial meningitis is spread by droplet infection, and the organism lodges and multiplies in the nasopharnynx. It enters the bloodstream giving rise to a generalized septicaemia, pyrexia, malaise, and rigors. Signs of cerebral irritability include photophobia, increased tendon reflexes, vomiting, and convulsions.

Kernig's sign (Fig. 34.6) may be positive, i.e. pain on passively extending `the knee with the hips fully flexed. A petechial rash may occur, especially with meningococcal meningitis.

In tuberculous meningitis, symptoms may initially be non-specific with malaise, anorexia, headache, and a variable mild pyrexia. These symptoms may persist for days but gradually an unremitting deterioration occurs. There may be personality changes and intermittent dulling of consciousness before signs of meningism are obvious. The appearance of focal neurological signs suggests a complication, e.g. venous sinus thrombosis, cerebral oedema, or hydrocephalus.

Differential diagnosis

Any cause of headache (Chapter 15) or infection should be considered. Of particular note are severe migraine, acute encephalitis, and SAH.

Investigations

Blood should be taken for FBC, U&Es, glucose , and culture. Cultures should also be taken from the urine and nose. A skull X-ray should be obtained with a history of head injury.

Lumbar puncture is the key investigation and should be performed as soon as possible. If the patient is profoundly ill, intravenous antibiotics should be given first.

A CT scan should be carried out if raised intracranial pressure is suspected or if there are focal neurological signs, to rule out a space-occupying lesion. If normal, a lumbar puncture should be performed.

CSF changes in meningitis are summarized in Fig. 34.7.

Treatment

High doses of appropriate antibiotics should be given immediately a lumbar puncture is performed, or before it if the patient is very ill. The treatment of viral meningitis is supportive. Causative organisms include echovirus, mumps, coxsackievirus, herpes simplex and zoster, measles and influenza. Other causes of aseptic meningitis include SLE, syphilis, Lyme disease, leptospirosis, *Listeria*, *Brucella*, and partially treated bacterial meningitis.

Gram-staining of CSF may demonstrate organisms Pneumococcus is a Gram-positive intracellular diplococcus, and meningococcus (*Neisseria meningitidis*) is a Gram-negative coccus. Ziehl–Neelsen staining may show acid-fast bacilli suggesting tuberculosis.

If bacterial meningitis is suspected, high doses of intravenous antibiotics should be started. If the organism is not known, adults should be given intravenous benzylpenicillin 2.4 g 4 hourly and i.v. chloramphenicol 50–100 mg/kg 6 hourly, in liaison with the microbiologist. If the organism is known, specific antibiotics can be given (Fig. 34.8).

Changes in the cerebrospinal fluid in meningitis				
	Normal	**Viral**	**Bacterial**	**Tuberculous**
appearance	clear	clear/turbid	turbid	turbid/fibrinous
predominant cell	<5 mononuclear cells/mL	10–100 mononuclear cells/mL	200–3000 polymorphs/mL	10–300 mononuclear cells/mL 0–300 polymorphs/mL
protein	0.2–0.4 g/L	0.4–0.8 g/L	0.5–5 g/L	0.5–5 g/L
glucose	>2/3 plasma level	>2/3 plasma level	<2/3 plasma level	<2/3 plasma level

Fig. 34.7 Changes in the cerebrospinal fluid in meningitis.

Causative organisms

This is likely to vary with the patient's age:

- In neonates: *E. coli* and β-haemolytic streptococci are common.
- In children: *Haemophilus influenzae* and meningococcus predominate.
- Young adults: prone to meningococcus.
- Older adults: prone to pneumococcus (*Streptococcus pneumoniae*).
- Immunocompromised patients and the elderly: prone to pneumococcus, *Listeria*, Gram-negative organisms, and cryptococcus.

Pain is treated with opiates and an appropriate antiemetic. Intravenous fluids are given if the patient is shocked, aiming to increase blood pressure and urine output.

Contacts of patients with meningitis due to *N. meningitidis* or *H. influenzae* should be given rifampicin for 2 days.

Cases of meningitis must be reported to the Department of Public Health.

EPILEPSY

Epilepsy refers to a group of conditions in which paroxysms of abnormal electrical activity of cerebral neurones results in seizures. As many as 1 in 20 of the general population have a fit at some time in their lives, and at any one time around 200 000 people in the UK are taking antiepileptic drugs.

Classification

Seizure disorders can be divided into two main groups: idiopathic generalized epilepsies, and localization-related epilepsies.

Idiopathic generalized epilepsies

These are mostly genetic in origin and are often associated with a characteristic spike and wave on electroencephalogram (EEG).

Tonic–clonic (grand mal) fits

Before the fit the patient may be irritable and experience minor disturbances such as myoclonic jerks. There may be a strange feeling (aura) before the fit, which has a sudden onset. The tonic phase involves

Fig. 34.8 Treatment of meningitis.

Treatment of meningitis	
Organism	**Treatment**
Neisseria meningitidis	benzylpenicillin or cefotaxime rifampicin 2 days before discharge
Streptococcus pneumoniae	cefotaxime benzylpenicillin if organism is penicillin sensitive add vancomycin if organism is highly resistant to penicillin or cephalosporins
Haemophilus influenzae	choramphenicol or cefotaxime for *H. influenzae* type B give rifampicin for 4 days before discharge
Listeria	amoxycillin and gentamicin
Escherichia coli	amoxycillin
Staphylococcus aureus	benzylpenicillin and flucloxacillin or vancomycin
Mycobacterium tuberculosis	isoniazid, rifampicin, pyrazinamide, and ethambutol pyridoxine prevents the neurotoxic effects of isoniazid
Cryptococcus neoformans	amphotericin B and flucytosine

powerful muscular contractions. The patient is struck unconscious and falls rigidly to the ground. Teeth are clenched; cyanosis may occur. After about a minute, the clonic phase starts, consisting of violent convulsive movements. There may be tongue biting and urinary or faecal incontinence. The patient then becomes drowsy or will sleep for several hours. The reflexes are depressed, with a positive Babinski sign. The patient may be confused on waking (post-ictal confusion).

Absence attacks (petit mal)
These start in childhood and are accompanied by a characteristic EEG pattern of three spike-and-wave discharges per second. It is due to a congenital neuronal instability. There are brief interruptions of consciousness, sometimes accompanied by rhythmical blinking of the eyelids. To an observer, the child may appear to be dazed or daydreaming. Recovery is immediate and there are no sequelae.

Myoclonic epilepsy
This is a form of idiopathic epilepsy developing in early childhood. Various types of generalized fits occur including sudden jerking movements of the limbs (myoclonus).

Localization-related epilepsy
These have a focus of activity, e.g. a tumour, or scar tissue caused by trauma or a stroke, from which epileptic activity begins and then spreads. They may lead to generalized tonic–clonic seizures. The nature of the attack varies according to the primary site of the lesion. Examples include focal motor attacks, focal sensory attacks, and temporal lobe epilepsy.

Focal motor attacks
These arise in the precentral motor cortex and consist of clonic movements in localized groups of muscles such as the hand or face. They may continue for hours, in which case it is called epilepsia partialis continuans. The discharge may spread along the precentral gyrus causing a march of clonic movements throughout the body (Jacksonian seizure). After the seizure, there may be a short-lived weakness of the affected parts of the body (Todd's paresis).

Focal sensory attacks
These start in the postcentral sensory cortex, and either localized or spreading paraesthesiae occur.

Temporal lobe epilepsy
This may consist of hallucinations of any of the five senses and of memory. Gustatory and olfactory hallucinations are usually unpleasant. *Jamais vu* is a sudden feeling of unfamiliarity while the patient is in his or her own environment and *déjà vu* is a vivid sense of familiarity with the current situation.

In automatism, the patient remains conscious but 'dreamy' and may continue with normal activities. The patient cannot remember these events after the attack.

Aetiology
Although most fits are idiopathic, a cause for the epilepsy and precipitating factors should be looked into. These include the following:
- Metabolic causes: hypoxia, hyper- or hypoglycaemia, hypocalcaemia, uraemia, alcoholism, hypo- and hypernatraemia, liver failure, pyridoxine deficiency.
- Drugs and toxins: alcohol, lead, and drugs, e.g. phenothiazines, monoamine oxidase inhibitors, tricyclic antidepressants, amphetamines, lidocaine, nalidixic acid.
- Trauma and surgery, e.g. perinatal trauma or head injury.
- Space-occupying lesions.
- Cerebral infarction.
- Other organic brain diseases: SLE, PAN, sarcoidosis, vascular malformations.
- Infections: encephalitis, syphilis, and human immunodeficiency virus.
- Degenerative brain disorders: Alzheimer's disease, Creutzfeld–Jacob disease.

Precipitants of epilepsy
Fits may be precipitated by flashing lights. Other possible precipitants include fever, irregular meals, menstruation, hyperventilation leading to alkalosis, lack of sleep, emotional disturbances, and pregnancy.

Differential diagnosis
When taking a history it is important to keep in mind a differential diagnosis of conditions causing transient loss of consciousness. These include the following:
- Syncope: this is due to cerebral ischaemia. The onset is gradual and the patient slips to the floor. Recovery occurs after 1–2 minutes and is gradual. The patient is back to normal within a few minutes.

- Drop attacks: this involves a sudden weakness of the legs making the patient fall. It is most commonly due to vertebrobasilar artery insufficiency.
- Hypoglycaemia: the onset is prolonged and the patient is confused, sweating, and light-headed. A time relationship to meals may be established.
- Narcolepsy: irresistible diurnal attacks of sleepiness. The patient may experience visual or auditory hallucinations when falling asleep (hypnogogic hallucinations). The patient wakes within a few minutes feeling well.
- Cataplexy: a sudden loss of muscle tone so that the patient crumples to the ground.
- Micturition, defecation, and cough syncope: fainting after the respective acts.
- Carotid sinus syncope: this is due to supersensitivity of the carotid sinus to external pressure.
- Postural hypotension: either autonomic or secondary to drugs.
- TIAs, especially in the posterior cerebral circulation.
- Cardiac arrhythmias: due to impaired cardiac output; the loss of consciousness is sudden and the patient goes pale; there may be flushing on regaining consciousness.
- Psychogenic (hysterical fits): there is usually some apparent gain for the patient, although he or she is seldom aware of the motivation. The fits usually only occur in front of an audience. There is often active opposition on attempting to examine the patient. There may be strange cries and flailing limbs in an attempt to mimic true epilepsy.

Investigations
In the UK, a single seizure in a young person who recovers fully (pseudoseizures) is not usually pursued. Investigation is reserved for those who do not recover fully, or who have had two or more seizures within 1 year. After a careful history and examination to consider differential diagnoses, blood tests include FBC, U&Es, serum calcium, liver function tests, and glucose. A CXR and ECG should be performed.

The diagnosis should not be based solely on the EEG because 10–15% of the general population may have an 'abnormal' EEG, and approximately 15% of people with epilepsy never have specific epileptiform discharges.

CT scanning as the sole basis of diagnosis is also unreliable. The frequency of abnormalities found in CT scans in people with epilepsy varies greatly. A CT scan is indicated in a patient with late-onset epilepsy who has focal seizures, because it may detect a tumour.

Treatment
The aims of drug treatment are to prevent seizures whilst keeping the patient free of side effects. Antiepileptic drugs should be prescribed singly using the lowest dose to obtain complete seizure control with minimum side effects. A single drug will suffice in approximately 80% of patients, the remainder needing a second drug to achieve acceptable control. Localization-related epilepsy is more likely to be refractory.

Carbamazepine, phenytoin, and barbiturates all induce hepatic enzymes and therefore speed up the metabolism of oestrogens and progestogens making the oral contraceptive pill unreliable. Sodium valproate does not affect oral contraceptive efficacy.

First-line drugs
Idiopathic generalized epilepsy
Sodium valproate is often recommended as the treatment of choice because carbamazepine is ineffective for the treatment of absence or myoclonic seizures. They are equally as effective for idiopathic generalized tonic–clonic seizures. Common unwanted effects of sodium valproate include weight gain, hair thinning, and tremor. Hepatotoxicity, thrombocytopenia, and pancreatitis may occur. Ethosuximide is a useful alternative in children with absence seizures only.

Localization-related epilepsies
Carbamazepine, sodium valproate, phenytoin and phenobarbitone are all equally effective. However, they differ in their side effect profiles and ease of use, and because of this carbamazepine and sodium valproate have become the drugs of first choice. Carbamazepine may cause CNS side effects, e.g. dizziness, nausea, headaches, and drowsiness, which may be avoided by slowly increasing the dose. It induces hepatic microsomal enzymes and so increases the metabolism of phenobarbitone, sodium valproate, lamotrigine, corticosteroids, oral contraceptives, theophylline, and warfarin. It also inhibits the metabolism of phenytoin. Idiosyncratic reactions include the Stevens–Johnson syndrome, exfoliative dermatitis, and hepatitis.

Second-line drugs
Phenytoin is useful but often difficult to use because of its unpredictable pharmacokinetics and so the best dose

UK advice on epilepsy and driving is as follows:
First/solitary fit:
○ 1 year off driving (must be fit free) with medical review before restarting.
If another fit occurs during this time, the patient must wait a year from
that fit before review.

Loss of consciousness without known cause:
○ As above.

Seizures during sleep:
○ After one seizure, regulations as above. If all attacks for at least 3 years have
been during sleep, and the patient has never had an attack while awake, driving is
allowed.

Withdrawal of antiepileptic medication:
○ Advise patient not to drive (but this is not a legal obligation on the patient's part)
for 6 months from the time of withdrawal. Clearly, if further seizures occur, the
above regulations apply.

is difficult to determine. Phenobarbitone affects cognition and behaviour and is no longer considered a first-line drug. Primidone is partly metabolized in the liver to phenobarbitone and is no longer recommended.

Add-on drugs
Vigabatrin, lamotrigine, and gabapentin are used as add-on therapies for partial or secondarily generalized seizures. They are equally effective. Vigabatrin may cause drowsiness, fatigue, irritability, weight gain, and psychosis. Lamotrigine can precipitate carbamazepine toxicity, so if unwanted effects such as diplopia occur, the dose of carbamazepine should be reduced. It causes a mild maculopapular rash in 5% of patients, the incidence of which can be reduced by starting at a low dose. Gabapentin is renally excreted so the dose should be reduced in patients with renal impairment. The most common side effects are somnolescence, dizziness, and ataxia.

The benzodiazepines, clobazem and clonazepam, may also be used. Clobazem can be used as an add-on for people with refractory epilepsy. Taken continuously it can cause dependence. Clonazepam is useful in children with myoclonic or tonic–clonic seizures. Sedation and tachyphylaxis are common, and withdrawal seizures may occur. It should be used only rarely.

Epilepsy can have profound social consequences including discrimination and exclusion from certain jobs, e.g. the armed forces. Personal implications include feelings of insecurity. There are also restrictions on driving. Patients can obtain information about epilepsy from the British Epilepsy Association.

INTRACRANIAL TUMOURS

Cerebral tumours represent about 10% of all malignancies. They may be primary or secondary mainly from the bronchus, breasts, kidneys, colon, ovary, prostate, or thyroid. The main sites of origin of brain tumours are shown in Fig. 34.9. Other tumours are rare.

Clinical features
Symptoms arise from the direct effects of the mass on surrounding structures, the effects of raised ICP, or by provoking seizures. Similar symptoms may be produced by any mass lesion, e.g. haematomas, aneurysms, abscesses, tuberculomas, granulomas, and cysts.

Direct effects depend on the site of the tumour:
• Frontal lobe: personality changes, apathy, and

The origins of brain tumours	
Site	**Example of tumour derived**
glia	gliomas (50%), oligodendrogliomas, ependymomas
meninges	meningiomas (25%)
blood vessels	angiomas, angioblastomas
the Schwann cells of the cranial nerves	acoustic neuromas
pituitary gland	craniopharyngioma

Fig. 34.9 The origins of brain tumours.

impairment of intellectual function. There may be anosmia, contralateral hemiparesis, or dysphasia (Broca's area).

- Parietal lobe: contralateral homonymous field defects and hemisensory loss. There may be apraxia, spatial disorientation, and dysphasia if the temporoparietal region is affected. Signs include 'parietal drift' or falling of the outstretched contralateral arm, asteriognosis (inability to recognize an object placed in the hand), and sensory inattention.
- Temporal lobe: symptoms and signs are those of temporal lobe epilepsy (see p. 304).
- Occipital lobe: contralateral hemianopia.
- Cerebellopontine angle: there is progressive ipsilateral perceptive deafness, numbness of the ipsilateral side of the face, facial weakness, vertigo, and ipsilateral cerebellar signs (see p. 299).

Raised intracranial pressure

Symptoms include a throbbing headache (which is worse in the morning and with stooping, coughing, and sneezing), nausea and vomiting, and papilloedema. A shift of intracranial contents produces symptoms similar to direct mass effects. There may be impairment of consciousness progressing to coma, respiratory depression, and 'false localizing signs', e.g. a 6th nerve lesion, as it is compressed on the petrous temporal bone.

Investigations

The main investigations are a skull X-ray, EEG, CT brain scan, and MRI. If metastases are suspected,

investigations for the primary neoplasm should be carried out. Lumbar puncture is contraindicated because of the risk of herniation of the cerebellar tonsils through the foramen magnum ('coning'). Biopsy should be considered, especially if an abscess is suspected.

Management

This is by surgical excision if possible. Radiotherapy is usually recommended for gliomas and for radiosensitive metastases. Dexamethasone will reduce cerebral oedema. Epilepsy is treated with anticonvulsants.

Prognosis

The overall 1-year survival for patients with primary intracerebral tumours is less than 50%. There may be complete recovery from meningiomas if they are removed completely.

MISCELLANEOUS NEUROLOGICAL DISORDERS

Motor neurone disease

This is a disease of unknown cause involving progressive degeneration of the anterior horn cells, lower cranial nuclei (hence the external ocular movements are normal), and neurones of the motor cortex and pyramidal tracts. Both upper and lower motor neurones can be affected but there are no sensory abnormalities.

It is slightly more common in men with a peak incidence between the ages of 50 and 70 years. The prevalence in the UK is about 6 in 100 000. Clinically there are three classical patterns of disease:

- Amyotrophic lateral sclerosis (50%): combined lower motor neurone wasting and upper motor neurone spasticity and hyperreflexia. Weakness starts in the legs and spreads to the arms.
- Progressive muscular atrophy (25%): anterior horn cell involvement leading to lower motor neurone weakness, wasting, and fasciculation of distal muscles, which spreads proximally.
- Progressive bulbar palsy (25%): lower motor neurone weakness and wasting of the tongue and pharynx leading to dysarthria and dysphagia.

Combinations of the above may occur.

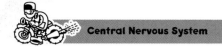

Causes of peripheral neuropathy	
Cause	**Example**
idiopathic	
drugs and chemicals	isoniazid, amiodarone lead, mercury
metabolic	diabetes mellitus amyloidosis uraemia acute intermittent porphyria
deficiency states	deficiencies of vitamin B_{12}, B_1 (beriberi) and niacin (pellagra) alcoholism
infections	leprosy diphtheria tetanus botulism
miscellaneous	Guillain–Barré syndrome collagen diseases, e.g. PAN, RA malignancy sarcoidosis myxoedema
congenital	rare hereditary ataxias and neuropathies

Fig. 34.10 Causes of peripheral neuropathy (PAN, polyarteritis nodosa; RA, rheumatoid arthritis).

Management

Management is symptomatic. The aim is help the patient with activities of daily living and to reduce symptoms. Opiates should be considered for joint pains and distress. Death usually occurs between 2 and 5 years after diagnosis.

Peripheral neuropathy

The causes of peripheral neuropathy are summarized in Fig. 34.10. The four most common causes are DM, malignancy, vitamin B_{12} deficiency, and drugs. Treatment is aimed at the underlying cause.

Guillain–Barré syndrome

This condition (also called acute postinfective polyneuropathy) affects motor nerves more than sensory nerves, and follows days or weeks after an infectious illness such as cytomegalovirus and Epstein–Barr virus. There is inflammation, oedema, and demyelination of peripheral nerves and roots. Clinically, there is parasthesia and numbness followed by a flaccid paralysis, which is progressive and ascending, but may come on rapidly and affect all four limbs simultaneously. The trunk, respiratory, and cranial nerves may be affected. Complications include respiratory failure, pulmonary embolism, and cardiac dysrhythmias.

Investigations

The CSF shows a very high protein concentration (up to 10 g/L) with a normal cell count. The vital capacity should be measured 4–6 hourly to anticipate respiratory depression.

Management

Treatment is supportive. Attention should be paid to fluid balance and nutrition, and prevention of pressure sores, deep vein thrombosis, and pneumonia (physiotherapy). Ventilation may be necessary if respiratory failure occurs. Around 90–95% of patients recover within 3–6 months.

Muscle disorders

For more on muscle disorders, see polymyositis on pp.350–351.

Myasthenia gravis

This is an autoimmune disease with a reduction in the number of functioning postsynaptic acetylcholine receptors leading to muscle weakness. About 90% of patients have detectable antiacetylcholine receptor antibodies. It is associated with thymic tumours, hyperthyroidism, rheumatoid arthritis, and SLE.

Clinical features

The condition affects young adults and women twice as commonly as men. There is painless muscle weakness, which worsens on repetitive contraction. It is usually most marked in the face and eyes producing ptosis, diplopia, and a 'myasthenic snarl' on smiling. The voice may weaken on continued speaking and dysphagia may occur. Proximal muscles and upper limbs are more often affected than distal muscles and lower limbs. Reflexes tend to be brisk.

Investigations

Edrophonium (Tensilon®) 10 mg is given intravenously (with cardiac monitoring and resuscitation facilities). This improves muscle power for 3–4 minutes. It is an anticholinesterase, which enhances neuromuscular transmission in myasthenia gravis. It prolongs the action of acetylcholine by inhibiting the action of the enzyme acetylcholinesterase. There is raised antiacetylcholine receptor antibody.

Management

Symptomatic control is with a longer-acting anticholinesterase, e.g. pyridostigmine or neostigmine. The dose is slowly titrated against muscle power. Side effects include nausea, vomiting, increased salivation, diarrhoea, and abdominal cramps. In overdosage there may be excessive bronchial secretions and sweating, involuntary defecation and micturition, bradycardia, agitation, and weakness eventually leading to fasciculation and paralysis. Thymectomy increases the percentage of patients in remission.

Immunosuppression with prednisolone on alternate days may achieve remission. If there is no remission and weakness is severe, azathioprine may be helpful. In intractable cases, plasmaphoresis gives about weeks of benefit. The condition is usually relapsing or slowly progressive, and respiratory muscle involvement can lead to death. The 5-year survival with a thymoma about 30%.

Myotonic dystrophy (myotonia dystrophica)

This is an autosomal dominant condition characterized by myotonia, i.e. the inability of the muscles to relax normally after contraction. The peak onset is between the ages of 20 and 30 years, and the incidence in the UK is about 5 in 100 000. There is muscle wasting and weakness of the facial muscles with frontal balding, ptosis, a wry smile or 'sneer' and a 'hound dog' appearance.

There is also weakness of the shoulder girdle and quadriceps, cataracts, testicular or ovarian atrophy, cardiomyopathy with conduction disturbances, and mental impairment. Reflexes are lost. The myotonia increases with fatigue, cold, and stress. It may improve with procainamide or phenytoin and there may be associated DM.

Muscular dystrophies

These are a group of genetically determined diseases characterized by progressive degeneration and weakness of certain muscle groups.

Duchenne muscular dystrophy (pseudohypertrophic)

This is the commonest type and is sex-linked recessive. The incidence is 25 in 100 000 male births. The condition presents at around 5 years of age with clumsiness in walking and difficulty in climbing stairs Examination reveals a lordotic posture and 'waddling' gait due to proximal muscle weakness. The calves are hypertrophied. Investigations show a markedly raised creatine kinase concentration. Electromyography and muscle biopsy show characteristic changes. Death usually occurs before the age of 20 years from intercurrent illnesses, e.g. chest infection. There is no specific treatment.

Fascioscapulohumeral dystrophy (Landouzy–Dejerine syndrome)

This is autosomal dominant. The onset is around puberty with wasting and weakness of the upper limb girdle and face. Life expectancy is normal.

Limb girdle dystrophy (Erb's syndrome)

This is autosomal recessive and presents at around 20–40 years. The shoulders and muscles of the pelvic girdles are affected, and the condition is progressive with death in middle age.

Disorders of the spinal cord
Syringomyelia
This is due to a longitudinal cyst in the cervical cord. As it enlarges it may extend into the dorsal horns and white matter. Clinical features are insidious and include the following:

- Weakness and wasting of the small muscles of the hand.
- Dissociated sensory loss in the hand: loss of pain and temperature sensation only. This may involve the trunk and arm may be involved.
- Trophic changes, e.g. ulceration and scarring, and swollen fingers due to subcutaneous hypertrophy.
- Loss of tendon reflexes.
- Pain in the arm.
- Spastic paraplegia: upper motor neuron signs.
- Charcot's joints in the upper limbs: destruction of the joints by too great a range of movement when normal sensation is lost.

Treatment is by surgical decompression or aspiration.

Syringobulbia
This is usually due to the extension of the cyst into the midbrain. It may involve the trigeminal nerve root, the motor nuclei of the lower cranial nerves, and the cervical sympathetic tract. Symptoms include the following:

- Facial pain or sensory loss: 5th cranial nerve.
- Vertigo and nystagmus: 8th cranial nerve.
- Facial, palatal, or laryngeal palsy: 7th, 9th, 10th, and 11th cranial nerves.
- Wasting of the tongue: 12th cranial nerve.
- Horner's syndrome: sympathetic tract.

Subacute combined degeneration of the cord
This is due to vitamin B_{12} deficiency and refers to demyelination of the posterior and lateral columns. The onset is usually insidious and associated with a sensory peripheral neuropathy. Clinical features include the following:

- Loss of vibration and proprioception senses, and positive rombergism: posterior columns.
- Weakness, hypertonia, and extensor plantars: upper motor neuron.
- Absent knee jerks and reduced touch sensation: peripheral neuropathy.

Treatment is with vitamin B_{12} injections intramuscularly.

Spinal cord compression
Spinal cord compression is a medical emergency. Symptoms include root pain often precipitated by movement or straining, spastic paraparesis with upper motor neurone signs and weakness, sensory loss, with sphincter disturbances at a later stage. Investigation is by X-ray of the spine, and CT or MRI to show the spinal cord. Investigations should also include those of the underlying cause.

Treatment is by decompression, which should be performed as soon as possible to prevent irreversible damage. Radiotherapy may be useful in malignant disease.

Causes of spinal cord compression are summarized in Fig. 34.11.

Causes of spinal cord compression	
Cause	**Example**
vertebral (extradural)	collapsed vertebrae, e.g. metastatic cancer (bronchus, breast, thyroid, kidney, prostate), osteoporosis, myeloma spondylosis with disc prolapse Pott's disease (tuberculosis) Paget's disease abscess reticuloses
intradural, extramedullary	meningioma neurofibroma
intramedullary	glioma

Fig. 34.11 Causes of spinal cord compression.

DIABETES

Diabetes mellitus (DM) is a persisting state of hyperglycaemia due to diminished availability or effectiveness of insulin. The diagnosis is made on finding two random plasma glucose concentrations greater than or equal to 11.1 mmol/L, or two fasting plasma glucose levels greater than or equal to 7.8 mmol/L.

If the fasting glucose is at least 6 mmol/L but below 7.8 mmol/L there may be impaired glucose tolerance; this is an indication for an oral glucose tolerance test although this is rarely carried out in practice. The patient is given 75 mg of glucose. If the glucose after 120 minutes is above 7.8 mmol/L but below 11.1 mmol/L then the patient has impaired glucose tolerance.

The cause of diabetes is not known but it is partly genetic and partly environmental—30% of identical twins and 10% of siblings develop diabetes. There is an association with human leukocyte antigen (HLA)-D3 and HLA-DR4. Environmental triggers may include viral infections. Diabetes affects about 2% of the population.

Classification

Type I, or insulin-dependent diabetes mellitus (IDDM), usually starts in young people who are usually thin and have an abrupt onset of signs and symptoms associated with low circulating insulin. IDDM is due to autoantibodies to pancreatic β cells causing a low concentration of circulating insulin.

Patients with type II, or non-insulin-dependent diabetes mellitus (NIDDM), are usually older and overweight, and the onset is more insidious. NIDDM is due to reduced insulin production and reduced sensitivity of peripheral tissues to circulating insulin. Patients may require insulin if hyperglycaemia persists despite maximal doses of oral hypoglycaemic agents, and in times of stress such as severe infections or after myocardial infarction.

Secondary DM may be caused by the following:
Drugs, e.g. thiazide diuretics and steroids.
Gestational DM: patients develop impaired glucose tolerance or frank diabetes during pregnancy.
Pancreatic disease, e.g. pancreatectomy, carcinoma of the pancreas, pancreatitis, cystic fibrosis, haemachromatosis.
- Endocrine causes: Cushing's syndrome, acromegaly, phaeochromocytoma.

Clinical presentation

Diabetes may be asymptomatic and found on routine screening but about half of all diabetics are undiagnosed. Patients may present with non-specific symptoms such as weight loss and lethargy, and they are more prone to infection, e.g. carbuncles and thrush. Polyuria and polydipsia are characteristic. The patient may present for the first time with diabetic ketoacidosis, i.e. smelling of ketones, hyperventilating, dehydrated, and even drowsy, confused, or comatosed (Fig. 35.1).

Complications

The chronic complications of DM are summarized in Fig. 35.2.

Vascular system

Disease in both the large and small vessels is more common in people with diabetes and occurs in all vascular beds, leading to an increased incidence of myocardial infarction, stroke, renal failure, retinopathy, and peripheral vascular disease. It is therefore important to control other cardiovascular risk factors such as hypertension, smoking, and hyperlipidaemia. Myocardial infarction is twice as common in diabetics than in the general population.

In small vessel disease, pedal ischaemia and gangrene can occur despite the presence of palpable pedal pulses.

Eyes

Blindness occurs in up to 20% of patients with IDDM. Good diabetic control reduces the incidence of eye complications. Large fluctuations in blood glucose concentration (and hence the glucose concentration of the vitreous humour) cause osmotic shifts across the lens resulting in transiently blurred vision. This is common when the diabetes is first treated. Cataracts occur at a younger age in diabetics.

311

Background retinopathy

This is characterized by haemorrhages ('blots'), hard exudates, and microaneurysms ('dots'), which are bulges in the capillary walls. Vision is rarely affected unless macular oedema develops, in which case referral to an ophthalmologist should be made.

Preproliferative retinopathy

The above changes are usually more marked. In

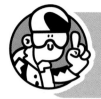

In a patient with gangrene and a palpable dorsalis pedis pulse, think of microvascular disease.

addition, there are soft 'cotton-wool' exudates, which are small deep retinal infarcts.

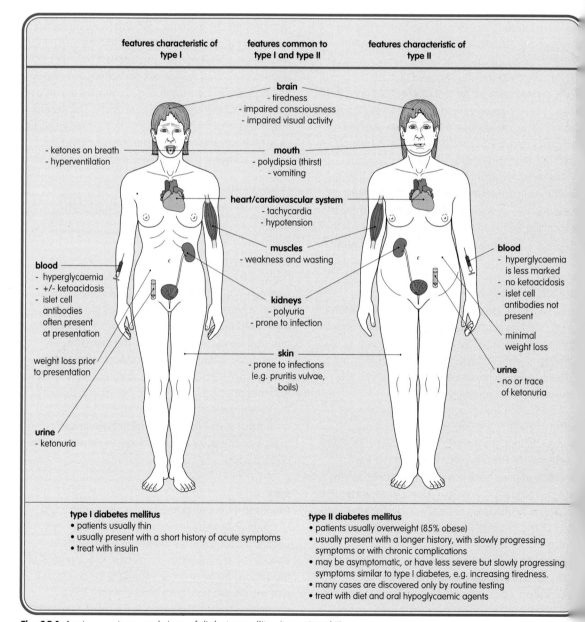

Fig. 35.1 Acute symptoms and signs of diabetes mellitus (types I and II).

Proliferative retinopathy

There is new vessel formation, mainly near the optic disc in response to relative hypoxia in the vitreous. Other features such as cluster haemorrhages and soft exudates are present. Urgent referral to an ophthalmologist for laser therapy should be made because the new vessels are fragile and may bleed into the vitreous leading to sudden blindness. Fibrosis then ensues and can lead to retinal detachment and thrombotic glaucoma.

Maculopathy

Although sometimes difficult to see on fundoscopy, this should be suspected if there is a decrease in visual acuity. Patients should visit an ophthalmologist.

Neuropathies

Somatic neuropathies

Somatic neuropathies may take the following forms:
- Peripheral neuropathies: this commonly affects the lower limbs, with numbness and parasthesiae of the

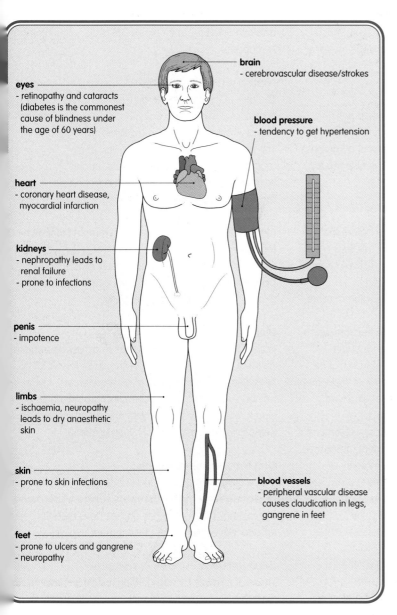

Fig. 35.2 Chronic complications of diabetes mellitus.

eyes
- retinopathy and cataracts (diabetes is the commonest cause of blindness under the age of 60 years)

heart
- coronary heart disease, myocardial infarction

kidneys
- nephropathy leads to renal failure
- prone to infections

penis
- impotence

limbs
- ischaemia, neuropathy leads to dry anaesthetic skin

skin
- prone to skin infections

feet
- prone to ulcers and gangrene
- neuropathy

brain
- cerebrovascular disease/strokes

blood pressure
- tendency to get hypertension

blood vessels
- peripheral vascular disease causes claudication in legs, gangrene in feet

feet, spreading up the leg. Symptoms are predominantly sensory with early loss of vibration sense and absent ankle jerks. In advanced cases, the loss of pain sensation may lead to the development of punched-out chronic ulcers at pressure points, in areas of thick callus. Foot pulses may be easily palpable; the foot may then become infected and eventually gangrenous.

- Mononeuritis: this is due to occlusion of an artery supplying the nerve. Commonly involved nerves include the 3rd cranial nerve, ulnar nerve, and lateral popliteal nerve. More than one nerve can be involved, hence mononeuritis multiplex.
- Diabetic amyotrophy: this is painful asymmetrical weakness and wasting of the quadriceps muscles. It may recover.

Autonomic neuropathies
This may lead to symptoms of postural hypotension, i.e. dizziness on standing, impotence, nocturnal diarrhoea, and urinary retention. There may be lack of awareness of symptoms of hypoglycaemia, which is also more frequent in patients on β-blockers.

Kidneys
About a quarter of diabetics diagnosed before the age of 30 years develop renal failure. Renal failure is hastened by concomitant poor blood pressure control. Predisposing factors include the following:

- Atherosclerosis and hypertension: leading to renal ischaemia.
- Infection: glycosuria predisposes to infection, which is more common throughout the urinary tract.
- Renal papillary necrosis: caused by infarction of the papillae resulting in haematuria and renal impairment. The papillae may slough and cause obstruction.

Most of the renal problems are secondary to glomerular lesions; there is thickening of the basement membrane. This may be diffuse and present in the majority of diabetics, or nodular as in the Kimmelstiel–Wilson lesion, which is pathognomonic of DM and consists of homogenous, acellular, eosinophilic nodules.

Skin
Complications occurring in the skin include the following:

- Lipoatrophy: this is fat necrosis at insulin injection sites. The patient should be advised to vary the injection sites because the absorption of insulin at sites of atrophy is unpredictable. Transfer to human insulin may help.
- Necrobiosis lipoidica diabeticorum: these are yellowish areas on the skin with telangiectasia. Biopsy shows atrophy of subcutaneous collagen. They are pathognomonic of diabetes.
- Infections, such as boils, are more common.
- Granuloma annulare.

Infections
Common infections are of the urinary tract and skin, and candidiasis. Tuberculosis (TB) is also more common in diabetics.

Management of diabetes
The aim of treatment is to achieve the best possible control of plasma glucose without making the patient obsessional, and avoiding disabling hypoglycaemia. The patient is best managed as part of a multidisciplinary team with doctors, nurses, ophthalmologists, dieticians, and chiropodists. A good rapport should be established and the patient should be educated about good diabetic control, how to abort hypoglycaemic attacks, and the symptoms to watch out for with hyperglycaemia.

New patients may be deliberately made hypoglycaemic so that they know what symptoms to expect, and how to abort the attack.

Diet
Calorie intake should be adjusted to achieve or maintain an ideal body weight. The diet should be low in fat (to help delay the progression of atherosclerosis), low in refined sugars but high in complex carbohydrates like starch, and high in fibre which, among other benefits, helps to lower postprandial hypoglycaemia.

Oral hypoglycaemic agents
These drugs should be used in addition to, not instead of, diet. The two main classes are sulphonylureas and biguanides, although other classes have recently been introduced, with more in development.

Sulphonylureas
These act mainly by augmenting insulin secretion and therefore some residual pancreatic β-cell activity is

required. There are several sulphonylureas but all are probably equally as effective. Chlorpropamide however has more side effects and a very prolonged duration of action leading to possible hypoglycaemia in some. It may also cause facial flushing after alcohol. Elderly patients are particularly prone to the dangers of hypoglycaemia when long-acting sulphonylureas are used, and so chlorpropamide and glibenclamide should be avoided and replaced by shorter-acting drugs.

The sulphonylureas tend to encourage weight gain. Caution is needed in the elderly and those with hepatic and renal insufficiency because of the hazard of hypoglycaemia. Side effects are generally mild and infrequent and include gastrointestinal (GI) disturbances and headache. Some patients acquire sensitivity reactions which include transient rashes, rarely progressing to erythema multiforme and exfoliative dermatitis.

Biguanides

Metformin is the only available biguanide. It exerts its effect mainly by decreasing gluconeogenesis and by increasing peripheral utilization of glucose. Some residual islet cell function is required. It is usually reserved for people with NIDDM who are overweight and in whom diet and sulphonylureas fail to control diabetes adequately, but it may be used as a first-line agent in overweight patients; hypoglycaemia is not usually a problem. GI side effects are common and lactic acidosis may also occur, although usually only in patients with renal impairment, in whom it should not be used.

Other agents

Acarbose, an inhibitor of intestinal α-glucosidases, delays the digestion of starch and sucrose and hence the increase in blood glucose levels which follow a carbohydrate-containing meal.

Guar gum can reduce postprandial plasma glucose concentrations in diabetes, probably by retarding carbohydrate absorption. It is also used to relieve symptoms of the dumping syndrome.

Insulin

Approximately 25% of diabetics require treatment with insulin (a polypeptide hormone). It is inactivated by GI enzymes and must therefore be given by injection, usually subcutaneously. Mixtures of available insulin

preparations may be required to maintain good control, and these will vary for individual patients. Requirements may be affected by variations in lifestyle, infections, and concomitant drugs.

Patients should aim for blood glucose concentrations between 4–10 mmol/L for most of the time, while accepting that on occasions they will be above or below these values. They should be advised to look for 'peaks' and 'troughs' of blood glucose, and to adjust their insulin dosage only once or twice weekly. Overall it is ideal to aim for an glycosylated haemoglobin (HbA_{1c}) level of below 7% (normal range is 4–6%) or an HbA_1 of below 8.8% (normal range is 5.0–7.5%).

The insulin preparations may be short, intermediate, or long-acting. Most patients are best started on insulins of intermediate action twice daily; a short-acting insulin can later be added to cover any hyperglycaemia which may follow breakfast or evening meals (Fig. 35.3).

Continuing assessment

The aims of continued assessment of diabetics are education, assessment of glycaemic control, and assessment of complications.

Many patients now monitor their own blood glucose concentrations using blood glucose strips, preferably with an electronic meter. These records should be examined, together with any hypoglycaemic symptoms, and HbA_{1c}. Visual acuity should be checked, together with an examination of the optic fundi (after dilatation of the pupils with tropicamide) for retinopathy. The feet should be examined for neuropathy, ischaemic changes, and infection. Nephropathy should be looked for by monitoring the urea and electrolytes (U&Es) and by testing for albuminuria.

Diabetes and surgery

Diabetic patients should be first on the operating list, and fasted on the morning of surgery. Oral agents should be stopped 24 hours before surgery, and restarted postoperatively unless the patient is ill or the blood glucose is very high, necessitating a period on insulin.

For patients already on insulin, the usual insulin should be given the night before the operation. An intravenous infusion of 500 mL of 5% glucose with 10 mmol KCl should be started early on the day of the operation and run at a constant rate to the patient's fluid requirements. A

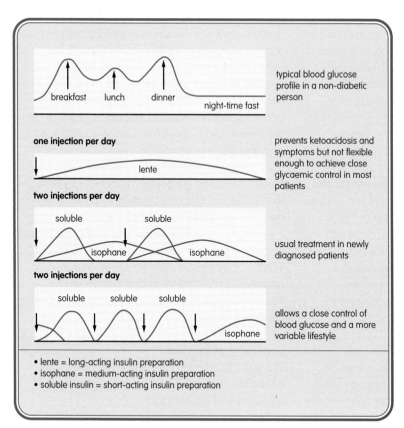

Fig. 35.3 Examples of different insulin regimens.

typical blood glucose profile in a non-diabetic person

one injection per day

lente

prevents ketoacidosis and symptoms but not flexible enough to achieve close glycaemic control in most patients

two injections per day

soluble   soluble

isophane   isophane

usual treatment in newly diagnosed patients

two injections per day

soluble   soluble   soluble

isophane

allows a close control of blood glucose and a more variable lifestyle

• lente = long-acting insulin preparation
• isophane = medium-acting insulin preparation
• soluble insulin = short-acting insulin preparation

1 unit/mL solution of soluble insulin in 0.9% saline should also be infused intravenously using a syringe pump. The rate varies according to the patient's blood glucose concentration, which should be measured every 2 hours until stable and every 6 hours thereafter.

When the patient starts to eat and drink, he or she may be restarted on the normal insulin regimen.

Diabetic coma
Hypoglycaemia
Symptoms of hypoglycaemia include sweating, hunger, and tremor. Very low glucose concentrations may cause drowsiness, fits, transient neurological symptoms, and loss of consciousness.

Aetiology
The aetiology of hypoglycaemia includes the following:
• Drugs: excessive insulin or sulphonylureas (especially chlorpropamide). Large doses may be taken deliberately, particularly by medical and paramedical staff. Alcohol binges, especially with decreased food intake, may also lead to hypoglycaemia.

• Endocrine causes: pituitary insufficiency, Addison's disease, and insulinomas.
• Post-gastrectomy and functional hypoglycaemia.
• Liver failure.
• Inherited enzyme defects.
• Neoplasms, e.g. retroperitoneal fibrosarcomas.
• Immune hypoglycaemia, e.g. anti-insulin receptor antibodies in Hodgkin's disease.
• Malaria.

Investigations
Blood glucose and simple tests to exclude possible causes, e.g. liver function tests (LFTs), and thick and thin blood films for malaria.

Insulinoma can be confirmed by infusing intravenous insulin and measuring C peptide. Normally insulin suppresses C peptide but this suppression does not occur in patients with insulinomas.

Management
If the patient is conscious, three or four lumps of sugar should be given with a little water, and this

should be repeated as necessary. If unconscious, 50 mL of 50% glucose should be given intravenously. Glucagon intramuscularly can be given as an alternative—this is a polypeptide hormone produced by the α-cells of the pancreatic islets of Langerhans. It increases plasma glucose by mobilizing glycogen stored in the liver.

For patients who have taken a long-acting preparation, a continuous intravenous glucose infusion for 24 hours may be required. If an underlying cause is found it should be treated on its own merits.

Diabetic ketoacidosis

Diabetic ketoacidosis usually presents as a gradual deterioration over hours or days, often precipitated by an infection such as pneumonia or urinary tract infections. The patient may be an undiagnosed diabetic. The patient is dehydrated and may be confused, vomiting, and hypotensive. The breath has a characteristic smell of ketones (like nail-polish remover).

Management

Dehydration, hypoglycaemia, electrolyte imbalances, and infections should be treated. Blood should be taken for glucose, U&Es, full blood count (FBC), blood cultures, and arterial blood gases (ABGs), and the urine should be tested for ketones and sent for microscopy and culture. A chest X-ray (CXR) should be requested.

A nasogastric tube may be passed to prevent gastric dilatation and aspiration, and 0.9% saline iv should be started immediately. Large volumes of fluid may be required as patients are usually 6–9 L fluid depleted, and the infusion should be started at 1 L per half hour in young people. The potassium may be low, and intravenous insulin will exacerbate this by shifting potassium into cells—intravenous fluids should therefore be supplemented with potassium.

Electrolytes should be checked hourly, aiming for a plasma potassium concentration between 4 and 5 mmol/L. Soluble insulin mixed with normal saline should be given intravenously by syringe pump. The rate is usually 4–12 units per hour according to the blood glucose level. When the blood glucose level has normalized and the patient is rehydrated and eating, the patient may be returned to subcutaneous insulin.

Urine output, blood glucose, blood pressure, pulse, and U&Es are monitored hourly. Patients are at risk of

deep vein thrombosis (DVT), so prophylactic subcutaneous heparin, such as heparin 5000 units b.d. or enoxaparin 20 units daily, may be given. Some centres give bicarbonate if the acidosis is very severe. However the acidosis will resolve with the above treatment, and its administration is potentially dangerous because it may exacerbate hypokalaemia. A source of infection should always be sought, with a low threshold for treatment.

Hyperglycaemic hyperosmolar non-ketotic coma

The onset of this is gradual over days. The patient is often elderly and may not be a known diabetic. Polyuria leads to dehydration. The blood glucose is very high and plasma osmolality is increased. There is no acidosis or ketonuria as there is no change to ketone metabolism. Patients require small doses of intravenous insulin and hypotonic saline, although long-term insulin may not be required. Central venous pressure monitoring may be required. Patients are at a high risk of DVT and are given prophylactic subcutaneous heparin. The mortality rate is up to 50%.

LIPID DISORDERS

Hypercholesterolaemia is widely prevalent in Western societies, particularly in the UK, where over 50% of the population older than 45 have serum total cholesterol concentrations above 6.5 mmol/L. There is a positive association between serum cholesterol and coronary heart disease, although cholesterol concentration alone is of limited predictive value. Of more importance is the patient's overall coronary risk, of which cholesterol is one risk factor. Hence some patients will have 'normal' cholesterol concentrations but may be at high coronary risk by virtue of additional risk factors such as diabetes or left ventricular hypertrophy. Conversely, some patients, notably young women, will be at low coronary risk even with 'high' cholesterol concentrations.

There is now good evidence that lowering serum cholesterol in high-risk patients leads to a reduction in coronary events, and these people should therefore be targeted for treatment. Drug treatment of people at low risk is undesirable as the adverse effects of treatment may outweigh any potential benefits.

317

Lipids are insoluble in water, and so cholesterol and triglyceride are transported in the bloodstream bound to proteins as lipoproteins. There are five principal types of protein in the blood, and they can be separated in the laboratory by their density and electrophoretic mobility.

Chylomicrons are very large particles, mainly containing triglyceride. They provide the main mechanism for transporting the digestion products of dietary fat to the liver and peripheral tissues. The endothelial enzyme lipoprotein lipase removes triglyceride from the particle. The remaining chylomicron remnant is taken up by the liver.

Very low density lipoproteins (VLDL) are synthesized and secreted by the liver and contain most of the endogenously synthesized triglyceride. As they pass round the circulation, triglyceride is progressively removed by lipoprotein lipase leaving a particle called an *intermediate density lipoprotein* (IDL).

IDLs can bind to the hepatocyte and be catabolized, or have further triglyceride removed producing *low density lipoprotein* (LDL) particles.

LDLs are the main carrier of cholesterol, and deliver it to both the liver and to peripheral cells. The circulating LDL concentration is regulated by hepatic LDL receptors, and by the rate limiting enzyme in the cholesterol synthetic pathway, 3-hydroxy-3-methylglutaryl coenzyme A (HMG-CoA) reductase. Some cholesterol synthesized by the liver is converted into bile salts and excreted in the bile, where they are reabsorbed through the terminal ileum and recirculated.

High density lipoproteins (HDLs) are produced in both the liver and intestine. They take up cholesterol from cell membranes in peripheral tissues to the liver by 'reverse cholesterol transport'. HDL cholesterol therefore has a cardioprotective effect and concentrations are inversely proportional to coronary risk.

Classification of hyperlipidaemia

The most common form of hyperlipidaemia is polygenic with high serum cholesterol concentrations and normal triglyceride concentrations. Other forms are much less common.

Familial combined hyperlipidaemia has a prevalence of 1 in 200 and is associated with high cholesterol and triglyceride concentrations.

Familial hypercholesterolaemia has an autosomal dominant inheritance and is due to LDL receptor deficiency resulting in an increase in LDL particles in the circulation. The prevalence is about 1 in 500. Homozygotes can have serum cholesterol levels of up to 30 mmol/L or more and may develop coronary artery disease in their teenage years.

Familial hypertriglyceridaemia is also an autosomal condition and can cause pancreatitis. Patients may have eruptive xanthomata. Triglyceride may also be raised in diabetes, alcoholism, and obesity.

Other classes of dyslipidaemia are rare.

Secondary hyperlipidaemia

Causes include DM, excess alcohol, hypothyroidism, cholestasis, chronic renal impairment, nephrotic syndrome, and synthetic oestrogens.

Management

Causes of secondary hyperlipidaemia should be treated. Where there is no secondary cause dietary measures should be tried first. However, the average fall in total cholesterol concentration with a general lipid lowering diet is only 2%. Drug treatment is aimed at high-risk patients. For every 1% reduction in total cholesterol concentration (by diet or drug treatment), coronary heart disease risk is reduced by 1–2%.

Drugs
Statins

The statins—atorvastatin, cerivastatin, fluvastatin, pravastatin, and simvastatin—competitively inhibit HMG-CoA reductase, an enzyme involved in cholesterol synthesis, especially in the liver. There is evidence that statins produce important reductions in coronary events in high-risk patients, and their use is outlined below. They should be used with caution in those with a history of liver disease. Side effects include reversible myositis.

Treatment should be stopped if there are symptoms of myopathy and creatinine phosphokinase is markedly elevated. Patients should therefore be advised to report unexplained muscle pain, tenderness, and weakness. Other side effects include headache, altered LFTs and effects, e.g. abdominal pain, nausea, and vomiting.

Fibrates

Examples include clofibrate, bezafibrate, ciprofibrate, fenofibrate, and gemfibrozil. Their main action is to decrease serum triglyceride but they also tend to reduce LDL cholesterol and raise HDL cholesterol. They can all cause a myositis-like syndrome, especially in patients with impaired renal function. Also, clofibrate predisposes to gallstones by increasing biliary cholesterol excretion. It should therefore only be prescribed to patients who have had a cholecystectomy.

Anion-exchange resins
These include cholestyramine and colestipol, and act by binding bile acids, preventing their reabsorption; this promotes hepatic conversion of cholesterol into bile acids. They reduce LDL cholesterol but can aggravate hypertriglyceridaemia. Anion-exchange resins interfere with the absorption of fat-soluble vitamins. Supplements of vitamins A, D, and K, and of folic acid may be required when treatment is prolonged.

Side effects are mainly GI effects and include change in bowel habit, nausea, vomiting, and abdominal pain. Other drugs should be taken at least 1 hour before, or 4–6 hours after cholestyramine or colestipol to reduce possible interference with absorption.

Nicotinic acid group
The value of nicotinic acid is limited by its side effects, especially vasodilatation. In high doses it lowers both cholesterol and triglyceride concentrations by inhibiting synthesis. It also increases HDL cholesterol.

Fish oils
These may be useful in hypertriglyceridaemia. They can however aggravate hypercholesterolaemia.

Ispaghula
Ispaghula husk is a form of soluble fibre and can be used as an adjunct to a lipid-lowering diet in patients with mild hypercholesterolaemia. It probably acts by reducing reabsorption of bile acids. Plasma triglycerides remain unchanged.

The use of statins
Before considering treatment with statins, other methods to reduce the risk of coronary heart disease (CHD) should be instigated. This includes stopping smoking, dietary advice to control weight and lower lipids, advice on regular physical activity, control of hypertension, and other pharmacological measures, such as aspirin therapy, where appropriate. Current recommendations for lipid lowering with statins in the UK is to prioritize patients according to risk.

Secondary prevention
The first priority is patients who have had a myocardial infarction with serum cholesterol ≥4.8 mmol/L or LDL ≥3.2 mmol/L. The second priority is patients with angina or other clinically overt atherosclerotic disease who have total cholesterol ≥5.5 mmol/L. This includes patients with peripheral vascular disease or symptomatic carotid disease or who have had a bypass or angioplasty. These two priority groups encompass about 4.8% of the UK population aged 35–69 years.

Primary prevention
The third priority is treatment of people without clinically apparent vascular disease but who nevertheless have a high risk of developing overt CHD, equivalent to those requiring secondary prevention (that is a risk of major CHD events of 3% per year or more) and with total cholesterol ≥5.5 mmol/L based on the average of at least two measurements taken several weeks apart.

People may have this level of risk because of a combination of other CHD risk factors, particularly diabetes or hypertension. Formal estimation of CHD risk is essential when identifying subjects for primary prevention of CHD. One means of assessing this level of risk is shown in Fig. 35.4. This group for primary prevention encompasses a further 3.4% of the population aged 35–69 years. At present there is little evidence of benefit or harm from starting statin treatment in people over the age of 70 years. Treatment of people free of vascular disease with a risk of developing overt CHD of less than 3% a year and a total cholesterol of ≥5.5 mmol/L would entail treating a high proportion of adults. At present cost-effectiveness is low.

Treatment should be started at a low dose and increased as necessary to reduce total cholesterol to 5.0 mmol/L or by 20–25% in high-risk patients who have serum cholesterol below 6.3 mmol/L before starting treatment.

METABOLIC BONE DISEASE

Vitamin D metabolism is shown in Fig. 35.5.

Osteoporosis
Bone normally consists of 60% mineral and 40% matrix or organic matter. In osteoporosis there is a loss of

Sheffield table for primary prevention of coronary heart disease
Showing serum cholesterol concentration conferring an estimated risk of coronary events of 3.0% per year

Men: cholesterol concentration (mmol/L)

Hypertension	Yes	Yes	Yes	Yes	Yes	No	Yes	Yes	No	No	Yes	No
Smoking	Yes	Yes	No	No	Yes	Yes	Yes	No	Yes	No	No	No
Diabetes	Yes	No	Yes	No	Yes	Yes	No	Yes	No	Yes	No	No
LVH on ECG**	Yes	Yes	Yes	Yes	No	No	No	No	No	No	No	No
Age (years)												
70	5.5	5.5	5.5	5.5	5.5	5.5	5.5	5.5	5.5	6.0	6.5	7.7
68	5.5	5.5	5.5	5.5	5.5	5.5	5.5	5.5	5.6	6.4	6.9	8.2
66	5.5	5.5	5.5	5.5	5.5	5.5	5.5	5.7	5.9	6.8	7.3	8.7
64	5.5	5.5	5.5	5.5	5.5	5.5	5.5	6.1	6.3	7.3	7.8	9.3
62	5.5	5.5	5.5	5.5	5.5	5.5	5.6	6.5	6.7	7.8	8.3	
60	5.5	5.5	5.5	5.5	5.5	5.6	6.0	6.9	7.2	8.3	8.9	
58	5.5	5.5	5.5	5.5	5.5	6.1	6.5	7.4	7.7	8.9		
56	5.5	5.5	5.5	5.5	5.5	6.5	7.0	8.0	8.3			
54	5.5	5.5	5.5	5.5	5.9	7.0	7.5	8.6	9.0			
52	5.5	5.5	5.5	5.5	6.3	7.6	8.1	9.3				
50	5.5	5.5	5.5	5.7	6.9	8.2	8.8					
48	5.5	5.5	5.5	6.2	7.5	8.9						
46	5.5	5.5	5.5	6.8	8.2							
44	5.5	5.5	5.8	7.4	9.0							
42	5.5	5.6	6.4	8.2								
40	5.5	6.1	7.1	9.0								
38	5.5	6.8	7.9									
36	6.0	7.6	8.8									
34	6.7	8.6										
32	7.6											
30	8.7											
<29												

Notes on use of table

Do not use for decisions on secondary prevention: patients with myocardial infarct, angina, peripheral vascular disease, or symptomatic cartoid disease already have high CHD risk. At this risk (3% events per year) treatment with a statin (but not necessarily other drug classes) is justifiable. Use the table after appropriate advice on smoking, diet, and control of systolic blood pressure to < 160mmHg. Use the average of two or more cholesterol concentrations. The table may underestimate CHD risk in some individuals;
- British Asians
- those with low HDL cholesterol
- those with very strong family history of premature CHD
- those with familial hyperlipidaemia

Women: cholesterol concentration (mmol/L)

Hypertension	Yes	Yes	Yes	Yes	Yes	No	Yes	Yes	No	No	Yes	No
Smoking	Yes	No	Yes	Yes	Yes	Yes	No	Yes	No	Yes	No	No
Diabetes	Yes	Yes	No	Yes	Yes	Yes	Yes	No	Yes	No	No	No
LVH on ECG**	Yes	Yes	Yes	No	No	No	No	No	No	No	No	No
Age (years)												
70	5.5	5.5	5.5	5.8	6.3	6.9	8.5	9.8				
68	5.5	5.5	5.5	5.8	6.4	7.0	8.6	9.9				
66	5.5	5.5	5.5	5.9	6.5	7.1	8.7	10.0				
64	5.5	5.5	5.5	6.1	6.6	7.2	8.9					
62	5.5	5.5	5.5	6.2	6.8	7.4	9.1					
60	5.5	5.5	5.5	6.4	7.0	7.7	9.4					
58	5.5	5.5	5.5	6.7	7.3	8.0	9.8					
56	5.5	5.5	5.5	7.0	7.7	8.4						
54	5.5	5.5	5.5	7.4	8.1	8.9						
52	5.5	5.5	5.9	7.9	8.7	9.4						
50	5.5	5.5	6.4	8.5	9.3							
48	5.5	6.0	6.9	9.3								
46	5.5	6.7	7.7									
44	5.5	7.5	8.6									
42	5.8	8.5	9.8									
40	6.7	9.9										
35	8.0											
36	9.7											
<35												

Instructions

Choose the table for men or women
Identify the correct column for smoking, hypertension and diabetes
In normotensive subjects assume LVH absent. In those with hypertension, LVH is diagnosed by ECG showing increased voltage and flat or inverted T waves in the left precordial leads. If no ECG is available, assume LVH is absent
Identify the row showing the age of the subject
Read off the cholesterol concentration at the intersection of the appropriate column and row:
If there is no entry, cholesterol need not be measured
If there is an entry, measure serum cholesterol
If the average cholesterol on repeated measurement is at or above the level shown, the CHD event risk is 3.0% per year consider treatment
The table can be used to look forward to need for measurement or treatment at an older age

**HYPERTENSIVE SUBJECTS ONLY
LVH = left ventricular hypertrophy;
CHD = coronary heart disease;
ECG = electrocardiograph

References: Haq IU et al. Lancet 1995, 346: 1467–71;
Ramsay LE et al. Lancet 1996, 348: 387–88; Haq IU et al. Clin Sci 1996, 91: 399–413

Fig. 35.4 Sheffield table for primary prevention of coronary heart disease.

bone matrix and reduction in bone mass, although the deposition of calcium salts, or mineralization, occurs normally. There is therefore a reduction in the amount of bone mineral per unit volume of anatomical bone. This prevalence increases with age, and overall affects about 5% of the population.

Aetiology

There are a number of risk factors associated with osteoporosis. They can be divided into physiological and pathological factors, as follows.

Physiological

- Age.
- Early menopause.
- Immobility.
- Smokers.
- Thin people.
- Excess alcohol intake.

Pathological

- Steroids.
- Cushing's disease.

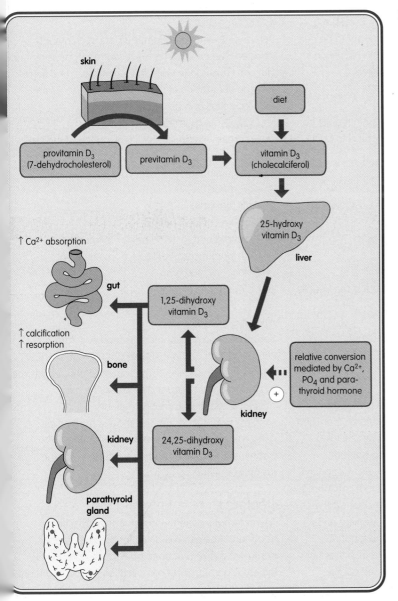

Fig. 35.5 Metabolism of vitamin D.

- Multiple myeloma.
- Thyrotoxicosis.
- Hypogonadism.
- Primary biliary cirrhosis.
- Rheumatoid arthritis.

Osteoporosis is sometimes subclassified into two types. Individuals with type I (postmenopausal osteoporosis) are middle-aged. Trabecular bone is more commonly affected leading to crush fractures of the vertebrae. It is principally due to oestrogen deficiency.

In type II (senile osteoporosis), individuals are usually over 70 years old. Cortical bone is most commonly affected resulting in fractures of the long bones, e.g. of the femoral neck. The mechanism is thought to be due to secondary hyperparathyroidism due to reduction in calcium and vitamin D intake and synthesis.

Clinical features
Osteoporosis is not painful in itself; the pain results from fractures. Vertebral crush fractures may lead to back pain, loss of height, and kyphosis.

Investigations
The following investigations should be considered in osteoporosis:
- Serum calcium, phosphate, and alkaline phosphatase: normal.
- Bone X-rays: show skeletal rarefaction.
- Bone histology: may be carried out but is not usually necessary.
- Bone densitometry.
- Exclusion of other disease associated with osteoporosis.

Management
As there is no effective cure, prevention is the key to management. High-risk individuals should be identified. Hormone replacement therapy (HRT) is beneficial in high-risk postmenopausal women. A combined preparation should be given to women, as unopposed oestrogens increase the risk of endometrial carcinoma, while androgens should be given to hypogonadal men. Exercise should be encouraged and increasing dietary calcium intake may be beneficial. Bisphosphonates may be of benefit in preventing fractures in susceptible individuals. Calcitonin and fluoride may be useful, although they are not of proven benefit.

Paget's disease
In Paget's disease there is uncontrolled bone turnover with local excessive osteoclastic resorption. This is followed by disordered osteoblastic activity, leading to new bone formation, which is structurally abnormal and weak (Fig. 35.6). The aetiology is unknown although viruses have been implicated. The incidence increases with age—it is uncommon in the under 40s but by the age of 90 years about 10% of the population in temperate climates is affected. It is also commoner in Anglo-Saxons and there appears to be a familial incidence.

Clinical features
The axial skeleton and femur are most commonly affected. The condition is most commonly asymptomatic but can cause bone pain and tenderness, and there may be deformities of affected bones, such as an enlarged skull and bowed (sabre) tibia.

Complications include:
- Progressive occlusion of the foramina of the skull, e.g. deafness due to nerve compression, basilar invagination, and cervical cord stenosis with paraparesis.
- Optic atrophy.
- Fractures of long bones.
- Hypercalcaemia: if the patient is immobile.
- High-output cardiac failure from shunting.
- Osteogenic sarcoma.
- Osteoarthritis of related joints.

Investigations
Serum alkaline phosphatase is markedly raised but serum calcium and phosphate are normal; 24-hour urinary hydroxyproline output is raised and reflects the increased bone turnover. There may be mild hypercalcaemia in immobile patients.

X-rays of affected bones show a mosaic of osteolytic and sclerotic lesions, thickening of trabeculae, and thick cortices with an enlarged irregular outline.

Treatment
Asymptomatic patients do not require specific treatment. Analgesia is given for pain but specific treatment is given for bone pain, bone deformities, hypercalcaemia, or for complications. Drug treatment is with bisphosphonates or calcitonin.

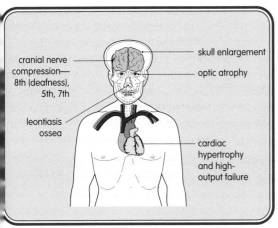

cranial nerve
compression—
8th (deafness),
5th, 7th

leontiasis
ossea

skull enlargement

optic atrophy

cardiac
hypertrophy
and high-
output failure

ig. 35.6 General features of Paget's disease of the bone.

Bisphosphonates

Bisphosphonates are adsorbed on to hydroxyapatite crystals, so slowing both their rate of growth and dissolution, and reducing the increased rate of bone turnover associated with the disease. Disodium etidronate is most commonly used. A single daily dose of 5 mg/kg is given for up to 6 months. This may be repeated after an interval of 3 months if there is evidence of reactivation. Side effects include focal osteomalacia and fractures.

Calcitonin

Calcitonin is involved with parathyroid hormone (PTH) in the regulation of bone turnover and hence in the maintenance of calcium balance and homoeostasis. The prolonged use of porcine calcitonin can lead to the production of neutralizing antibodies.

Salcatonin (synthetic salmon calcitonin) is less immunogenic and thus more suitable for long-term therapy. The dose for Paget's disease ranges from 50 units three times weekly up to 100 units daily, in single or divided doses. Treatment is for 3–6 months. Side effects include nausea, faintness, and flushing.

Osteomalacia

Osteomalacia results from inadequate mineralization of bone and occurs after fusion of the epiphyses. Rickets is the result if this occurs during the period of bone growth.

Aetiology

The aetiology of osteomalacia includes the following:
  Lack of dietary vitamin D.

- Ineffective conversion of 7-dehydrocholesterol (provitamin D_3) to previtamin D_3 by ultraviolet light in the dermis. This is due to lack of sunlight and, in the UK, is most commonly seen in Asians.
- Intestinal malabsorption, e.g. gluten-sensitive enteropathy and postgastrectomy states.
- Vitamin D resistance: chronic renal disease most commonly due to ineffective conversion of 25-hydroxyvitamin D_3 to 1,25-dihydroxyvitamin D_3, inherited deficiency of renal 1α-hydroxylase, or end-organ receptor abnormality (rare).
- Drug induced: chronic anticonvulsant therapy may induce liver enzymes, leading to the breakdown of 25-hydroxyvitamin D_3.
- Excessive renal phosphate loss due to Fanconi's syndrome or a specific defect in renal phosphate handling.

Clinical features

In patients with osteomalacia, there may be bone pain and tenderness. Fractures, especially of the femoral neck, may occur. There is a proximal myopathy resulting in a waddling gait and difficulty in rising from a chair.

In rickets, there are deformities of the legs (bow-legs and knock-knees), the chest (ricketic rosary), and the skull. There may also be features of hypocalcaemia, e.g. tetany.

Investigations
Biochemistry
- Serum calcium and phosphate: tend to be decreased.
- Serum alkaline phosphatase activity: increased.
- Urinary calcium excretion: low.
- Plasma 25-hydroxyvitamin D_3: low except in resistant cases.
- 1,25-dihydroxyvitamin D_3: low in renal failure.
- Parathormone is high because of secondary hyperparathyroidism due to hypocalcaemia.

X-rays
X-rays of bone in rickets show cupped, ragged metaphyseal surfaces. In osteomalacia, there is loss of cortical bone, and pseudofractures (Looser's zones), which are small translucent bands perpendicular to the bone and extending inwards from the cortex. They are best seen on the lateral border of the scapula, the femoral neck, and in the pubic rami.

Bone scan
A bone scan shows a generalized diffuse increase in uptake of isotope.

Treatment
Dietary vitamin D deficiency can be prevented by taking an oral supplement of 10 μg of ergocalciferol daily. Vitamin D deficiency caused by intestinal malabsorption or chronic liver disease usually requires vitamin D in pharmacological doses, such as calciferol tablets up to 1 mg (i.e. 10 000 units) daily. The hypocalcaemia of hypoparathyroidism often requires doses of up to 2.5 mg (100 000 units) daily in order to achieve normocalcaemia.

The newer hydroxylated vitamin D derivatives—alfacalcidol and calcitriol—have a shorter duration of action, and therefore have the advantage that problems associated with hypercalcaemia due to excessive dosage are shorter lived and easier to treat.

In patients with chronic renal impairment alfacalcidol or calcitriol should be prescribed. All patients receiving pharmacological doses of vitamin D should have their serum levels calcium checked at intervals, and whenever nausea and vomiting are present.

Breast milk from women taking pharmacological doses of vitamin D may cause hypercalcaemia if given to an infant.

Renal osteodystrophy
The term 'renal osteodystrophy' is used to cover the various forms of bone disease that develop in chronic renal failure. These include the following:

- Delayed epiphyseal closure in children and young adults.
- Rickets or osteomalacia.
- Osteitis fibrosa cystica (brown tumours) due to secondary or tertiary hyperparathyroidism.
- Generalized or localized osteosclerosis.

There is usually a metabolic acidosis. Serum calcium is low but serum ionic calcium is normal unless steps are taken to treat the acidosis actively. This can precipitate a severe attack of tetany. Serum phosphate and chloride are raised, which leads to ectopic calcification.

Management
Hydroxylation of 25-hydroxyvitamin D_3 is impaired and so treatment is with the hydroxylated derivatives of vitamin D. Phosphate binders, e.g. aluminium hydroxide, will lower serum phosphate and reduce the risk of metastatic calcification. Dialysis will help to return serum calcium and phosphate levels to normal.

Renal transplantation should restore calcium metabolism to normal although this may take some months as the parathyroid glands may not always switch off immediately after a long period of secondary hyperparathyroidism. Occasionally, subtotal parathyroidectomy is required.

HYPERPARATHYROIDISM

Hyperparathyroidism results from excess circulating parathyroid hormone (PTH), which increases serum calcium by increasing calcium absorption from the gut, increasing mobilization of calcium from bone, and reducing renal calcium clearance.

Primary hyperparathyroidism is usually due to a single benign adenoma but may less commonly be due to multiple adenomas, carcinoma, or hyperplasia. It may be associated with other endocrine abnormalities as part of the multiple endocrine neoplasia (MEN) syndromes. Ectopic PTH production may be produced by carcinoma from the lung and kidney.

Secondary hyperparathyroidism is due to raised PTH levels secondary to hypocalcaemia; the hypocalcaemic persists. Causes include chronic renal failure and deficiency of vitamin D, e.g. due to inadequate intake or malabsorption.

Tertiary hyperparathyroidism is the continued secretion of excess PTH after prolonged secondary hyperparathyroidism. The parathyroids act autonomously and cause hypercalcaemia, despite the absence of the original cause of the secondary hyperparathyroidism.

Clinical features
Symptoms may be due to bone disease and can result in fractures. There may be renal stones and nephrocalcinosis due to hypercalciuria, resulting in renal failure. Abdominal pain may be non-specific or due to constipation, peptic ulcer, or pancreatitis. Other features include anorexia, nausea and vomiting, thirst, polyuria, muscle fatigue, and psychiatric disorders including depression and confusion.

Investigations
In primary hyperparathyroidism serum calcium is raised. Fasting blood samples should be taken without venous compression. Serum phosphate is low and

For the clinical features of hypercalcaemia remember **bones** (bone pain), **stones** (renal stones), **groans** (peptic ulcer), and **moans** (psychiatric disease).

alkaline phosphatase is high, reflecting increased bone turnover. There is a mild renal tubular acidosis with a high serum chloride level, and serum PTH is raised. In secondary hyperparathyroidism of renal failure, serum calcium is low but phosphate is high.

X-rays show subperiosteal resorption, being most marked in the hands, and evidence of osteitis fibrosa cystica. A CXR should be done to look for bilateral hilar lymphadenopathy of sarcoidosis, or carcinoma producing PTH. A skull X-ray shows a 'pepperpot' appearance.

Treatment
Parathyroidectomy is indicated for persistent hypercalcaemia above 2.8 mmol/L or for symptomatic hypercalcaemia. The parathyroid glands may be localized by computed tomography (CT) scan or isotope scans. All four glands should be biopsied; single adenomas can be removed.

If the glands are hyperplastic, three-and-a-half are removed, leaving the last half *in situ*. Serum calcium and magnesium should be checked frequently postoperatively as removal of the glands may lead to rapid hypocalcaemia and hypomagnesaemia.

HYPOPARATHYROIDISM

Hypoparathyroidism is usually secondary to thyroid surgery. Primary (idiopathic) hypoparathyroidism is an autoimmune disorder associated with vitiligo, Addison's disease, pernicious anaemia, and other autoimmune diseases. The DiGeorge syndrome is a familial condition with parathyroid agenesis. It is associated with intellectual impairment, cataracts, and calcified basal ganglia.

Pseudohypoparathyroidism is a syndrome of end-organ resistance to PTH. It is associated with intellectual impairment, short stature, a round face, and short metacarpals and metatarsals.

Pseudopseudohypoparathyroidism describes the appearance present in pseudohypoparathyroidism but without the calcium abnormalities.

Clinical features
Circumoral paraesthesiae, cramps, anxiety, and tetany are followed by convulsions, laryngeal stridor, dystonia, and psychosis. Trousseau's sign may be present—carpopedal spasm when the brachial artery is occluded with a blood pressure cuff. Chvostek's sign may also be present—twitching of the facial muscles when the facial nerve is tapped.

Investigations
Serum calcium is low, phosphate is high, and alkaline phosphatase is normal. Additional tests include serum urea and creatinine, serum PTH level, parathyroid antibodies, and vitamin D metabolite levels.

X-rays of the hands show short fourth metacarpals in pseudohypoparathyroidism.

Treatment
Emergency treatment is with 10 mL 10% intravenous calcium gluconate, repeated as necessary. Intravenous magnesium chloride may also be required if there is hypomagnesaemia.

Long-term treatment is with alfacalcidol or calcitriol. Serum calcium should be monitored to prevent hypercalcaemia.

CRYSTAL ARTHROPATHY

Gout
Gout is a result of the deposition of sodium urate crystals in joints and soft tissues due to an abnormality of uric acid metabolism. It affects about 1 in 500 people in the UK. It is commoner in men, drinkers, and in higher socio-economic classes, and about a third have a positive family history. The underlying biochemical abnormality is an overproduction or underexcretion of uric acid resulting in hyperuricaemia. The main causes are given in Fig. 35.7.

Clinical features
Acute gout
This typically starts in the first metatarsophalangeal joint with an acute onset of a red, hot, swollen, extremely

painful big toe (Fig. 35.8). It may be precipitated by alcohol, diet, starvation, diuretics, or after surgery. Other commonly affected joints include the ankle, wrist, knees, and bursae. The patient may have high blood pressure, renal impairment, or peripheral vascular disease. The renal disease may be secondary to uric acid stones.

Chronic tophaceous gout

This leads to joint erosion and disruption leading to chronic disability. There are tophi in the ear lobes or around joints (particularly hands and elbows), which are soft tissue deposits of urate.

Causes of gout

- idiopathic
- drugs: diuretics, low-dose aspirin
- chronic renal impairment
- hypertension
- primary hyperparathyroidism
- hypothyroidism
- alcohol
- glucose-6-phosphate deficiency

rapid cell turnover:
- myeloproliferative disorders, e.g. polycythaemia rubra vera
- lymphoproliferative disorders, e.g. leukaemia
- severe psoriasis

Fig. 35.7 Causes of gout.

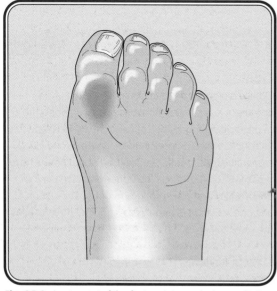

Fig. 35.8 Acute gout of the first metatarsophalangeal joint.

Investigations

The following investigations are important in patients with gout:

- Synovial fluid examined under polarized light microscopy shows needle-shaped, negatively birefringent crystals.
- X-rays may be normal in acute gout but show punched-out erosions and joint disruption in chronic gout.
- Serum uric acid may be high but there are a large number of false positive and false negative results. It is more useful for monitoring treatment.

Management
Acute attacks

These are normally treated with high doses of non-steroidal anti-inflammatory drugs (NSAIDs) such as naproxen 500 mg b.d. or ibuprofen 400 mg t.d.s. They should be used with care in patients with peptic ulcer disease, heart failure, hypertension, and renal impairment.

Colchicine is probably as effective as NSAIDs but excessive doses cause diarrhoea. Other common side effects include nausea and vomiting, and abdominal pain. They do not cause fluid retention and may be given to patients with hypertension, heart failure and renal impairment, and patients on anticoagulants.

Prophylactic treatment

The patient should be advised on weight reduction, reducing alcohol consumption, avoiding precipitating foods such as red meat, and avoiding precipitating drugs if possible.

Drug treatment should be continued indefinitely onc the decision to prevent further attacks had been made The initiation of treatment may precipitate an acute attack, therefore colchicine or NSAIDs should be used prophylactically for at least 1 month after the hyperuricaemia has been corrected.

Allopurinol inhibits xanthine oxidase, which catalyse the conversion of hypoxanthine to xanthine, and of xanthine to uric acid. It is especially useful in patients with renal impairment or urate stones where uricosuric agents cannot be used. It is usually given once daily (initially 100 mg after food) and gradually increased to maintenance dose of about 300 mg daily. Lower dose are given in patients with renal impairment. It may cause skin rashes.

Uricosuric drugs include probenecid and sulphinpyrazone. They may be used instead of allopurinol or with it in cases that are resistant to treatment. Aspirin antagonizes the effect of uricosuric drugs. It is important to ensure a good urine output as they may lead to crystallization of urate in the urine.

HYPERCALCAEMIA

The causes of hypercalcaemia have already been given in Fig. 29.22. The two commonest pathological causes are primary hyperparathyroidism and malignant disease. However the commonest cause of borderline hypercalcaemia is probably faulty technique, i.e. excessive venous stasis when collecting blood samples. An abnormally high result should therefore be repeated.

The physiologically relevant measurement is of ionized calcium. This can be determined by correcting serum total calcium levels for serum protein or albumin concentrations. The higher the protein concentration, the more calcium is protein bound, and the lower the proportion of ionized calcium.

Clinical features

These are discussed under hyperparathyroidism (see p.324–325).

Management

Severe hypercalcaemia is a medical emergency, and in extreme cases can lead to drowsiness, altered consciousness, and coma; adequate rehydration with intravenous saline is essential. Frusemide should also be given if necessary. Drugs that promote hypercalcaemia should be discontinued and dietary calcium should be restricted. Intravenous bisphosphonates are given for hypercalcaemia of malignancy, e.g. intravenous pamidronate 7.5 mg per kg per day for 3 days.

High-dose prednisolone is effective for hypercalcaemia secondary to myeloma, sarcoidosis, and excess vitamin D but otherwise is of little value. It may take some days to achieve the desired effect. Intravenous calcitonin has an acute but short-lived effect. It is rarely effective where intravenous bisphosphonates have failed to reduce serum calcium adequately. Sodium cellulose phosphate, which binds calcium in the gut, has been used but is rarely helpful, and any associated increase in serum phosphate may be harmful.

After treatment of severe hypercalcaemia the underlying cause must be established and treated appropriately.

PITUITARY DISORDERS

Non-functioning pituitary tumours and hypopituitarism

The incidence of pituitary tumours varies from 0.2–3 in 100 000 population, and the prevalence is about 9 in 100 000. Prolactin (PRL)- and adrenocorticotrophic (ACTH)-secreting tumours occur most commonly in 25–35 year olds, growth hormone (GH)-secreting tumours in 35–50 year olds, and non-functioning tumours usually present after the age of 60 years.

The signs and symptoms of functioning tumours are related to hormonal hypersecretion. They may cause acromegaly via GH, amenorrhoea–galactorrhoea syndrome via PRL, or Cushing's disease via ACTH. Non-functioning tumours can extend beyond the sella turcica and produce symptoms related to the mass of the tumour. These may be related to pressure on the anterior pituitary resulting in hypopituitarism, or symptoms related to extrasellar tumour growth resulting in headaches, bitemporal hemianopia due to pressure on the optic chiasma, other visual field defects and cranial nerve disturbances, personality changes, focal neurological symptoms and signs, and epilepsy.

Investigations include skull X-ray, magnetic resonance imaging (MRI), or CT scanning of the brain, and endocrinological assessment as outlined in Chapter 29.

Management may be surgical or medical. Trans-sphenoidal surgery improves visual field defects in up to 70% of patients. However, the recurrence rate of non-functioning tumours is about 20% after 5 years. Drug therapy includes dopamine receptor agonists, e.g. bromocriptine which inhibits PRL release and induces shrinkage of PRL-secreting adenomas. Somatostatin analogues inhibit GH release and induce a lesser degree of tumour shrinkage in most GH-secreting adenomas.

Hypopituitarism

This may result from hypothalamic or pituitary disease. The most common cause includes the mass effect of pituitary adenomas, with additional loss of pituitary function after surgery and pituitary irradiation. Other causes include hypothalamic tumours and cysts, peripituitary tumours, e.g. gliomas and meningiomas, craniopharyngiomas, infiltrative diseases, e.g.

sarcoidosis, and vascular and metastatic lesions in and around the pituitary fossa.

Clinical features

These can be worked out from knowledge of the effects of the various pituitary hormones:

- GH: fatigue, loss of energy, increased abdominal adiposity, and reduced muscle strength and exercise capacity.
- Luteinizing hormone (LH) and follicle-stimulating hormone (FSH): in women there is oligomenorrhoea, infertility, dyspareunia, breast atrophy, loss of pubic and axillary hair, and hot flushes; in men, there is loss of libido, impotence, infertility, flushes, regression of secondary sexual characteristics, soft testicles, and fine wrinkles on the face.
- Thyroid-stimulating hormone (TSH): fatigue, muscle weakness, sensitivity to cold, constipation, apathy, weight gain, and dry skin.
- ACTH: fatigue, anorexia, weight loss, pallor, weakness, nausea and vomiting, hypoglycaemia, apathy, and loss of pubic and axillary hair.
- Vasopressin: polyuria and polydipsia with nocturia.

Tests of pituitary function are given in Chapter 29.

Management

Hormone replacement involves the use of multiple hormones. Careful instruction and patient compliance are mandatory for long-term recovery.

Acromegaly

Acromegaly is an insidious disease resulting from excessive circulating levels of GH in adults. The incidence is about 5 per million per year, and the prevalence is 50 per million.

Acromegalic gigantism results from acromegaly in young individuals before epiphyseal fusion, and is very uncommon.

Aetiology

The commonest cause is a benign pituitary tumour secreting GH. Pituitary carcinoma is an uncommon cause. Carcinoid tumours which secrete hypothalamic GH-releasing hormone are another uncommon cause.

Clinical features

The clinical features of acromegaly are summarized in Fig. 35.9.

Facial appearance

Features are coarse, with enlargement of the supraorbital ridges, a broad nose, and thickening of the soft tissues. The lips are thick, with prognathism, and increased dental separation, and macroglossia. There is excessive sweating and in women there may be hirsutism.

Hands

The hands enlarge and become spade-like. Carpal tunnel syndrome may occur as a result of compression of the median nerve.

Arthritis

This occurs prematurely, especially in the spine and weight-bearing joints.

Cardiovascular problems

These are often the cause of mortality. Coronary artery disease, hypertension, and diabetes are more common than in the normal population. Cardiomyopathy may occur.

Effects of the pituitary tumour

Headaches, visual field defects, and cranial nerve palsies may occur. Hyperprolactinaemia is common and hypopituitarism can also occur.

Diagnosis

GH levels are elevated although they may rise with stress. Therefore, GH is measured during a glucose tolerance test. In healthy individuals, GH is undetectab during the test.

Other investigations include the following:

- Assessment of visual fields: bitemporal hemianopia.
- Skull X-ray, and CT or MRI of the brain.
- Hand X-ray: tufting of the terminal phalanges and increased joint spaces due to hypertrophy of the cartilage. The heel pad is usually thickened.

The diagnosis of acromegaly may become more obvious by comparing old photographs of the patient with their present appearance.

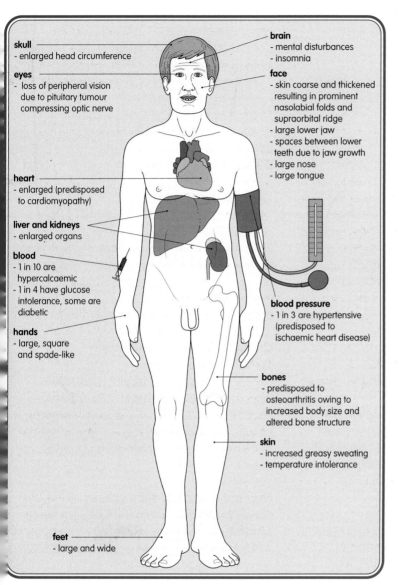

Fig. 35.9 Signs and symptoms of acromegaly (caused by excessive growth hormone secretion in adults).

skull
- enlarged head circumference

eyes
- loss of peripheral vision due to pituitary tumour compressing optic nerve

brain
- mental disturbances
- insomnia

face
- skin coarse and thickened resulting in prominent nasolabial folds and supraorbital ridge
- large lower jaw
- spaces between lower teeth due to jaw growth
- large nose
- large tongue

heart
- enlarged (predisposed to cardiomyopathy)

liver and kidneys
- enlarged organs

blood
- 1 in 10 are hypercalcaemic
- 1 in 4 have glucose intolerance, some are diabetic

hands
- large, square and spade-like

blood pressure
- 1 in 3 are hypertensive (predisposed to ischaemic heart disease)

bones
- predisposed to osteoarthritis owing to increased body size and altered bone structure

skin
- increased greasy sweating
- temperature intolerance

feet
- large and wide

• Glucose or glucose tolerance test.
• CXR and electrocardiogram (ECG): left ventricular hypertrophy secondary to hypertension.

Management

The aim of treatment is to relieve symptoms, reverse somatic changes, and reverse metabolic abnormalities. Treatment is by surgery, radiotherapy, or drugs.

Surgery

The trans-sphenoidal route is usually used. Up to 90% of microadenomas are cured. The success rate is lower for larger tumours. Complications include hypopituitarism, meningitis, intra-operative bleeding, and death.

Radiotherapy

This is often used if attempts at surgery do not reduce GH levels sufficiently. Hypopituitarism may occur, and regular tests of pituitary function should be performed.

Medical therapies

The most effective treatment is with octreotide, a somatostatin analogue. Somatostatin inhibits GH secretion. Side effects include colicky abdominal pain and diarrhoea but this usually settles with continued treatment. Gallstones occur in about a third of patients. Bromocriptine also reduces GH and PRL levels.

Prognosis

Untreated, mortality is more than twice that in healthy individuals. Death is secondary to cardiovascular and cerebrovascular disease.

Prolactin disorders

Prolactin (PRL) is the hormone most commonly secreted by pituitary tumours. Secretion of PRL is under tonic inhibitory control by hypothalamic dopamine, such that interruption produces hyperprolactinaemia. Thyrotrophin-releasing hormone and vasoactive intestinal polypeptide exert less important stimulatory effects on pituitary prolactin release. Elevation of serum prolactin occurs physiologically during pregnancy and lactation. Pathologically, hyperprolactinaemia is more common in women than men. Most are due to microprolactinomas.

Clinical features

In women, the commonest symptoms are oligomenorrhoea, galactorrhoea, infertility, and occasionally hirsutism. In men, symptoms include reduced libido, impotence, infertility, and galactorrhoea. Symptoms caused by large tumour size are more common in men and include headache, visual field defects, and cranial nerve palsies. Varying degrees of hypopituitarism may be present.

Aetiology

The causes of hyperprolactinaemia are summarized in Fig. 35.10.

Investigations

Elevated prolactin levels should be confirmed on repeat testing. Other blood tests include thyroid function tests (TFTs) and a pregnancy test in women. A careful drug history should always be taken.

Radiological assessment of the pituitary tumour should be carried out with skull X-rays, and MRI or CT scans of the brain. Full assessment of pituitary function should be undertaken if a macroadenoma is suspected, and visual fields should be assessed.

Management

The dopamine agonist bromocriptine is most commonly used, which produces a fall in serum PRL in more than

90% of patients and reduces tumour size in patients with macroadenomas.

Cabergoline and quinagolide are more recent longer-acting dopamine receptor agonists.

For patients intolerant of drugs, surgery and radiotherapy can be tried.

Tumours may enlarge rapidly in pregnancy. However, bromocriptine does not appear to have any adverse effects in mother or child when used before or during pregnancy.

Diabetes insipidus

This rare disease is due to deficiency of vasopressin—cranial diabetes insipidus. The differential diagnosis includes nephrogenic diabetes insipidus, i.e. a lack of renal response to adequate circulating vasopressin, and primary polydipsia or excessive drinking. Clinically the patient presents with polyuria, nocturia, and polydipsia. Investigation is outlined in Chapter 12.

Causes of diabetes insipidus

Cranial diabetes insipidus

Familial cranial diabetes insipidus is inherited as autosomal dominant or as part of the DIDMOAD syndrome (**d**iabetes **i**nsipidus, **d**iabetes **m**ellitus, **o**ptic **a**trophy, and **d**eafness).

Causes of acquired cranial diabetes insipidus are given in Fig. 35.11.

Nephrogenic diabetes insipidus

Familial nephrogenic diabetes insipidus is X-linked recessive and autosomal recessive.

Causes of acquired nephrogenic diabetes insipidus are given in Fig. 35.12.

Treatment

For cranial diabetes insipidus, desmopressin is the treatment of choice because it has minimal pressor activity but prolonged antidiuretic potency compared to native vasopressin. It may be administered orally, intranasally, or parenterally.

Metabolic and electrolyte disturbances should be corrected if they are responsible for nephrogenic diabetes insipidus. In familial forms, thiazide diuretics indomethacin can reduce urine output by up to 50%.

For patients with primary polydipsia, water restriction and treatment of any associated psychiatric disorder is required.

Fig. 35.10 Causes of hyperprolactinaemia.

Causes of hyperprolactinaemia	
Cause	**Examples**
physiological	pregnancy, lactation, stress
drugs	antiemetics, e.g. metoclopramide, prochlorperazine phenothiazines tricyclic antidepressants
primary hypothyroidism	—
pituitary tumours	prolactinoma growth-hormone secreting tumours non-functioning tumours
polycystic ovary syndrome	—
uncommon	sarcoidosis
hypothalamic lesions	Langerhans' cell histiocytosis hypothalamic tumours
chest wall stimulation	repeated self-examination of breasts post herpes zoster
liver or renal failure	—

Fig. 35.10 Causes of hyperprolactinaemia.

THYROID DISORDERS

For a diagram of the hypothalamus–pituitary–thyroid axis refer to Fig. 29.18.

Hypothyroidism

Hypothyroidism results from deficiency of thyroxine (T_4) or tri-iodothyronine (T_3). The prevalence is 15 in 1000 females and 1 in 1000 males.

Aetiology

Primary thyroid failure may take the following forms:
- Autoimmune (Hashimoto's thyroiditis): this is 15 times commoner in women than men, and tends to affect the middle aged and elderly. Patients may present with a firm, non-tender goitre, hypothyroidism, or both. It is associated with vitiligo, pernicious anaemia, IDDM, Addison's disease, and premature ovarian failure.
- Idiopathic atrophic hypothyroidism: incidence increases with age and is 10 times commoner in women than men. The aetiology is probably autoimmune.
- Previous treatment for hypothyroidism: operative or radioiodine.

Causes of acquired cranial diabetes insipidus	
Cause	**Examples**
trauma	head injury and neurosurgery
tumours	craniopharyngioma or secondary tumours
granulomas	tuberculosis, sarcoid, histiocytosis
infections	encephalitis or meningitis

Fig. 35.11 Causes of acquired cranial diabetes insipidus.

Causes of acquired nephrogenic diabetes insipidus
• metabolic: hypokalaemia, hypercalcaemia • chronic renal failure • lithium toxicity • postobstructive uropathy • diabetes mellitus

Fig. 35.12 Causes of acquired nephrogenic diabetes insipidus.

- Congenital hypothyroidism: the prevalence in the UK is 1 in 3500–4000 infants and is diagnosed in the first week of life by routine screening, measuring TSH or T_4. It is usually due to thyroid agenesis or dyshormonogenesis, which are both due to autosomal recessively inherited enzyme defects. The commonest is Pendred's syndrome, characterized by congenital hypothyroidism, goitre, and nerve deafness in homozygotes.
- Iodine-deficient hypothyroidism: this is a major cause of hypothyroidism and goitre worldwide, although most iodine deficient-people are euthyroid even though they have a goitre.
- Iatrogenic hypothyroidism: long-term iodine therapy, for example in expectorants, may result in hypothyroidism. Other drugs include amiodarone and lithium carbonate.

Secondary thyroid failure is caused by diseases of the hypothalamus or pituitary. These are very rare.

Clinical presentation
The onset is insidious and the symptoms often non-specific and vague. Common presenting symptoms include tiredness, lethargy, weight gain, cold intolerance, hoarseness, and dryness of the skin. However, virtually any organ system can be affected (Fig. 35.13).

Investigations
The following investigations are important in patients with hypothyroidism:
- Free or total T_4 are reduced, and serum TSH is high.
- T_4 may be normal with a high serum TSH. This indicates subclinical hypothyroidism.
- If secondary hypothyroidism is suspected, the free and total T_4 are reduced and the TSH is also low. This picture is also obtained in sick people without thyroid disease, and patients on steroids and anticonvulsants.
- Antibodies to thyroglobulin or thyroid peroxidase (microsomal antibodies): typically strongly positive in Hashimoto's thyroiditis.
- Cholesterol: raised.
- FBC: anaemia and raised mean corpuscular volume.
- ECG: sinus bradycardia, low voltage complexes.

Treatment
Thyroxine sodium is the treatment of choice for maintenance therapy. Usual maintenance doses are between 100–200 µg daily. The initial dose is usually 50 µg, increased as necessary over a few weeks, and even lower doses (25 µg) are started in elderly patients or patients with cardiac disease to avoid worsening angina or precipitating a myocardial infarction. Treatment is monitored by serum TSH and serum T_4 and is nearly always lifelong except in cases of subacute or silent thyroiditis.

Fig. 35.13 Effects of hypothyroidism by body system.

Effects of hypothyroidism by body system	
Body system	**Effects**
cardiovascular	bradycardia, hyperlipidaemia, angina, heart failure, pericardial and pleural effusions
neuromuscular	aches and pains, carpal tunnel syndrome, deafness, cerebellar ataxia, depression and psychoses, delayed relaxation of reflexes
haematological	iron-deficiency anaemia, macrocytic anaemia, pernicious anaemia, normochromic normocytic anaemia
dermatological	dry skin, myxoedema (which is local infiltration of the skin with mucopolysaccharides), erythema ab igne, vitiligo, alopecia
gastrointestinal	constipation, ileus, ascites
reproductive	infertility, menorrhagia, galactorrhoea
developmental	growth retardation, mental retardation, delayed puberty

Myxoedema coma
This is uncommon. It is typically seen in the elderly and precipitated by infection, treatment with sedatives, or inadequate heating in cold weather. Most patients have hypothermia and are hypotensive with heart failure, hyponatraemia, hypoxia, and hypercapnia.

Treatment is with T_3 intravenously because of its rapid action. Supportive measures are also needed including intravenous fluids, antibiotics, ventilation, and slow rewarming. T_4 can be substituted after 2–3 days if there is a clinical improvement.

Thyrotoxicosis
Thyrotoxicosis results from an excess of circulating free T_4 free T_3. It affects about 10 in 1000 women and 1 in 1000 men. Hyperthyroidism indicates thyroid gland overactivity, resulting in thyrotoxicosis.

Aetiology
Primary hyperthyroidism
Graves' disease
This accounts for 70–80% of all cases of hyperthyroidism. It is caused by the production of autoantibodies that stimulate the TSH receptor. There is painless diffuse goitre in more than 90% of patients. In addition to the general features of thyrotoxicosis, pathognomonic features include ophthalmopathy, pretibial myxoedema, and thyroid acropachy.

The ophthalmopathy includes grittiness and increased tear production, periorbital oedema, conjunctival oedema (chemosis), proptosis, diplopia, impaired visual acuity, and corneal ulceration. It is clinically obvious in 60% of patients with Graves' disease but subclinical ophthalmopathy can be detected in more than 90% by CT scan or MRI, revealing fusiform enlargement of the extraocular muscles caused by lymphocytic infiltration, oedema, and later fibrosis.

Pretibial myxoedema occurs in 1–5% of patients with Graves' disease and comprises of painless thickening of the skin in nodules or plaques, generally over the shin.

Thyroid acropachy occurs in less than 1% of patients and resembles finger clubbing.

Other causes of primary hyperthyroidism
Toxic multinodular goitre and toxic adenoma account for most of the remaining causes. Less common causes include metastatic thyroid cancer, genetic causes such

as the McCune–Albright syndrome and TSH receptor mutations, and ectopic thyroid tissue, e.g. struma ovarii.

Secondary hyperthyroidism
This is very uncommon. Causes include pituitary adenoma-secreting TSH, and trophoblastic tumours secreting human chorionic gonadotrophin.

Thyrotoxicosis without hyperthyroidism
This may occur with destructive thyroiditis such as in postpartum thyroiditis, subacute (de Quervain's) thyroiditis, and amiodarone-induced thyroiditis, and with excessive thyroxine administration, or self-administered thyroxine, particularly in doctors and nurses.

Clinical presentation
The symptoms and signs of Thyrotoxicosis are shown in Fig. 35.14. General symptoms include:
- Weight loss.
- Increased appetite.
- Heat intolerance and sweating.
- Fatigue and weakness.
- Hyperactivity, irritability.
- Tremor.

Less common symptoms include:
- Depression.
- Oligomenorrhoea.
- Pruritus.
- Diarrhoea.
- Polyuria.

Signs include:
- A goitre possibly with a murmur over it.
- Tremor.
- Tachycardia and atrial fibrillation.
- Warm moist skin.
- Lid retraction and lid lag.
- Muscle weakness.
- Proximal myopathy.
- Cardiac failure.

Investigations
In thyrotoxicosis TSH is suppressed. It can also be suppressed in euthyroid patients with Graves' ophthalmopathy, large goitres, recent treatment for thyrotoxicosis, or severe non-thyroid illness.

T_4 is raised although excess oestrogens, protein-losing states, drugs, and hereditary abnormalities can alter the binding of T_4 to thyroxine-binding globulin, making total T_4 levels inaccurate in these situations. Free T_4 assays are therefore preferable.

If the TSH is suppressed and free T_4 is normal, T_3 should be measured to diagnose T_3 toxicosis.

In Graves' disease, 80% of people have serum autoantibodies against thyroglobulin and thyroid peroxidase/microsomal antigen. However, these also occur in autoimmune thyroiditis, and in 15% of healthy women and 5% of healthy men.

Treatment

Treatment options include drugs, radioiodine, and surgery. Most patients under 50 years old receive a course of antithyroid drug as initial treatment. Patients with large goitres usually relapse after antithyroid drugs. Relapse after a period of drug therapy should be treated with ^{131}I or subtotal thyroidectomy; ^{131}I is generally given to older patients in whom recurrent thyrotoxicosis may be dangerous. Subtotal thyroidectomy is often recommended in young patients with large goitres to remove the neck swelling. All options should be discussed with the patient and a joint decision should be arrived at.

Antithyroid drugs

In the UK carbimazole is the most commonly used drug. Propylthiouracil (PTU) may be used in patients who suffer sensitivity reactions to carbimazole. Both

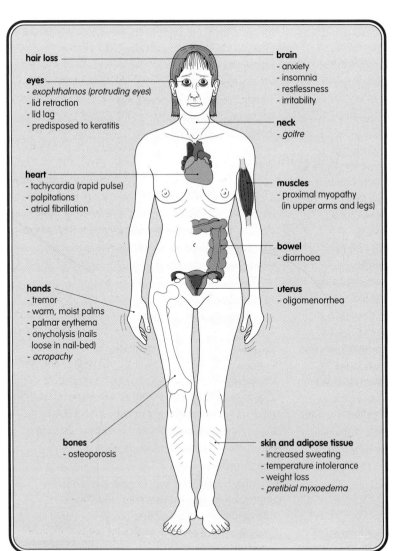

Fig. 35.14 Symptoms and signs of thyrotoxicosis (caused by hyperthyroidism). The features shown in italics are exclusive to thyrotoxicosis caused by Graves' disease.

hair loss

eyes
- *exophthalmos (protruding eyes)*
- lid retraction
- lid lag
- predisposed to keratitis

heart
- tachycardia (rapid pulse)
- palpitations
- atrial fibrillation

hands
- tremor
- warm, moist palms
- palmar erythema
- onycholysis (nails loose in nail-bed)
- acropachy

bones
- osteoporosis

brain
- anxiety
- insomnia
- restlessness
- irritability

neck
- *goitre*

muscles
- proximal myopathy (in upper arms and legs)

bowel
- diarrhoea

uterus
- oligomenorrhea

skin and adipose tissue
- increased sweating
- temperature intolerance
- weight loss
- *pretibial myxoedema*

drugs act primarily by interfering with the synthesis of thyroid hormones.

Carbimazole is given in a daily dose of 20–60 mg and maintained at this dose until the patient becomes euthyroid, usually after 4–8 weeks. The dose may then be progressively changed to a maintenance dose of 5–15 mg daily, adjusted according to response. Rashes are common and PTU may then be substituted. Pruritus and rashes can also be treated with antihistamines without discontinuing therapy, although patients should be advised to report any sore throat immediately because of the rare complication of agranulocytosis.

PTU is given in a dose of 300–600 mg daily and maintained at this dose until the patient becomes euthyroid. The dose is then lowered to a maintenance dose of 50–150 mg daily.

A combination of carbimazole, 20–60 mg daily with thyroxine 50–150 μg daily, may be used in a blocking replacement regimen. Treatment is usually for 18 months—this regimen is not suitable during pregnancy.

Iodine may be given 10–14 days before surgery in addition to carbimazole to assist control and to reduce vascularity of the thyroid.

Propanolol is useful for the rapid relief of thyrotoxic symptoms because antithyroid drugs may take several weeks to produce an improvement in symptoms. They are also useful for the control of supraventricular arrhythmias secondary to thyrotoxicosis.

Radioiodine
Radioactive sodium iodide (Na^{131}I) is concentrated by the thyroid and causes cell damage and cell death. Hypothyroidism may therefore develop at any stage after treatment, and so the patient should be under regular follow-up. It is used increasingly for the treatment of thyrotoxicosis at all ages, particularly where medical therapy or compliance is a problem, in patients with cardiac disease, and in patients who relapse after thyroidectomy. Contraindications include pregnancy and breastfeeding. Pregnancy is safe 6 months or more after treatment.

Subtotal thyroidectomy
The aim of surgery is to remove sufficient thyroid tissue to cure hyperthyroidism. One year later about 80% of patients are euthyroid, 15% hypothyroid, and 5% have relapsed. Complications include hypoparathyroidism,

recurrent laryngeal nerve damage, and bleeding into the neck causing laryngeal oedema.

Thyrotoxic crisis (thyroid 'storm')
This is an uncommon, life-threatening exacerbation of thyrotoxicosis with a mortality of 50%. Precipitating factors include thyroid surgery, radioiodine, withdrawal of antithyroid drugs, iodinated contrast agents, and acute illnesses, e.g. stroke, infection, trauma, and diabetic ketoacidosis. It requires emergency treatment with oxygen, intravenous fluids due to profuse sweating, propanolol (5 mg i.v.) for control of tachycardia, hydrocortisone (100 mg 6 hourly i.v.), which inhibits T_4 conversion to T_3 in the tissues, as well as oral iodine solution, which may need to be administered by nasogastric tube.

Subacute (de Quervain's) thyroiditis
Various viruses, e.g. enterovirus or coxsackievirus, can cause subacute thyroiditis. Patients present with a small, tender goitre and initially thyrotoxicosis caused by release of stored thyroid hormones. There may be a history of preceding 'flu-like' illness. Some weeks later there is a period of hypothyroidism followed by the recovery of normal thyroid function 3–6 months after onset.

The erythrocyte sedimentation rate is raised and there is low radioisotope uptake by the thyroid. Treatment is with NSAIDs for mild symptoms, and with high-dose prednisolone for moderate or severe thyroiditis. The dose is gradually tailed off in subsequent weeks.

Goitre and thyroid cancer
'Goitre' means an enlarged thyroid gland. Diffuse goitres can be due to simple, non-toxic goitres, Graves' disease, Hashimoto's thyroiditis, subacute thyroiditis, or thyroid lymphoma. Goitres with a single nodule may be due to adenoma or carcinoma, and multiple nodules secondary to multinodular goitre or Hashimoto's thyroiditis. Goitres are four times commoner in women than men, and are present in about 7% of the population. Aetiological factors include underlying autoimmune disease and iodine deficiency.

Clinical features
Most patients are asymptomatic. The history should include the following:
- Duration of goitre: long-standing goitres suggest benign disease.

The most common thyroid carcinoma is P-apillary (P-opular). It also has P-sammoma bodies on histology. It causes P-alpable lymph nodes (lymphatic spread).

- Goitrogenic drugs, e.g. lithium.
- Prior exposure to radiation: risk factor for benign and malignant thyroid nodules.
- Age: increased risk of cancer in the over 65s.
- Sex: thyroid cancer is more common in men than women.
- Family history: if positive for goitre, this suggests autoimmune thyroiditis. A positive family history for thyroid cancer suggests familial thyroid cancer or MEN.
- Tenderness: subacute thyroiditis.
- Local symptoms: dysphagia, dyspnoea, and hoarseness; all are uncommon.

Investigations

The following investigations are important in patients with goitre and thyroid cancer:

- TFTs: hyper- or hypothyroidism.
- Calcitonin secretion: increased in medullary thyroid cancer, and should be measured in patients with a positive family history.
- Thyroid size: assessed using plain X-rays, which may show tracheal deviation, or CT scan.
- Respiratory function tests: upper airways obstruction.
- Radionuclide imaging: can distinguish 'hot nodules' (high uptake of radioisotope) from 'cold nodules' (due to lack of concentration of radioisotope). Unfortunately there are no specific features that indicate the benign or malignant nature of a thyroid nodule. Malignant nodules are more likely to be cold than hot, although most cold nodules are benign. Even so, the presence of a hot nodule does not exclude malignancy.
- Ultrasound scan: differentiation of solid from cystic lesions of the thyroid; it cannot distinguish benign from malignant nodules, although a solid nodule is more likely to contain malignant cells.
- Fine-needle aspiration cytology: can be done in outpatients and is well tolerated; cytology is not completely reliable as false positive and false negative results occur.

Thyroid malignancy

Papillary thyroid carcinoma

This accounts for 70–80% of thyroid malignancies and is more common in women; the peak age of onset is 20–30 years. It may be locally invasive or multifocal, treatment is by surgical excision, and the 10-year survival rate is 95%.

Follicular thyroid carcinoma

This occurs in older people. Distant metastases develop in 20% of patients. Treatment is by thyroidectomy and radioiodine ablation of the thyroid remnant. The 10-year survival rate is 20%.

Anaplastic carcinoma

Anaplastic carcinoma is uncommon. The peak incidence is at 60–70 years. The mean survival is only 6 months from diagnosis.

Medullary thyroid carcinoma

This is rare. It secretes calcitonin and other hormones. It may be associated with phaeochromocytoma. The prognosis is poor. Family members should be screened.

Lymphoma

Lymphoma may be primary or as part of a systemic disease. There is an increased risk in patients with autoimmune thyroiditis. Radiotherapy is the treatment of choice.

DISORDERS OF THE ADRENAL GLANDS

Histologically, the adrenal glands are divided into the medulla, which secretes adrenaline and noradrenaline, and the cortex, which is divided into three zones:

- The inner zone or zona reticularis produces sex hormones.
- The middle zone or zona fasciculata produces cortisol. Production is stimulated by ACTH produced by the pituitary gland. In turn, cortisol influences, by negative feedback, both corticotropin-releasing hormone production in the hypothalamus and pituitary release of ACTH.

- The outer zona glomerulosa produces aldosterone which is regulated through the renin–angiotensin system.

Cushing's syndrome

Cushing's syndrome is the result of chronic exposure to excess glucocorticoid. This is most commonly iatrogenic secondary to glucocorticoid administration given to treat inflammatory diseases. Other causes include the following:

- As a result of ACTH hypersecretion by a pituitary corticotrophic adenoma (60–70%).
- Primary adrenocortical tumours (30%).
- Ectopic ACTH syndrome caused by a variety of ACTH-secreting non-pituitary tumours (5–10%), e.g. small cell lung carcinoma.

The annual incidence of spontaneous Cushing's syndrome is about 1 in 100 000 and is 3–5 times more common in women than men.

Clinical features

The clinical features of Cushing's syndrome include the following:

- Centripetal fat deposition producing the typical moon facies and buffalo hump (dorsocervical fat pad).
- Skin thinning, and purple striae over the abdomen and flanks. Bruising is common and wounds heal slowly.
- Lower limb oedema.
- Proximal muscle wasting.
- Osteoporosis, particularly of the vertebral bodies leading to compression fractures.
- Impaired defence against infections.
- Hypertension.
- Mild hirsutism in women.
- Amenorrhoea and infertility in women, and impotence in men.
- Electrolyte disturbances with hypernatraemia and hypokalaemia.
- Impaired glucose tolerance or frank diabetes.

Investigations

Investigations for Cushing's syndrome are discussed in Chapter 29. They include 24-hour urinary free cortisol measurement, dexamethasone suppression tests, assessment of corticotrophic function, and imaging techniques.

Management
Cushing's disease

Trans-sphenoidal surgery is the first line of treatment and is curative in about 80% of patients. Drugs are used if surgery fails. Metyrapone inhibits steroidogenesis and is the drug of choice. Op'DDD has a specific adrenolytic action and is used for patients intolerant to metyrapone.

Rarely, bilateral adrenalectomy is necessary although this has a risk of leading to Nelson's syndrome resulting in hyperpigmentation from excess β-lipotrophin activity (melanocyte-stimulating hormone and ACTH) which is not suppressed by a high blood cortisol.

Adrenocortical tumours

Surgical removal of an adrenocortical tumour is curative. Bilateral adrenalectomy necessitates replacement therapy with cortisol 20–40 mg daily and fludrocortisone 0.1 mg daily.

Ectopic ACTH syndrome

Surgical resection of the tumour cures the hypercortisolism, although this is often not possible.

Addison's disease

Addison's disease is primary adrenocortical failure. The prevalence is about 100 per million per year, and the incidence is about 5 per 1 million per year.

Causes

Causes of Addison's disease include the following:

- Autoimmune adrenal destruction: this accounts for up to 90% of cases. Women are affected 2–3 times more often than men. Patients may have other autoimmune endocrine deficiencies.
- Infections: especially tuberculosis; cytomegalovirus and fungal infections associated with AIDS are now becoming common.
- Adrenal haemorrhage/infarction: this may be associated with sepsis, particularly meningococcal septicaemia—the Waterhouse–Friderichsen syndrome. The presentation is usually acute.
- Metastatic carcinoma: especially from the breast.
- Inherited disorders: there are several familial disorders of adrenal function which are all rare.

Clinical features

Symptoms and signs of Addison's disease are predominantly caused by cortisol deficiency, although deficiencies of aldosterone and adrenal androgen will also be present to varying extents (Fig. 35.15). The main symptoms are insidious and non-specific: fatigue, weight loss, orthostatic dizziness, and anorexia. Patients may present with GI symptoms, e.g. abdominal pain, nausea, vomiting, and diarrhoea. Hyperpigmentation of the skin and mucous membranes may occur as a result of high ACTH concentrations.

Investigations

The following are important investigations in patient with Addison's disease:

- Serum cortisol concentration: low.
- Adrenal autoantibodies are detected in about 50% of patients.

- Serum ACTH levels: raised in Addison's disease and low in secondary failure.
- Serum electrolytes: usually normal but in an impending crisis there may be hyponatraemia, hyperkalaemia, and raised blood urea.
- Short and long synacthen tests: described in Chapter 29.
- TFTs: may show low thyroxine and raised TSH.
- Screening for other autoimmune diseases.

Management

In emergencies, intravenous saline and glucose are required. Intravenous hydrocortisone 100 mg 6 hourly is given. Underlying infection must be treated.

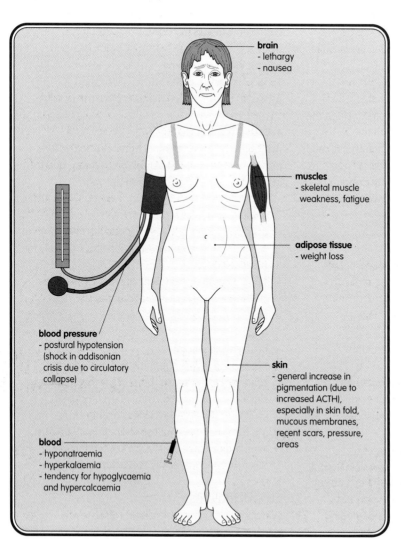

Fig. 35.15 Symptoms and signs of adrenal insufficiency. (ACTH, adrenocorticotrophic hormone.)

Maintenance therapy is with hydrocortisone, usually 20 mg in the mornings and 10 mg in the evenings. The dose of hydrocortisone should be increased during intercurrent illnesses and during surgery. Enzyme inducing drugs, e.g. phenytoin and rifampicin, may also increase patient requirements for hydrocortisone. Fludrocortisone is used to replace aldosterone because aldosterone taken orally undergoes first pass metabolism through the liver. The dose is adjusted to maintain blood pressure and potassium levels. The usual dose is about 0.1 mg daily.

Phaeochromocytoma

This is a rare tumour arising from the chromaffin tissues of the sympathetic nervous system, producing catecholamines. It may be associated with medullary carcinoma of the thyroid, parathyroid adenoma, and neurofibromatosis.

Clinical features

Symptoms and signs are due to the release of adrenaline and noradrenaline, and include episodic hypertension, cardiomyopathy, weight loss, and hyperglycaemia. During a period of crisis there may be pallor, palpitations, panic, sweating, nausea, tremor, pain (headache or chest pain), and rarely paroxysmal thyroid swelling. The blood pressure may rise to very high levels and may precipitate a cerebrovascular accident or myocardial infarction.

Investigations

Urine is collected for 24 hours for measurement of adrenaline and noradrenaline, or of their metabolites vanillylmandelic acid or hydroxymethylmandelic acid. An abdominal CT scan may show the tumour.

Treatment

This is by surgical removal of the tumour. The patient must be fully α-blocked with phenoxybenzamine or phentolamine, and β-blocked with propanolol before surgery to prevent the consequences of release of catecholamines during operation. Changes in pulse and blood pressure should be monitored closely.

Conn's syndrome (primary hyperaldosteronism)

This is a very rare condition, which is due to a unilateral adrenocortical adenoma in 75% of cases. Other causes include adrenal carcinoma or bilateral hyperplasia of the zona glomerulosa.

Clinical features

The clinical features are due to excess production of aldosterone. Hypokalaemia and muscle weakness occur during attacks, and polyuria and polydipsia are secondary to hypokalaemia. The diagnosis should be suspected in a patient with hypertension and hypokalaemia when not on a diuretic. Sodium tends to be mildly raised but there is usually no oedema.

Investigation

Serum potassium is low and should be measured whilst the patient is not on drugs. Urinary potassium is increased for serum blood level. There is usually a metabolic alkalosis. Serum sodium is raised.

Serum renin is low and 24-hour urinary aldosterone and serum aldosterone are raised.

Secondary hyperaldosteronism is a result of high circulating renin. Causes include nephrotic syndrome, heart failure, hepatic failure, and bronchial carcinoma.

Management

Tumours should be resected. Spironolactone is an aldosterone antagonist, which can be given in primary or secondary aldosteronism.

MISCELLANEOUS ENDOCRINE CONDITIONS

Multiple endocrine neoplasia

There are two main syndromes, both autosomal dominant and both rare. Tumours originate from two or more endocrine glands which produce peptide hormones.

MEN type I refers to benign adenomas of parathyroid, pancreatic islets, pituitary, adrenal cortex, and the thyroid.

In phaeochromocytoma 90% are benign, 90% are in the adrenal medulla, and 90% of these are unilateral.

MEN type IIa refers to the association of phaeochromocytoma, medullary carcinoma of the thyroid, and parathyroid adenoma or hyperplasia.

MEN type IIb is the same as IIa but with a Marfanoid phenotype and intestinal and visceral ganglioneuromas.

Family members should be screened. In type I, fasting serum calcium should be measured. In type II, pentagastrin and calcium infusion tests with measurement of serum calcitonin will pick up C-cell hyperplasia. Urinary metanephrines should be measured for phaeochromocytoma.

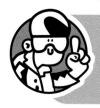

Multiple endocrine neoplasia is a common MCQ question. MEN I is three Ps (pituitary, parathyroid, and pancreas), MEN II is two Cs (catecholamines, i.e. phaeochromocytoma, and carcinoma of the medullary of the thyroid) and parathyroid (for MEN IIa) or mucocutaneous neuromas (for MEN IIb).

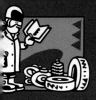

ARTHRITIS

Rheumatoid arthritis

Rheumatoid arthritis (RA) is a systemic disease producing a symmetrical inflammatory polyarthropathy with extra-articular involvement of many organs. It affects 2–3% of the population and is three times more common in women than men. The peak age of onset is between 30 and 40 years, although it can start at almost any age. There is often a family history and there is an association with HLA-DR4. The aetiology is unknown but it is thought to be autoimmune.

Clinical features

RA usually presents with an insidious onset of swollen, painful, and stiff hands and feet, progressing to involve the larger joints. Less common presentations include a relapsing and remitting monoarthritis of different large joints, a persistent monoarthritis, systemic features before joint problems are apparent, and an acute onset of widespread arthritis especially in the elderly.

General features of the disease include general malaise and fatigue; signs affecting the joints are described in Chapter 16. The metacarpophalangeal (MCP) joints, proximal interphalangeal (PIP) joints, and wrists are most commonly affected (Fig. 36.1). Initially there is joint swelling, which may progress to subluxation of joints and deformities. There is wasting of small muscles resulting from disuse atrophy, vasculitis and peripheral neuropathy. There may be tenosynovitis and bursitis; rheumatoid nodules are present in about 20% of patients. The feet are similarly affected.

Atlantoaxial subluxation may give rise to neurological signs, spinal cord compression and death. Other organs affected are summarized in Fig. 36.2.

Investigations

These are discussed in Chapter 16. They should include:

- Full blood count (FBC).
- Erythrocyte sedimentation rate (ESR).

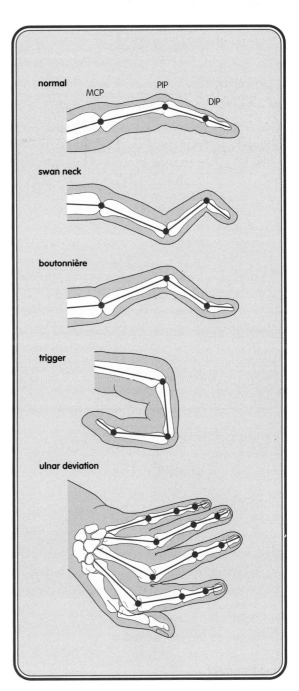

Fig. 36.1 Finger and hand abnormalities in rheumatoid arthritis (DIP, distal interphalangeal joint; MCP, metacarpophalangeal joint; PIP, proximal interphalangeal joint).

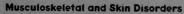
Organ systems affected by rheumatoid arthritis	
Organ system	**Effects**
eyes	Sjögren's syndrome occurs in 15% of patients scleritis causes a painful red eye, and may lead to uveitis and glaucoma scleromalacia perforans is an uncommon complication where a rheumatoid nodule in the sclera perforates
nervous system	carpal tunnel syndrome (most common) peripheral neuropathy causing glove and stocking sensory loss and occasionally motor weakness mononeuritis multiplex due to vasculitis of vessels supplying nerves atlantoaxial subluxation resulting in spinal cord compression
lymphoreticular system	generalized lymphadenopathy and splenomegaly may be present Felty's syndrome
blood	normochromic normocytic anaemia or iron-deficiency anaemia (see Chapter 25) ESR and CRP are raised thrombocytosis may be found
respiratory system	pleural effusions (commoner in men) rheumatoid nodules diffuse fibrosing alveolitis Caplan's syndrome (the presence of large rheumatoid nodules and fibrosis in patients with RA exposed to various industrial dusts)
cardiac	pericarditis and pericardial effusions may occur
skin	vasculitis may produce nail-fold infarcts, ulcers, and digital gangrene peripheral oedema may be present and is due to increased vascular permeability
kidneys	secondary amyloidosis may affect the kidneys leading to proteinuria, nephrotic syndrome, and renal failure

Fig. 36.2 Organ systems affected by rheumatoid arthritis (CRP, C-reactive protein; ESR, erythrocyte sedimentation rate; RA, rheumatoid arthritis).

- Rheumatoid factor and other autoantibodies.
- Joint X-rays.
- Aspiration of synovial fluid, if appropriate.

Management

The aims of treatment are to control symptoms, to maintain a normal life and to modify the underlying disease process and inflammation. Physiotherapy will help to keep joints mobile, strengthen muscles, and prevent deformities. Surgery may be required to correct deformities, e.g. the repair of tendons, joint prostheses, and arthrodeses. Resting the joints will relieve pain, and splints can help prevent deformities.

Drug treatment

Initial measures should include analgesia with paracetamol alone or with a low dose of an opioid analgesic. The pain and stiffness due to inflammation responds to non-steroidal anti-inflammatory drugs

(NSAIDs) (see below). Drugs are available that may affect the disease process itself and favourably influence the outcome. These include penicillamine, gold salts, antimalarials, immunosuppressants, and sulphasalazine. They are sometimes referred to as disease-modifying antirheumatic drugs or DMARDs. Corticosteroids may also be able to reduce the rate of joint destruction.

Non-steroidal anti-inflammatory drugs

About 60% of patients will respond to any NSAID, and those who do not may well respond to another. An analgesic effect should be obtained within a week, whereas an anti-inflammatory effect may not be achieved for up to 3 weeks. If appropriate responses are not obtained within these times, another NSAID should be tried.

The main differences amongst the NSAIDs are in the incidences and types of side effect; efficacy should always be weighed against possible side effects. They should be used with caution in the elderly, during pregnancy and breastfeeding, and in coagulation defects.

NSAIDs may cause deterioration of renal function and may worsen cardiac failure via fluid retention. They should not be used in patients with active peptic ulceration. Common side effects include gastrointestinal (GI) discomfort, nausea, diarrhoea, and peptic ulceration.

Corticosteroids

Treatment with corticosteroids should be reserved for specific indications, e.g. when other anti-inflammatory drugs are unsuccessful. Prednisolone 7.5 mg/day may substantially reduce the rate of joint destruction in moderate to severe RA of less than 2 years' duration. This dose should only be maintained for 2–4 years, after which treatment should be tapered off to avoid possible long-term adverse effects. Corticosteroids may also be given intra-articularly to relieve pain, increase mobility, and reduce deformity in one or a few joints.

Disease-modifying antirheumatic drugs

Disease-modifying antirheumatic drugs (DMARDs) do not produce an immediate therapeutic effect but require 4–6 months' treatment for a full response. If there is no objective benefit within 6 months they should be stopped. The drugs may also improve extra-articular manifestations of RA, e.g. vasculitis. Some may retard erosive damage as judged radiologically. The drugs are normally used in RA where treatment with NSAIDs alone provides inadequate control.

Gold salts

These are given intramuscularly or orally. They should be discontinued in the presence of blood disorders or proteinuria. Blood and urine tests should therefore be carried out regularly when on treatment. Rashes with pruritus may occur after some months of intramuscular treatment and may necessitate discontinuation of treatment. The most common side effect of oral therapy is diarrhoea, which may respond to bulking agents or a temporary reduction in dosage.

Penicillamine

Penicillamine has a similar action to gold salts. Blood counts and urine tests should be checked frequently.

Side effects include:
- Thrombocytopaenia.
- Neutropaenia.
- Aplastic anaemia.
- Proteinuria associated with immune complex nephritis.
- Nausea
- Anorexia.
- Fever.
- Skin reactions.
- Taste loss.

Antimalarials

Chloroquine and hydroxychloroquine have a similar action to gold salts and penicillamine and are better tolerated. Retinopathy is a rare side effect.

Sulphasalazine

This has a beneficial effect in suppressing the anti-inflammatory activity of RA. Side effects include rashes, GI intolerance, and occasionally bone marrow suppression.

Immunosuppressants

These are useful in patients who do not respond to the drugs above. Agents include azathioprine, methotrexate, cyclosporin, and cyclophosphamide.

OSTEOARTHRITIS

Osteoarthritis (OA) is the commonest joint condition and affects about half of the population by the age of 60 years; it is more common in women. OA is a degenerative disorder affecting mainly the weight-bearing joints, e.g. the hips and knees. It is a disease of cartilage, which becomes eroded and progressively thinned as the disease proceeds. Risk factors include age, family history, obesity, and systemic features, e.g. sex and growth hormones. It may also be secondary to other joint conditions and trauma.

Clinical features

Clinical signs and symptoms are described in Chapter 16. Joints commonly affected by OA are summarized in Fig. 36.3. There is pain in affected joints, which is worse with movement and towards the end of the day, superimposed on a background of pain at rest.

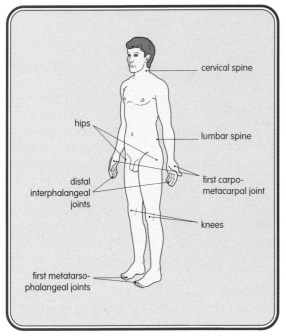

Fig. 36.3 Joints commonly affected by osteoarthritis.

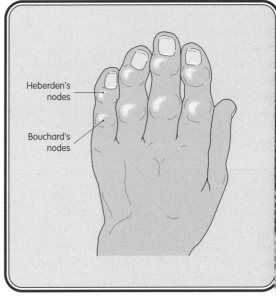

Fig. 36.4 Osteoarthritis in a hand, showing Heberden's nodes at the distal interphalangeal joints and Bouchard's nodes at the proximal interphalangeal joints.

The joints are stiff, immobile, and deformed.

On examination, there may be swelling due to bony protuberances or joint effusions, crepitus on movement, signs of inflammation, limited joint movement, and deformities. The pattern of joint involvement tends to be asymmetrical. In the hands, the most commonly affected joints are the distal interphalangeal (DIP) joints (Heberden's nodes), proximal interphalangeal (PIP) joints (Bouchard's nodes), and first carpometacarpal joints giving an appearance of 'square hands' (Fig. 36.4). Unlike RA, there is no systemic illness or extra-articular manifestations of the disease.

Investigations
There are no biochemical abnormalities. Diagnosis is based on clinical findings and radiological changes of loss of joint space, subchondral sclerosis and cysts, and marginal osteophytes.

Management
Treatment options include combinations of drugs, physical treatments (e.g. weight reduction and heat application), exercises, hydrotherapy, aids (e.g.

walking sticks and special shoes), and surgery (e.g. arthrodesis, arthroplasty, joint replacement). Initially, simple analgesics, e.g. paracetamol, should be prescribed for the pain. NSAIDs are given if simple analgesia is not effective. Intra-articular corticosteroids can be used for inflammatory exacerbations.

Spondyloarthropathies
This term describes a group of related diseases with some common features. There is an association with HLA-B27 with familial clustering of cases. Common features include:
- Ankylosing spondylitis.
- Reiter's syndrome and reactive arthritis.
- Enteropathic arthropathies.
- Psoriatic arthritis.
- Juvenile chronic arthritis.
- Undifferentiated spondyloarthropathy.

Ankylosing spondylitis
This most commonly affects young men with a prevalence of about 1 in 2000. HLA-B27 is present in over 90% of patients.

Clinical features

The onset is insidious with sacroiliitis causing pain in the buttocks radiating down the back of the legs. There is progressive spinal fusion with loss of movement, low back pain, and morning stiffness. Eventually the patient has a fixed kyphotic spine, hyperextended neck and spinocranial ankylosis, and a reduction in chest expansion leading to a 'question mark' posture (Fig. 36.5). Peripheral joints may be affected and tend to affect larger joints in an asymmetrical distribution. Other features include:

- General malaise.
- Uveitis: in about one-third of cases.
- Ulcerative colitis: more common than uveitis.
- Aortic regurgitation: due to aortitis.
- Respiratory failure: secondary to kyphoscoliosis and fibrosing alveolitis.

Investigations

The following investigations should be performed in the patient with ankylosing spondylitis:

- ESR and C-reactive protein (CRP): often raised.
- HLA-B27: provides useful supporting evidence but it is also present in the normal population.
- X-rays: sacroilitis indicated by irregular margins and sclerosis of adjacent bone; 'bamboo' spine with squaring of the vertebrae and calcification and ossification of intervertebral ligaments.

Management

Treatment includes analgesia with NSAIDs. Patients should be encouraged to exercise to prevent deformity, and to maintain movement and relieve symptoms—sulphasalazine improves symptoms due to peripheral arthritis. Radiotherapy may be tried in a minority of patients with intractable symptoms, although the majority of patients will be able to maintain a normal lifestyle. The disease may be progressive, it may remit, or there may be recurrent episodes. In extreme cases, ventilation may be impaired due to immobility of the spine and rib cage.

Reiter's syndrome

Reiter's syndrome consists of the triad of seronegative arthritis, non-specific urethritis (NSU), and conjunctivitis. It is 20 times more common in men than women and usually affects young adults. It follows NSU with a history of unprotected sexual intercourse about 1 month prior to presentation. Less commonly, it may follow GI infection with *Shigella*, *Salmonella*, *Yersinia*, or *Campylobacter*.

Clinical features

The arthritis is often of acute onset, polyarticular, and asymmetrical, particularly affecting the lower limbs. It may be associated with non-articular inflammatory

36.5 Advancing ankylosing spondylitis. Eventually the ...nk may become fixed in a fully flexed position, so that the ...tient cannot see directly ahead—the classic 'question ...ark' posture.

lesions including plantar fasciitis and Achilles tendinitis. Other clinical features include:

- Urethritis: associated with penile discharge and dysuria; there may be circinate balanitis (an erythematous circular lesion on the penis with a pale centre).
- Conjunctivitis: usually mild and bilateral; iritis and anterior uveitis may also occur.
- Mouth ulcers.
- Keratoderma blennorrhagica: a pustular hyperkeratotic lesion on the soles of the feet.
- Nail dystrophy and subungual keratosis.
- General malaise.
- Low-grade fever.Cardiovascular, respiratory, and neurological complications are rare.

Investigations
The diagnosis is clinical and autoantibodies are negative. HLA-B27 is positive in 60% of patients.

Management
Treatment is symptomatic with analgesia, e.g. NSAIDs, and rest of affected joints. Effusions can be aspirated. In chronic cases, sulphasalazine or azathioprine can be tried. In most cases, the acute arthritis settles within 1–2 months; about 50% of patients develop recurrent symptoms.

Reactive arthritis
This term describes arthritis following enteric or venereal infection as in Reiter's syndrome, but the other features of Reiter's syndrome are absent.

Psoriatic arthritis
This is a seronegative arthritis occurring in 10% of patients with psoriasis. The commonest pattern is involvement of the small joints of the hand, particularly the DIP joints, in an asymmetrical pattern (Fig. 36.6). Other variants are described in Chapter 16. There is nail pitting and onycholysis.

Treatment is with analgesia and anti-inflammatory drugs. Immunosuppressive drugs may be effective and are used in severe cases.

Enteropathic arthropathies
This occurs in patients with inflammatory bowel disease and usually affects the knees and ankles as a monoarthritis or asymmetrical oligoarthritis. The aetiology is unknown but immune complexes in the joint may play a part. Management should be aimed at the underlying bowel disease, which will improve the arthritis. NSAIDs and joint aspiration will provide symptomatic relief.

SYSTEMIC LUPUS ERYTHEMATOSUS

Systemic lupus erythematosus (SLE) is a multisystem, autoimmune connective tissue disorder. The prevalence in the UK is about 1 in 10 000. It is nine times commoner in women, and also more common in Black people. The peak age of onset is between 20 and 40 years. The aetiology is unknown but is probably multifactorial. Predisposing factors include genetic predisposition, and environmental triggers, e.g. drugs such as hydralazine, ultraviolet light, viral infections, and immunological mechanisms.

Clinical features
SLE is characterized by vasculitis—the clinical features of the disease are mainly due to the effects of the

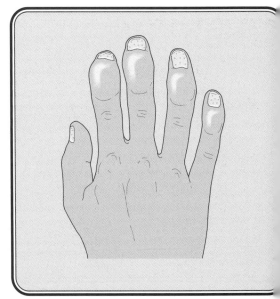

Fig. 36.6 Psoriatic arthritis involving the distal interphalangeal joints. There is 'pitting' of the nails, and there may be anycholysis.

vasculitis in different body systems. The commonest early features are fever, arthralgia, malaise, tiredness, and weight loss. The following systems may be involved.

Musculoskeletal system
This is involved in over 90% of cases. There is arthralgia, the symptoms of which are clinically similar to RA although examination is often normal. There may be myalgia and myositis, and rarely there is a deforming arthropathy due to capsular laxity (Jaccoud's arthropathy). Aseptic necrosis affecting the hip or knee may also rarely occur.

Cutaneous system
This is involved in about 80% of cases. Classically there is a 'butterfly' rash over the bridge of the nose and spreading over both cheeks (Fig. 36.7). Other features include photosensitivity, alopecia, livedo reticularis, Raynaud's phenomenon, nail-fold infarcts, purpura, urticaria, and oral ulceration.

Discoid lupus is a benign variant of SLE, with skin involvement only. There are discoid erythematous plaques on the face that progress to scarring and pigmentation. Patients with widespread skin disease may develop SLE.

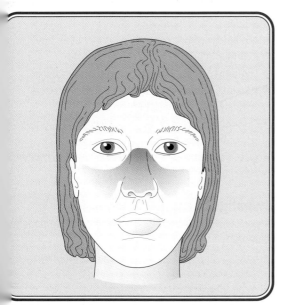

Fig. 36.7 Systemic lupus erythematosus showing the classic 'bat' or 'butterfly wing' rash.

Central nervous system
The central nervous system (CNS) is involved in 60% of cases. Psychiatric disturbances include depression and occasionally psychosis. Other features include:
- Epilepsy.
- Cerebrovascular accidents.
- Cranial nerve lesions.
- Cerebellar ataxia.
- Aseptic meningitis.
- Peripheral neuropathies.

The effects are due to arteritis and ischaemia or immune complex deposition.

Respiratory system
The respiratory system is involved in about 50% of cases. Pulmonary manifestations include:
- Pleurisy with pleural effusions.
- Pneumonia and atelectasis.
- Restrictive defects with diffuse reticular–nodular shadowing on the chest X-ray.

Renal system
The renal system is involved in about 50% of cases. This is associated with a poor prognosis. Proteinuria is common. There may be minimal change, and membranous or proliferative glomerulonephritis. Clinically, the patient may present with nephrotic or nephritic syndrome, hypertension, or chronic renal failure.

Cardiovascular system
The cardiovascular system is involved in 40% of cases. There may be:
- Pericarditis with pericardial effusion.
- Myocarditis with consequent heart failure.
- Aortic valve lesions.
- Non-bacterial endocarditis of the mitral valve (Libman–Sacks endocarditis).

Blood and lymphatic systems
The ESR is markedly raised. There may be:
- Normochromic normocytic anaemia.
- Haemolytic anaemia.
- Leucopenia.
- Thrombocytopenia.
- Generalized lymphadenopathy.
- Hepatosplenomegaly.

Drug-induced lupus

Drug-induced lupus may occur with hydralazine in slow acetylators, and with procainamide, isoniazid, chlorpromazine, and anticonvulsants. It remits when the drug is stopped. Renal and CNS involvement is rare.

Investigations

The following investigations are important in patients with SLE:

- ESR: raised.
- CRP: usually normal.
- There may be anaemia, leucopenia, or thrombocytopenia.
- Antinuclear antibody: positive in almost all cases; antidouble-stranded DNA is present in about 75% of cases and is specific for SLE.
- Serum complement levels: reduced; immunoglobulins raised.
- Renal biopsy: if there is involvement of the kidneys, renal biopsy shows characteristic histological changes.

Management

Patients with mild disease can be managed with aspirin or NSAIDs for joint pain. Anaemia can be corrected with transfusion, and sun block will protect from photosensitivity. For acute exacerbations, steroids are given in high doses and gradually tailed off depending on symptoms, signs, and changes in ESR.

Immunosuppressive drugs are used for patients with more serious disease, e.g. if there is renal or CNS involvement, as they have a steroid-sparing effect. Drugs used include azathioprine, chlorambucil and cyclophosphamide.

In some patients in whom NSAIDs are ineffective in controlling joint pain, or in whom skin manifestations predominate, the antimalarial drug chloroquine may be useful. It can cause irreversible retinal degeneration so vision should be formally assessed at regular intervals.

Some women are prone to recurrent abortions, which are associated with lupus anticoagulant. Specialist care should therefore be available in pregnancy.

POLYMYALGIA RHEUMATICA

Polymyalgia rheumatica (PMR) is a clinical syndrome characterized by proximal muscle pain and stiffness.

The incidence increases with age and the prevalence is as much as 2% in patients aged over 60 years. It is 2–3 times commoner in women than men, more common in Northern Europe than Southern Europe, and is rare in non-Whites. PMR and giant cell arteritis (see p. 295) are closely linked, but either can occur in isolation.

Clinical features

Discriminating characteristics for PMR include:

- Bilateral shoulder pain with or without stiffness.
- Bilateral upper arm tenderness.
- Illness of less than 2 weeks' duration.
- Morning stiffness that lasts for more than 1 hour.
- Depression with or without weight loss.
- Age greater than 65 years.
- An initial ESR of at least 40 mm/hour.

The distribution tends to be symmetrical, and systemic features such as sweating and malaise are common. True weakness does not occur, although power and range of movement may be limited by pain.

Differential diagnosis

The differential diagnosis of PMR includes:

- Late-onset RA.
- OA.
- Soft tissue rheumatic conditions: rotator cuff disease, non-specific back pain, trochanteric bursitis.
- Multiple myeloma (due to elevated ESR): however, stiffness is not usually a major feature.
- Hypothyroidism: due to myalgia and malaise.
- Parkinson's disease: may occasionally cause confusion due to loss of mobility.
- Connective tissue diseases, polymyositis, and proximal myopathy.
- Occult malignancy if systemic features are marked.
- Infection.

Investigations

The following investigations are important in patients with PMR:

- ESR: usually over 40 mm per hour; very high values can occur.
- Acute phase proteins: increased, e.g. CRP.
- Alkaline phosphatase: raised in about 30% of patients

- Platelets: tend to be increased.
- Mild normochromic normocytic anaemia: common.
- Temporal artery biopsy: rarely helpful.
- Tests to exclude conditions capable of mimicking PMR: rheumatoid factor, myeloma screen, thyroid function tests, creatine kinase if muscle weakness is suspected, autoantibodies if there are features suggesting connective tissue disease.

Management

Eighty percent of symptoms improve within a few days with corticosteroids. The ESR falls to normal within 2–3 weeks and the CRP becomes normal within 1 week. An initial daily dose of 15–20 mg of prednisolone is usually adequate to control symptoms. The dose should be continued for 1 month and slowly reduced over the following month to about 10 mg daily.

There is no indication for prophylactic high-dose steroids to prevent blindness as with giant cell arteritis. Patients should, however, be warned to look out for additional symptoms such as headache or blurred vision. Steroids should be reduced slowly over the subsequent months.

Approximately 50% of patients manage to discontinue steroids within 2 years. Management should be based mainly on the clinical picture, although a rise in ESR in someone who is otherwise well should prompt more frequent monitoring. Relapses are most common in the first year but the incidence falls steadily thereafter, and they are often associated with a reduction in steroid dose. Adding a NSAID to cover aching and stiffness may be of help.

In patients who are becoming cushingoid, a steroid-sparing immunosuppressant, e.g. azathioprine, should be considered under expert supervision. In a few patients, it is impossible to withdraw steroids altogether and so it is acceptable to maintain them indefinitely on prednisolone 2–3 mg/day.

Prognosis

The prognosis is good provided the steroid dosage is not excessive. Most patients can be reassured that treatment can usually be discontinued after 2–4 years with a low rate of recurrence thereafter.

OTHER CONNECTIVE TISSUE DISORDERS

Systemic sclerosis

Systemic sclerosis is a multisystem disease that mainly occurs in middle-aged women. It presents with Raynaud's phenomenon in more than three-quarters of cases. The aetiology is unknown. Familial cases occur with HLA-B8 and HLA-DR3 at increased frequency. There are abnormalities of both humoral and cellular immunity. Early in the disease the skin is oedematous and the blood vessels show arteritis and thickening. There is an increase in collagen and progressive fibrosis of viscera.

Clinical features

There is general malaise, lassitude, fever, and weight loss. The following systems may be involved.

Cutaneous system

Systemic sclerosis is also termed scleroderma, reflecting the thickening and hardening of the skin associated with increased collagen content. Patients classically have a beaked nose, telangiectasia, and tight skin around the mouth causing difficulty in opening the mouth wide (Fig. 36.8). The skin becomes smooth and waxy, and atrophic with pigmentation or depigmentation. There is sclerodactyly and the fingers are 'sausage shaped'. Raynaud's phenomenon is common. There may also be subcutaneous calcification.

Morphoea is a benign condition affecting only the skin, especially on the the trunk and limbs. Plaques evolve to produce waxy, thickened skin and induration. These may enlarge or new lesions may appear over time. Resolution is associated with hyperpigmentation. Only rarely does morphoea proceed to systemic sclerosis.

Gastrointestinal system

Oesophageal involvement is very common. There is delayed peristalsis, dilatation or stricture formation leading to dysphagia or heartburn in about half of affected patients. Dilatation and atony of the small bowel may lead to bacterial overgrowth, and hence malabsorption and steatorrhoea.

Respiratory system

There is interstitial fibrosis, which either affects the lower lobes of the lungs or is diffuse. This may cause a restrictive defect and may progress to respiratory failure. There may be aspiration pneumonia and pulmonary hypertension.

Musculoskeletal system
There may be polyarthralgia and flexion deformities due to fibrosis of tendons. Myopathy and polymyositis can occur.

Cardiovascular system
Myocardial fibrosis can cause arrhythmias and conduction defects. Pericardial effusions can occur and cardiomyopathy can lead to heart failure.

Renal system
Renal involvement due to an obliterative endarteritis of renal vessels can lead to progressive renal failure and hypertension, which may be fatal.

Eyes
Sjögren's syndrome may occur.

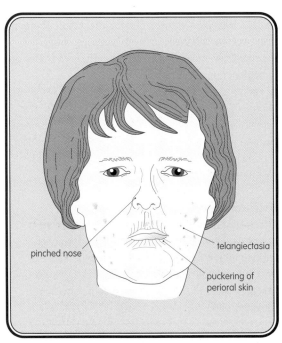

Fig. 36.8 Systemic sclerosis, showing pinched nose, multiple telangiectasia, and tightening of the skin around the mouth. The skin may also be waxy and shiny.

pinched nose

telangiectasia

puckering of perioral skin

The CREST syndrome
The CREST syndrome is a form of systemic sclerosis including **c**alcinosis of subcutaneous tissues, **R**aynaud's phenomenon, (o)**e**sophageal dysmotility, **s**clerodactyly, and **t**elangiectasia. The prognosis is generally better than systemic sclerosis *per se*. It is associated with anticentromere antibodies.

Investigations
The following investigations are important in patients with systemic sclerosis:
- Antinuclear antibodies: present in 80% of patients; rheumatoid factor is positive in 30%.
- ESR: often raised.
- FBC: may show a normochromic normocytic anaemia or a haemolytic anaemia.
- Hand X-rays: may show calcinosis.
- Barium swallow or oesophageal manometry: motility problems.

Management
Treatment is symptomatic. Electrically heated gloves may help with Raynaud's phenomenon. Antacids, H_2 receptor-antagonists, or proton pump inhibitors will help relieve heartburn. Physiotherapy may help when joints are affected, and NSAIDs can be given for joint pain.

Prognosis
The course of the disease is variable but is usually slowly progressive. Death usually occurs from lung or cardiac complications. The overall mean 5-year survival is about 70%.

Polymyositis and dermatomyositis
Polymyositis is a disorder of muscle and is of unknown aetiology. Immunological and viral factors have been suggested. Pathologically there is necrosis of muscle fibres with regeneration and inflammation. When accompanied by a rash, it is known as dermatomyositis. It can occur at any age, with a peak incidence at around 50 years old, with women twice as likely to be affected as men. About 20% of cases are associated with an underlying malignancy of bronchus, breast, stomach, or ovary. The incidence of malignancy increases with age and is more common in men.

Clinical features

The clinical feature of polymyositis and dermatomyositis include the following:

- Muscle weakness and proximal muscle wasting.
- Onset: acute or chronic with progressive weakness.
- Muscle pain and tenderness: about 50% of patients.
- Fibrosis: flexion deformities of the limbs.
- Arthralgia and arthritis: about 50% of patients.
- Skin involvement: purple 'heliotrope' colour around the eyes, and sometimes the rest of the face; violaceous, oedematous lesions over the knuckles; telangiectasia, nail-fold infarcts.
- Muscle involvement: can affect the oesophagus leading to dysphagia.
- Raynaud's phenomenon.
- Lung fibrosis.
- Cardiomyopathy.
- Sjögren's syndrome.

> **The risk of underlying malignancy with dermatomyositis or polymyositis is 30% at age 30, 40% at age 40, etc.**

Investigation

- Muscle enzymes: creatine phosphokinase and aldolase are raised, and can be used to follow the course of the disease.
- Characteristic electromyographic changes.
- Muscle biopsy: necrosis of muscle fibres with swelling and disruption of muscle cells; fibrosis, thickening of blood vessels, and inflammatory changes.
- ESR: usually raised and there may be a normochromic normocytic anaemia; antinuclear antibodies and Pos-1 antibodies may be positive.
- Investigations for underlying malignancy

Management

High-dose steroids should be prescribed in the acute phase. These can be gradually tailed off.

Immunosuppressive drugs, e.g. methotrexate or azathioprine, may be required if there is a poor response to steroids. Physiotherapy may help to restore muscle power.

Prognosis

Adults fare better than children unless there is an underlying malignancy. The disease may be progressive, or may wax and wane. Death usually occurs from respiratory or cardiac failure.

Sjögren's syndrome

This is the association of a connective tissue disease with keratoconjunctivitis sicca (dry eyes) or xerostomia (dry mouth). There is an association with HLA-B8 and HLA-DR3. Involvement of other secretory glands may cause dyspareunia, dry skin, dysphagia, otitis media, and pulmonary infection. Other features include:

- Arthralgia and polyarthritis.
- Raynaud's phenomenon.
- Oesophageal motility abnormalities and dysphagia.
- Renal tubular defects.
- Pulmonary fibrosis.
- Polyneuropathy.
- Hepatosplenomegaly.
- Vasculitis.

There is an increased incidence of lymphoma. It is associated with other organ-specific, autoimmune diseases, e.g. thyroid disease, myasthenia gravis, primary biliary cirrhosis and chronic active hepatitis.

Pathologically there is a lymphocytic and plasma cell infiltrate of the secretory glands.

Investigations

The following investigations are important in patients with Sjögrens syndrome:

- Anti-Ro and anti-La antibody titres: high levels.
- Immunoglobulins: raised.
- Rheumatoid factor: always present.
- Schirmer's test: this is a method of quantifying conjunctival dryness. A strip of filter paper is put under the lower eyelid and the distance along the paper that tears are absorbed is measured. This should be more than 10 mm in 5 minutes.

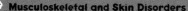

Immunological tests	
Test	**Associated disorder**
antinuclear factor (ANA)	SLE: fits, confusion, neuropathy, aseptic meningitis Sjögren's syndrome: gritty eyes, neuropathies, MCTD
anti double-stranded DNA antibodies	SLE
rheumatoid factor	rheumatoid arthritis: cervical spine subluxation, neuropathies, vasculitis, SLE, MCTD
anti-Ro (SSA), anti-La (SSB) antibodies	Sjögren's syndrome
antiphospholipid antibodies (e.g. anticardiolipin)	antiphospholipid syndrome
anti ribonucleoprotein antibodies	MCTD; myositis, trigeminal nerve palsies
Jo-1 antibodies	polymyositis
antineutrophil cytoplasmic antibodies (ANCA)	pANCA (peripheral): polyarteritis nodosa cANCA (classical): Wegener's granulomatosis
antiacetylcholine receptor antibodies	myasthenia gravis
anti-GM1 antibodies	multifocal motor neuropathy, Guillain–Barré syndrome
anti-GAD antibodies	stiff-man syndrome

Fig. 36.9 Immunological tests. (ANA, antinuclear antibody; GAD, glutamate decarboxylase; MCTD, mixed connective tissue disease; SLE, systemic lupus erythematosus.

Mixed connective tissue disease

This is a term used when the symptoms and signs do not fit neatly into one of the well-defined syndromes. It affects women more than men, and presents in young adults. There are high titres of antibody to an extractable nuclear antigen such as ribonucleoprotein (RNP). The condition may respond to steroids. Immunological tests for this disorder and others are summarized in Fig. 36.9.

Polyarteritis nodosa

Polyarteritis nodosa (PAN) is one of the 'vasculitides'. It is a necrotizing vasculitis which causes aneurysms of medium-sized arteries. It is four times more common in men than women, and the peak incidence is between the ages of 20 and 50 years. The association with hepatitis B surface antigen suggests that the vasculitis is secondary to deposition of immune complexes.

Clinical features
Clinical features include the following:
- General: fever, malaise weight loss, myalgia.

- Renal: the main cause of death. Patients may present with hypertension, proteinuria, an acute nephritic syndrome, nephrotic syndrome, or renal failure.
- Cardiac: this is the second commonest cause of death. Coronary arteritis may lead to angina and myocardial infarction. There may be pericarditis.
- Pulmonary: pulmonary infiltrates and late-onset asthma. The Churg–Strauss syndrome is associated with allergic angiitis and granuloma formation accompanied by an intense eosinophilic infiltration that affects the pulmonary arteries and causes asthma and pneumonia.
- GI tract: abdominal pain from visceral infarction; malabsorption from chronic ischaemia.
- CNS: mononeuritis multiplex, sensorimotor polyneuropathy, fits, subarachnoid haemorrhage, psychoses.
- Skin: tender nodules, nail-fold infarcts, urticaria, purpura, livedo reticularis.
- Joints: arthralgia or a non-deforming polyarthritis.

Investigations

Investigations include:

- ESR and CRP: usually raised; normochromic normocytic anaemia, leucocytosis, and eosinophilia in 30% of cases.
- Biopsy: affected organs may be biopsied demonstrating fibrinoid necrosis and cellular infiltration in the arteries.
- Angiography: may demonstrate microaneurysms in affected viscera.

Management

Treatment is symptomatic, and with steroids and immunosuppressive agents. The course of the disease may be rapidly or slowly progressive. Renal failure is the main cause of death. The overall 5-year survival is 40%.

PRIMARY SKIN DISEASES

Psoriasis

Psoriasis is a papulosquamous, proliferative, inflammatory skin disease that affects 2% of the population. It may present at any age with a peak incidence in the late-20s. Triggers include stress, trauma, infection, and drugs, e.g. lithium, chloroquine and β-blockers.

The main lesion in plaque psoriasis is a salmon-pink plaque topped by a silvery scale, most frequently found over the extensor surfaces of the limbs, e.g. elbows and knees. Involvement of the scalp with a thickened hyperkeratotic scale is also common. Plaques may be round or 'guttate' (like rain drops), geographical or circinate (ring like). Removal of the scales leaves pinpoint bleeding sites (Auspitz's sign).

In flexural psoriasis, lesions have a pinkish glazed appearance, are clearly demarcated, and are non-scaly. The commonest sites of involvement are the groin, perianal and genital regions, and inframammary folds.

Pustular psoriasis affects the palms or soles with well-demarcated scaling and erythema. The pustules are white, yellow, green, or brown when dried.

Arthropathy occurs in about 10% of patients. Other extradermal manifestations include nail pitting, corneal nodules, oedema, and liver damage.

Management

For mild conditions, treatment other than reassurance and an emollient may be unnecessary. In more troublesome cases, local application of salicylic acid, coal tar, calcipotriol or dithranol may have a beneficial effect.

Salicylic acid

This enhances the rate of loss of surface scale. Side effects include irritation or toxicity when large areas are treated.

Coal tar

Coal tar has anti-inflammatory and antiscaling properties but its use is limited by its unpleasant appearance and odour, and it may not be used on the face. However, when the lesions are extensive, coal tar baths are useful.

Dithranol

This is very effective in psoriasis. It can cause severe skin irritation, and should therefore be started at low concentrations and gradually built up.

Ultraviolet B radiation therapy

This is helpful in mild-to-moderate, guttate or chronic plaque psoriasis.

Calcipotriol

Calcipotriol is a vitamin D derivative that can be applied topically for mild-to-moderate psoriasis. It does not have an unpleasant odour.

Photochemotherapy using psoralens with long-wave ultraviolet irradiation

Photochemotherapy using psoralens with long-wave ultraviolet (UV) irradiation (or PUVA) is effective in some patients. Special lamps are required, and short-term side effects include burning; long term, there may be cataract formation, accelerated ageing of the skin (solar elastosis), and the development of skin cancer.

Acitretin

This is a retinoid (vitamin A derivative) given orally for severe resistant or complicated psoriasis. Side effects include dry and chapped lips, mild transient increase in the rate of hair fall, pruritus, paronychia, and nose bleeds. It is teratogenic.

Cytotoxic drugs

Cytotoxic drugs, e.g. methotrexate and cyclosporin, can be used for severe resistant psoriasis.

Eczema (dermatitis)

The terms eczema and dermatitis are often used interchangeably. It affects 10% of the population. Clinically, lesions are often vesicular, rupturing to leave a raw weeping surface. They may be diffuse, irritating, and sometimes painful. There may be itching and secondary infection. Lesions can be chronic and scaling with lichenification.

Atopic eczema

This often starts in infancy with the vast majority growing out of it by the age of 12. Breastfeeding may help prevent atopic eczema. Clinically, there is itching and inflammation. Investigations include prick tests to common allergens, and raised serum IgE.

Irritant contact dermatitis

The hands are often affected by erythema, vesiculation, and fissuring. Irritants include detergents, bleaches, soaps, etc. It may be a problem in certain occupations, e.g. hairdressers and engineers.

Allergic contact dermatitis

This requires previous sensitization. Patch testing produces a marked, prolonged response even to dilute quantities of the allergen. The pattern of eczema depends on the site of contact. There is often a sharp cut-off where contact ends although spread to other sites may occur (autosensitization). Thin, moist skin is the most vulnerable. Common allergens include:

- Dyes.
- Nickel: buttons and zips.
- Chromates: cement and leather.
- Lanolin: cosmetics.
- Rubber.
- Resins: glues.
- Plants.
- Topical antibiotics.
- Antiseptics.

Seborrhoeic dermatitis

This is a scaly, crusty, red, itchy eruption appearing on oily areas of the skin, e.g. the face, flexures, and scalp (dandruff).

Management

Where possible, the cause should be established and removed. A patient with suspected contact dermatitis should be patch tested to establish the diagnosis. Atopic eczema usually requires the regular application of an emollient with short courses of a mild-to-moderate topical corticosteroid, the least potent that is effective. In more severe eczema, more potent steroids may be needed, and if itching is a major problem consideration should be given to the administration of antihistamines and possibly antibiotics to prevent secondary bacterial infection.

For dry, fissured, scaly lesions, treatment is with emollients, and emulsifying ointment as soap substitutes. For weeping eczema, treatment is with topical corticosteroids, wet dressings of potassium permanganate, and topical antibacterials. Coal tar is used occasionally in chronic atopic eczema. Cyclosporin may be used for severe resistant atopic dermatitis.

Acne vulgaris

This is a papulopustular inflammatory condition, usually affecting the face and trunk, which affects about 90% of adolescents. Overproduction of sebum leads to blockage of the sebaceous duct producing the primary lesion (the comedo or 'blackhead'). Colonization by *Propionibacterium acnes* is probably an important factor. Healing may leave residual scarring.

Management

A sympathetic approach is needed. Dispel myths that the patient is dirty or that acne is caused by eating chocolate or greasy food. Advise on washing the face with soap and water frequently to degrease the skin. Both comedones and inflamed lesions respond well to benzoyl peroxide or azelaic acid.

Topical antibiotics are used for mild-to-moderate acne and include erythromycin, tetracycline, and clindamycin. Prolonged periods of oral antibiotics, e.g.

Lichen planus is summed up by **four Ps: peripheral, pruritis, polygonal, and purple.**

for 6 months, are also effective. Isotretinoin is a retinoid used for severe acne unresponsive to systemic antibiotics. It acts primarily by reducing sebum secretion. The drug is teratogenic.

Lichen planus

Lesions are purple, polygonal, and planar or flat-topped papules. The cause is unknown but may be related to disturbances of immune function. Lichen planus-like reactions occur with certain drugs, such as sulphonamides, sulphonylureas, methyldopa, thiazides, ß-blockers, and drugs that alter immune function (e.g. antimalarials, gold salts, penicillamine).

The distribution of lesions is mainly peripheral and symmetrical. Scarring occurs with chronic disease. Linear lesions may follow trauma or scratching (Koebner's phenomenon). Lesions may occur on the buccal mucosa or in the nails. The presence of Wickham's striae help to distinguish the disease. These are fine white lacy lines coursing over the papule. Postinflammatory hyperpigmentation is also a useful diagnostic sign.

The lesions usually last for 12–18 months if untreated. Systemic steroids may be required to suppress intractable itching. Less acute disease can be managed with topical corticosteroids with an antihistamine at night to control the itching.

Pityriasis rosea

This is a self-limiting, non-recurrent, scaling, maculopapular eruption occurring mainly in children and young adults. The cause is probably viral, and some drugs may produce similar features, e.g. gold salts or penicillamine. It is preceded by a red oval lesion 2–6 cm in diameter–this is the herald patch. The rash that follows may cover the entire trunk, upper thighs, and arms. The reddish-brown discrete macules tend to follow the lines of the ribs in a linear fashion. The eruption is only mildly pruritic, and usually clears within 6–8 weeks without treatment.

Rosacea

This is a chronic inflammatory eruption over the flush areas of the face (cheeks, nose, and chin) with erythema, papules, pustules, and telangiectasia. It mainly affects fair-skinned, middle-aged women and can be triggered by hot drinks, stress, sunlight, spicy foods, alcohol, and topical steroids.

Management is by avoiding these precipitating factors and taking oxytetracycline for at least 3 months. Metronidazole may be of help if tetracycline is not effective. Isotretinoin can be tried in resistant cases.

SKIN MANIFESTATIONS OF SYSTEMIC DISEASE

Erythema nodosum

These are painful, nodular lesions usually on the anterior shins which go through similar colour changes to a bruise. New crops of lesions emerge while earlier lesions are fading. It is five times more common in women, with a peak incidence between 20 and 50 years.

Causes of erythema nodosum

- Sarcoidosis.
- Drugs, e.g. sulphonamides, oral contraceptive pill, dapsone.
- Bacterial infections, e.g. streptococcus, tuberculosis.
- Crohn's disease and ulcerative colitis.
- Behçet's disease.
- Leptospirosis.
- Fungal infections, e.g. *Histoplasma*.
- Viral infections.

Erythema multiforme

These are 'target' lesions, or circular lesions in a symmetrical distribution with central blistering. It usually occurs on the limbs. The lesions may be preceded by a prodrome of fever, sore throat, headache, arthralgia, and gastroenteritis.

In Stevens–Johnson syndrome there is systemic illness, and lesions are present in the mouth, eye, and genital regions.

Causes of erythema multiforme

- Drugs, e.g. barbiturates, sulphonamides, penicillin, salicylates.
- Systemic infections, especially viral, e.g. herpes simplex.
- Vitamin deficiency, especially niacin, and vitamins A and C.
- Collagen disorders.

355

Erythema marginatum

This is associated with rheumatic fever. There are pink rings on the trunk which come and go.

Specific diseases with skin manifestations

Ulcerative colitis

There may be pyoderma gangrenosum, i.e. ulcers on the back, thigh, and buttocks with a bluish edge.

Crohn's disease

This is associated with pyoderma gangrenosum and erythema nodosum. There may be perianal and perivulval ulcers.

Diabetes mellitus

Skin manifestations include recurrent infections, ulcers, necrobiosis lipoidica diabeticorum (shiny area on the shins with a yellowish colour and telangiecstasia), granuloma annulare (purplish patches with the skin surface remaining intact), and fat necrosis at the site of injections.

Coeliac disease

Coeliac disease is associated with dermatitis herpetiformis. There are pruritic symmetrical clusters of urticarial lesions, particularly in the gluteal region and extensor aspects of the elbows and knees. They progress to vesicles and bullae. There may be secondary bacterial infection. Treatment is with dapsone.

Hyperthyroidism

Look for pretibial myxoedema or red oedematous swellings above the lateral malleoli, which progress to thickened oedema of the legs and feet.

Neoplasia

Features may include the following:

- Acanthosis nigricans (especially with gastric carcinoma): these are areas of pigmented rough thickening of the skin in the axillae or groin with warty lesions.
- Dermatomyositis (see p.350).
- Secondary skin metastases.
- Acquired ichthyosis: dry, scaly skin (vaguely resembling that of a fish), associated with lymphoma.

- Thrombophlebitis migrans (especially with pancreatic carcinoma): successive crops of tender nodules affecting blood vessels throughout the body.
- Chronic myeloid leukaemia: skin infiltration.
- Herpes zoster.

Herpes zoster is often present in any debilitating disease or immunosuppressed patient. The appearance is of groups of vesicles on an inflamed base which are painful. It is due to the virus varicella zoster which remains latent in dorsal root ganglia after infection with chicken pox. Diminished resistance allows reactivation. The lesions heal leaving scarring and pigmentation. Postherpetic neuralgia may be severe and difficult to treat.

Liver disease

Look for palmar erythema, spider naevi, gynaecomastia, and decrease in secondary sexual hair. For details of this, see Chapters 10 and 32.

Sarcoidosis

Lupus pernio may be present, i.e. a diffuse bluish plaque with small papules within the swelling, affecting the nose.

Neurofibromatosis

This condition is autosomal dominant and may include the following features:

- *Café-au-lait* spots (light brown macules).
- Axillary freckling.
- Violaceous dermal neurofibromata.
- Subcutaneous nodules.

Porphyria

This condition involves light sensitivity and blistering.

Lyme disease

Cutaneous signs are erythema chronicum migrans. This starts off as a small red papule which gradually enlarges to form a ring with a raised border. It lasts for 2 days to 3 months. Lyme disease is caused by *Borrelia burgdorferi*, a spirochete spread by ticks from deer and rodents. Other features include:

- Malaise.
- Migratory arthralgia.
- Neck stiffness.

- Lymphadenopathy.
- CNS abnormalities, e.g. meningitis and peripheral neuropathies.
- Cardiac disease with conduction disturbances.
- Myopericarditis.

Treatment is with tetracycline, penicillin, or third generation cephalosporin, e.g. cefotaxime.

Xanthomatosis

Tendon xanthomata are associated with familial hypercholesterolaemia (see p.318). Eruptive xanthomata occur with greatly elevated serum lipid concentrations. Xanthelasmata are yellow plaques commonly found on the eyelids. They may indicate hyperlipidaemia.

Behçet's disease

This is a recurrent progressive systemic disease of unknown aetiology with painful ulceration of the oral and genital regions. Other features of Behçet's disease may include:

- Iritis.
- Keratitis.
- Hypopyon and retinal vein occlusion.
- Arthritis.
- CNS complications, e.g. meningoencephalitis, parkinsonism, dementia, thrombophlebitis.

Treatment is with steroids for ulcers and systemic features. In resistant cases colchicine or cytotoxic drugs, e.g. azathioprine, may be needed

MALIGNANT SKIN TUMOURS

Basal cell carcinoma

This is the commonest skin tumour and is frequently seen in elderly, fair-skinned people. Lesions mainly occur on the face, especially at the side of the nose or periorbital skin. They may be flesh-coloured papules or plaques with superficial dilated blood vessels over the surface. There may be central necrosis with ulceration or crusting and a pearly rolled edge. They may also be pigmented or cystic. They tend to be locally invasive (hence the alternative name rodent ulcer) but metastases are rare. Treatment is by surgical excision, cryotherapy, or radiotherapy.

Squamous cell carcinoma

This tumour arises from the epidermis or skin appendages, and is most commonly seen on damaged or chronically irritated skin. It is invasive and can metastasize. Viral disease, e.g. human papilloma virus, may be a predisposing factor. Tumours are hyperkeratotic, crusted and indurated, and may ulcerate. Treatment is by excision or radiotherapy.

Malignant melanoma

This tumour is increasing in incidence and occurs particularly in fair-skinned people with exposure to UV light. Some melanomas arise in pre-existing moles. Malignancy should be expected if a pigmented lesion shows the following:

- Rapid enlargement.
- Bleeding.
- Increasing variegated pigmentation, particularly blue-black or grey.
- Ulceration.
- An indistinct border.
- Persistent itching.
- Small 'satellite' lesions around the principal lesion.

The prognosis is related to the thickness of the tumour assessed histologically. The 5-year survival for patients with a tumour less than 1 mm thick is greater than 90%. If the thickness is greater than 3.5 mm the 5-year survival rate is less than 35%.

Beware of the man with a big liver and a glass eye— think of metastatic ocular melanoma

Sites of malignant melanoma with a poor prognosis are BANS: back of the arm, neck, and scalp.

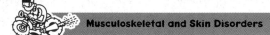

Patients with lesions on the limbs have a better prognosis than those with truncal lesions who, in turn, have a better prognosis than those with facial lesions. Interferon may slow progression of metastases. There is currently much work being done looking at the use of tumour vaccines.

Management
People should avoid exposure to direct sunlight and should use sunscreen lotions. Self-examination should be practised, and people should be aware of the warning signs and symptoms listed above. Treatment is by wide excision with skin grafting if necessary.

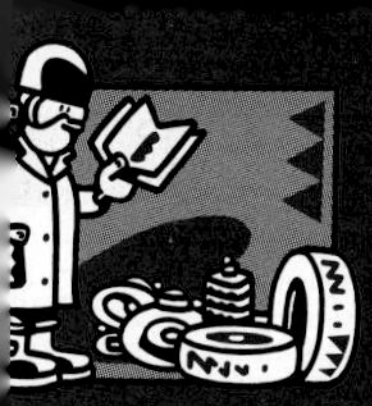

ANAEMIA

Anaemia is a common clinical problem as it is the end result of many different pathological processes. The aetiology, clinical evaluation, complications, and investigation policy have been considered in Chapter 25. The general approach to management is outlined first, and then specific conditions are discussed in detail.

General approach to the management of anaemia

What is the underlying cause of anaemia?

Remember that there may be more than one cause of anaemia in any one patient and this can catch out the unwary! For example, folate and iron deficiency may both be present in coeliac disease.

Fig. 37.1 shows possible causes of anaemia in rheumatoid arthritis.

Treat the underlying cause (where possible)

The anaemia will recur if the underlying problem persists, e.g. peptic ulceration or colonic neoplasm.

Correct the anaemia

The method of correction will depend on the type of anaemia and presence of complications. In general, iron, vitamin B_{12}, and folate should only be prescribed when the patient has been appropriately investigated and shown to have a deficiency.

Causes of anaemia in rheumatoid arthritis

- anaemia of chronic disease
- hypersplenism due to splenomegaly (Felty's syndrome if also neutropaenic)
- chronic blood loss from peptic ulceration due to steroid and NSAID administration
- bone marrow suppression by disease modifying drugs such as gold and penicillamine
- folate deficiency (increased utilization of folate)

Fig. 37.1 Causes of anaemia in rheumatoid arthritis. (NSAID, non-steroidal anti-inflammatory drug.)

Iron replacement

Oral iron replacement therapy, e.g. ferrous sulphate 200 mg t.d.s., should be continued for 3 months after the haemoglobin returns to normal to replace iron stores. Side effects include nausea, change in bowel habit, and abdominal pain. (Note that stool colour becomes very dark or black.) If side effects occur, reduce dose to once or twice daily. Intramuscular iron can be given but only if there is poor patient compliance with oral therapy, severe gastrointestinal (GI) disturbance with oral therapy, or malabsorption.

Vitamin B_{12} replacement

Most causes of vitamin B_{12} deficiency are due to malabsorption and so vitamin B_{12} is given by intramuscular injection. Stores are replaced by giving hydroxocobalamin 1 mg repeated every 2–3 days for a total of 6 doses. Maintenance therapy is 1 mg every 3 months, which needs to be lifelong in most patients.

Folate replacement

Oral folic acid 5 mg daily for 4 months corrects anaemia and replaces folate stores (a higher dose may be needed in malabsorption states). Oral folic acid 400 µg daily should be given as prophylaxis against neural tube defects to women prior to conception and throughout the first 12 weeks of pregnancy.

It should not be given in malignancy unless essential, as some tumours are dependent on folate, and it should not be given alone in megaloblastic anaemia unless vitamin B_{12} status has been shown to be normal, as it can precipitate the neurological complications of vitamin B_{12} deficiency (subacute combined degeneration of the cord).

Blood transfusion

Whole blood should only be administered when there is hypovolaemia in addition to anaemia, as occurs in massive acute haemorrhage. In an emergency, where time does not allow crossmatching, O Rhesus-negative blood can be given safely. In chronic symptomatic anaemia, which cannot be corrected by folate, vitamin B_{12} or iron therapy, matched packed red blood cells

(RBCs) may be given. Fig. 37.2 summarizes the complications of transfusion.

Splenectomy

Splenectomy is useful in hereditary spherocytosis and autoimmune haemolytic anaemia that is refractory to steroids or immunosuppressive therapy. Other indications for splenectomy include trauma, refractory idiopathic thrombocytopenic purpura, and symptomatic splenomegaly, e.g. myelofibrosis, lymphoma, chronic lymphocytic leukaemia (CLL), or chronic myeloid leukaemia (CML). Complications of splenectomy include thrombocytosis and increased susceptibility to infection with encapsulated bacteria (pneumococcus and *Haemophilus influenzae* type B). Patients should be immunized with vaccines against these two organisms. Dental treatment should be covered by antibiotic prophylaxis and any febrile episode treated quickly.

Sideroblastic anaemia

Aetiology

Sideroblastic anaemia can be congenital or acquired:
- Congenital: X-linked.
- Acquired: primary—refractory anaemia with ring sideroblasts (this is a subgroup of myelodysplasia); secondary—drugs (e.g. isoniazid, pyrazinamide), alcohol, lead poisoning, myeloproliferative disease, connective tissue disease.

Pathology
- Haem cannot be incorporated into protoporphyrin to form haemoglobin.
- Erythropoiesis becomes disordered.
- Iron accumulates in the marrow.

Presentation
- Symptoms and signs of anaemia.
- No specific clinical features.

Complications of blood transfusion	
Complication	**Cause**
haemolytic reaction	ABO incompatibility (severe), extravascular haemolysis (mild/clinically silent)
anaphylaxis	hypersensitivity to plasma proteins
febrile reaction	antibodies to white cells
volume overload	particularly the elderly and in megaloblastic anaemia
coagulopathies	platelets and clotting factors are reduced by a dilutional effect in massive transfusion
infection	virus (HIV, hepatitis B and C, EBV, CMV) Gram-negative bacteria (uncommon)
haemosiderosis	with repeated transfusions
alloimmunization	antibodies may develop to red cells, leukocytes, platelets and plasma proteins despite receiving compatible blood; this may cause problems the next time the patient receives a transfusion
graft versus host disease	uncommon: preventable by using irradiated blood (important in transplant recipients)
air embolism	particularly if given via central lines
thrombophlebitis	at cannula site

Fig. 37.2 Complications of blood transfusion. (CMV, cytomegalovirus; EBV, Epstein–Barr virus; HIV, human immunodeficiency virus.)

Complications
- Those of anaemia (see Chapter 25).
- Primary refractory anaemia with ring sideroblasts may progress to acute myeloid leukaemia (AML).
- Haemosiderosis if recurrent transfusions are given.

Investigations
- Dimorphic RBCs on blood film with normochromic and hypochromic cells.
- Mean corpuscular volume: low, normal, or slightly raised.
- Ferritin is raised.
- Ring sideroblasts in the marrow (these are erythroblasts where haem has accumulated in the mitochondria, causing granules which stain with Prussian blue and are situated in a perinuclear ring).

Treatment
- Withdraw any possible aetiological agents, such as drugs, as the anaemia may resolve.
- Pyridoxine 50–200 mg daily given orally in hereditary sideroblastic anaemia.
- Folate orally may also help.
- Blood transfusion.

Lead poisoning
Aetiology
- In adults, usually due to industrial exposure, e.g lead smelting.
- Exposure in children is mostly from old toys (as toy paints used to contain lead).

Pathology
- Absorbed from the lungs or GI tract.
- Most profound effects on bone marrow, nervous system, and kidneys.
- Also deposited in bones, teeth, nails, and hair.

Presentation
- Nausea, vomiting, and colicky abdominal pain.
- Altered conscious level, irritability, and seizures if encephalopathic (more common in children).
- Foot drop or wrist drop (usually adults).
- Burton's line (blue line on the gums).

Complications
- Peripheral motor neuropathy.
- Encephalopathy.

- Sideroblastic anaemia.
- Haemolytic anaemia.
- Fanconi's syndrome (lead nephropathy).

Investigations
- Blood lead levels >50mg/dL.
- Lead lines on X-ray: dense metaphyseal lines in children (wrists and knees) due to lead and calcium deposition.
- Hypochromic anaemia with basophilic stippling of RBCs (RNA deposition).
- May be evidence of haemolysis (see Chapter 25).
- Ring sideroblasts may be present in bone marrow.
- Free RBC protoporphyrin is raised.

Treatment
- Discuss with poisons information services.
- Treat with sodium calcium edetate (drug of choice), dimercaprol or penicillamine.

Anaemia of chronic disease
Aetiology and pathology
For the aetiology, see Fig. 25.2. The pathology is multifactorial, with inappropriate erythropoeitin production, poor release of iron from macrophages, and reduced RBC survival.

Presentation and complications
Presentation is with the symptoms and signs of anaemia (see p. 25), and of the primary disease. The complications are those of anaemia (see p. 25) and the underlying disease.

Investigations
Characteristic findings are:
- Normochromic normocytic anaemia (may be hypochromic, microcytic).
- Serum iron low.
- Serum ferritin high (can be normal).
- Increased storage iron in bone marrow.
- A raised erythrocyte sedimentation rate (ESR), neutrophil leucocytosis, and thrombocytosis, in addition to the anaemia constitutes a 'reactive' blood picture reflecting the primary pathology.

Treatment
- Treat the underlying disease.
- If mild and asymptomatic no treatment is necessary.

- If symptomatic, consider transfusion and rarely recombinant erythropoietin therapy.

Hereditary spherocytosis

Hereditary spherocytosis is an inherited disease (autosomal dominant), with an incidence of 1 in 5000.

Pathology

- Deficiency or defect of RBC membrane protein (probably spectrin).
- RBCs are normally shaped when released from the bone marrow.
- Circulating cells lose membrane due to instability of the lipid layer and become dehydrated (increased permeability to sodium).
- RBCs become spherical. They are no longer deformable and become trapped in the spleen where they are haemolysed.
- Severity is variable.

Presentation

- Jaundice can develop at any age depending on severity.
- Splenomegaly is usually present.
- Signs of complications may also be present.

Complications

- Gallstones (pigmented) due to increased unconjugated bilirubin in the bile.
- Aplastic crises due to parvovirus infection.
- Megaloblastic anaemia due to increased folate utilization, particularly during pregnancy (see Fig. 25.4).

Investigations

- Anaemia, which may not be present if bone marrow compensates for haemolysis.
- Spherocytosis and reticulocytosis (polychromasia) on blood film.
- Mean corpuscular haemoglobin concentration (MCHC) often increased.
- Erythroid hyperplasia in bone marrow (to compensate for increased breakdown).
- Increased unconjugated bilirubin.
- Increased lactate dehydrogenase (LDH).
- Reduced haptoglobin.
- Increased urinary urobilinogen.
- Increased osmotic fragility.

Treatment

- No treatment if the haomolysis is mild or if the patient is very young.
- Splenectomy in moderate to severe disease.
- Folate supplementation.
- Screen family members.

Note that hereditary elliptocytosis is an autosomal dominant condition with a similar but milder presentation to that of hereditary spherocytosis. The RBCs are elliptical on the blood film. Most cases require no treatment but the severity is variable, and severe forms may also require splenectomy and folate supplementation.

Glucose-6-phosphate dehydrogenase deficiency

Glucose-6-phosphate dehydrogenase (G6PD) deficiency occurs in 300 million people worldwide. It is an inherited (X-linked recessive) condition.

Pathology

- G6PD is an important enzyme in the hexose monophosphate shunt pathway.
- Glutathione is kept in a reduced state by this pathway and provides protection against oxidative stress.
- If erythrocytes deficient in G6PD are exposed to oxidative stress, haemoglobin becomes oxidized, and forms precipitates called Heinz bodies which stick to the RBC membrane. The cells lose deformability and become trapped and destroyed in the spleen.

Presentation

- The disease affects males in the Middle East, South East Asia, West Africa, the Mediterranean, and Southern Europe.
- The severity of disease varies, being most severe in the Mediterranean type.
- Acute episodes of intravascular haemolysis are precipitated by intercurrent illness (particularly infection), drugs (e.g. antimalarials, nitrofurantoin, sulphonamides), and the ingestion of fava beans (favism).
- The patient is usually completely well in between episodes.

- In severe deficiency, chronic haemolysis with splenomegaly may occur.
- Icterus neonatorum may occur and lead to kernicterus.
- Female heterozygotes have improved resistance to *Falciparum* malaria.

Complications
These include anaemia, kernicterus (icterus neonatorum), and shock, which can be fatal (particularly in favism).

Investigations
- Between episodes: G6PD assays (concentration or activity) show deficiency; other tests are normal.
- During acute episode; the blood film shows 'bite' cells, 'blister' cells, Heinz bodies, and reticulocytosis. Features of haemolysis will be present: increased unconjugated bilirubin, reduced haptoglobin, and increased urinary urobilinogen.

Treatment
- Avoiding or stopping precipitating drugs.
- Treating any underlying infection.
- Transfusion for severe, symptomatic anaemia.
- Considering exchange transfusion and phototherapy in icterus neonatorum.

Pyruvate kinase deficiency
This is an inherited condition (autosomal recessive).

Pathology
- Pyruvate kinase is an important enzyme in the glycolytic (Embden–Meyerhof) pathway.
- In deficiency, ATP production is reduced.
- Abnormal erythrocytes are removed by the spleen.
- 2,3-DPG increases, shifting the oxygen dissociation curve to the right, resulting in better toleration of anaemia.

Presentation
This condition presents with symptoms of anaemia, jaundice and gallstones; splenomegaly is common. Severity is variable.

Complications
Complications include anaemia and gallstones.

Investigations
- Blood film: poikilocytosis (with 'prickle' cells) and reticulocytosis.
- Autohaemolysis: abnormal.
- Pyruvate kinase: assay demonstrates deficiency.

Treatment
Treatment is by blood transfusion for severe anaemia; consider splenectomy if requiring multiple transfusions.

Sickle cell anaemia
Sickle cell anaemia occurs in 8% of Black Americans. It is an inherited (autosomal recessive) condition which most commonly affects Afro-Caribbeans but is also found in the Middle East and Mediterranean. The condition provides advantage in infection with *Falciparum* malaria.

Pathology
- A single base mutation in the DNA on chromosome 11 causes substitution of glutamic acid for valine at position 6 in the β-haemoglobin chain (HbS).
- When HbS becomes deoxygenated it aggregates in an organized fashion forming polymers within the RBCs which are less soluble and less deformable.
- As a result the erythrocyte shape becomes distorted and changes from a biconcave disc to a sickle shape.
- The sickle cells cannot readily pass through the microcirculation and become trapped in small vessels (causing infarction) and in the spleen (where they are destroyed—haemolysed).

Presentation
In the homozygote, severity is variable, and the disease may present from the third month onwards (as haemoglobin F levels fall). There is chronic haemolysis with intermittent crises and complications.

Types of sickle cell anaemia crisis
There are four types of sickle cell anaemia crisis:
- Aplastic: due to parvovirus infection of RBC precursors. Profound anaemia and reticulocytopenia. Self-limiting but transfusion may be required.
- Sequestration: sequestration may occur in the spleen, liver, and lungs. The haemoglobin drops rapidly with a compensatory increase in reticulocytes. Splenic sequestration is seen only in

children as the spleen is usually infarcted by 6 years old. Exchange transfusion may be required.

- Haemolytic: may be precipitated by infection. Seen particularly in cases with coexistent G6PD deficiency. The haemoglobin drops rapidly with a compensatory increase in reticulocytes.
- Painful: due to vascular occlusion. Can be precipitated by dehydration, hypoxia, infections, and cold exposure. Almost any organ can be affected. Small bones of the hands and feet most often affected in childhood ('hand–foot syndrome'). In older patients, the lungs, hips, shoulders, and spine are more commonly involved.

Complications
- Anaemia.
- Infection: pneumonia (*Streptococcus pneumoniae, H. influenzae*), ostomyelitis (*Salmonella*).
- Vessel occlusion: retinopathy (proliferative with vitreous haemorrhage and retinal detachment), splenic infarction (resulting in predisposition to infection), renal papillary necrosis, priapism, aseptic necrosis of the femoral head, transient ischaemic attacks, strokes, placental infarction, and spontaneous abortion.
- Gallstones.
- Leg ulceration.

Investigations
- Normochromic normocytic anaemia.
- Reticulocytosis, sickle cells, and target cells on film (features of hyposplenism may also be present following splenic infarction; Fig. 25.7).
- Haemoglobin electrophoresis demonstrates HbS.
- Leucocyte and platelet counts may also be raised.
- Prenatal diagnosis can be made using PCR (polymerase chain reaction) techniques on chorionic villous samples.

Treatment
- Prophylactic folate (increased folate utilization because of haemolysis).
- Immunization against pneumococcus and *H. influenzae* (increased risk of these because of hyposplenism secondary to splenic infarction).
- Prophylactic penicillin in children.
- Supportive care during crises.
- Prophylactic exchange transfusions if recurrent crises or significant organ damage.

Prognosis
There is a 5% mortality in the first 10 years of life.

Note that in the sickle cell trait (a heterozygous carrier state), the disease is much milder with no anaemia and a normal blood film. Crises may be caused in extreme conditions. The most common complication is renal disease.

Thalassaemia
Normal haemoglobin synthesis is summarized in Fig. 37.3.

Prevalence and aetiology
The prevalence of thalassaemia is 2.5–15% in the 'thalassaemia belt' (see below). It is an inherited condition.

Pathology
- Reduced production of one or more of the haemoglobin chains (most importantly α or β), which results in a relative excess and accumulation of the other chain (called 'imbalanced globin chain synthesis').
- The unstable haemoglobin precipitates, causing ineffective erythropoiesis and haemolysis.
- There is deficiency of α chains in α-thalassaemia and of β chains in β-thalassaemia.

Presentation
- α-Thalassaemia is found in populations in the Mediterranean, Africa, the Middle East and South-East Asia.
- β-Thalassaemia affects those in China, the Mediterranean, the Middle East and India.
- The clinical presentation is dependent on the underlying defect as shown in Figs 37.4 and 37.5.
- Thalassaemia provides an advantage in infection with *Falciparum* malaria.

Treatment
- Transfusion to maintain an adequate haemoglobin (>10 g/dL) during childhood to ensure normal growth and development.
- Iron chelation to prevent haemosiderosis using desferrioxamine.
- Oral vitamin C also increases iron excretion.
- Splenectomy can reduce transfusion

requirements but should be avoided where possible because of the increased susceptibility to infection.

- Prophylactic folate supplementation in severe disease (β-thalassaemia major).
- Endocrine therapy may be necessary in haemosiderosis.
- Bone marrow transplantation may be curative in some patients with β-thalassaemia major.
- Current research emphasis is on the prospect of using gene therapy techniques.
- Prenatal diagnosis and genetic counselling should be available.

Pernicious anaemia
Incidence and aetiology
This is an autoimmune condition and has an incidence of 2 per 10 000.

Pathology
- Immunoglobulin G (IgG) autoantibodies are produced against gastric parietal cells and intrinsic factor.
- This causes gastric mucosal atrophy with loss of parietal cells and achlorhydria.
- Intrinsic factor, necessary for vitamin B_{12} absorption, is not produced.

Normal haemoglobin synthesis

- normal haemoglobin is composed of four polypeptide chains (tetramer)
- at various stages of development, different polypeptide chains are produced (ζ, ε, α, γ, δ and β)
- in the embryo (first 8 weeks' gestation), three different haemoglobins are produced by the yolk sac, Hb Gower-1 (ζ_2, ε_2), Hb Gower-2 (α_2, ε_2) and Hb Portland (ζ_2, γ_2)
- fetal haemoglobin (HbF) is composed of two α chains and two γ chains (α_2, γ_2) and is the major haemoglobin of intrauterine life. It declines rapidly around birth and constitutes less than 1% haemoglobin by 6 months of age. HbF is produced predominantly made by the liver until 30 weeks, after which the bone marrow takes over. It has an avid affinity for oxygen
- production of β chains increases rapidly at 36 weeks' gestation; 96% adult haemoglobin is HbA (α_2, β_2), 3.5% is HbA_2 (α_2, δ_2) with the remainder being HbF
- the genes for the globin chains α and ζ are found clustered on chromosome 16. The genes for the remaining chains are located in a cluster on chromosome 11
- each person has four α genes (two on each chromosome 16) and two β genes (one on each chromosome 11)

Fig. 37.3 Normal haemoglobin synthesis.

Characteristic features of the α-thalassaemias

Subtype	Silent carrier	α-Thalassaemia trait	HbH disease	Hydrops fetalis
genetic abnormality	one α gene deleted	two α genes deleted	three α genes deleted	four α genes deleted
clinical features	asymptomatic	usually asymptomatic	haemolytic anaemia splenomegaly bone changes	hepatosplenomegaly gross oedema hypoalbuminaemia extramedullary haemopoiesis
haematological findings	no abnormality	hypochromia microcytosis	hypochromia microcytosis reticulocytosis HbH (β_4) on electrophoresis inclusion bodies with cresyl blue	hypochromia microcytosis reticulocytosis target cells nucleated red cells Hb Bart's (γ_4) on electrophoresis
survival	normal	normal	variable	stillborn or death shortly after birth

Fig. 37.4 Characteristic features of the α-thalassaemias. (HbH, haemoglobin H.)

Characteristic features of the β-thalassaemias			
Subtype	β-Thalassaemia minor	β-Thalassaemia intermedia	β-Thalassaemia major
genetic abnormality	heterozygous abnormality in β globin gene	homozygous or mixed heterozygous abnormality in β globin gene	homozygous abnormality in β globin gene

clinical features	usually asymptomatic	variable
		extramedullary haematopoiesis
		  hepatosplenomegaly
		skeletal deformity
		gallstones
		leg ulcers
			failure to thrive (3–6 months)
			jaundice
			extramedullary haematopoiesis
			  hepatosplenomegaly
			skeletal deformity
			haemosiderosis
			recurrent infections
			cardiac failure
			gallstones
			leg ulcers

haematological findings	mild anaemia
	microcytosis
	hypochromia
	target cells
	poikilocytosis
	HbA_2 high
	HbF may be raised
		moderate anaemia but not
		  transfusion dependent
		microcytosis
		hypochromia
		target cells
		poikilocytosis
			transfusion-dependent severe anaemia
			microcytosis
			hypochromia
			target cells
			anisopoikilocytosis
			reticulocytosis
			nucleated RBCs
			basophilic stippling
			inclusion bodies on supravital staining with
			  methyl violet
			HbA absent or very low
			HbF high

survival	normal	survive to adulthood even
		  without treatment
			death in childhood without treatment; bone
			  marrow transplantation may be curative

Fig. 37.5 Characteristic features of the b-thalassaemias. (Hb, haemoglobin; RBC, red blood cell)

Presentation

- The onset is usually insidious and is more common after the age of 50, affecting females more than men.
- Higher prevalence in Scandinavian populations (fair hair and blue eyes).
- Strong association with other autoimmune diseases and blood group A.
- Symptoms include those of anaemia and the neurological complications of vitamin B_{12} deficiency.
- Examination may reveal anaemia, glossitis, lemon tint (increased bilirubin due to breakdown of abnormal RBCs), low-grade pyrexia, mild splenomegaly, and neurological signs.

Complications

- Complications of anaemia (see Chapter 25).
- Neurological abnormalities from vitamin B_{12} deficiency (dementia, optic atrophy, peripheral neuropathy, subacute combined degeneration of the cord).
- Gastric carcinoma.

Investigation

- Macrocytic anaemia with typical blood film (see Fig. 25.7).
- White cell and platelet counts: may be low.
- Serum vitamin B_{12}: low, with abnormal Schilling test.
- Megaloblastic bone marrow.
- Bilirubin: increased.
- LDH: increased (also due to breakdown of abnormal RBCs).
- Parietal cell antibody in 90% (can be seen in normal elderly).
- Intrinsic factor antibody in 50%.
- Thyroid antibodies in 50%.
- Gastroscopy should be performed to exclude gastric carcinoma.

Treatment

- Lifelong vitamin B_{12} replacement as on page 359.
- Initial response to treatment can be demonstrated by an increase in reticulocyte count.

LEUKAEMIAS

The leukaemias are a group of conditions characterized by the malignant proliferation of leucocytes in the bone marrow. The cells spill out into the blood stream and may infiltrate other organs.

In the acute leukaemias, there is a proliferation of early lymphoid and myeloid precursors (called blasts) which do not mature. The clinical course is very aggressive and rapidly fatal without treatment.

The chronic leukaemias have a more indolent course and are characterized by the proliferation of lymphoid and myeloid cells, which reach maturity (lymphocytes and neutrophils respectively).

Acute lymphoblastic leukaemia

Epidemiology and aetiology
Acute lymphoblastic leukaemia (ALL) is the second most common malignancy in children under 15. Its aetiology is unknown but is probably multifactorial.

Pathology
- Lymphoblasts accumulate in the bone marrow, and can cause bone marrow failure.
- Lymphoblasts circulate in the blood stream and can infiltrate the lymph nodes, liver, spleen, kidneys, testicles, and central nervous system (CNS).
- Classified according to the French–American–British (FAB) system (Fig. 37.6).

Presentation
- Peak incidences at age 4 and over 65 years.
- The history is usually short as the disease is so aggressive (days to a few weeks).
- Symptoms are due to rapidly expanding tumour cells in the bone marrow causing bone pain or bone marrow failure (Fig. 37.7).

- There is fever, lymphadenopathy, and hepatosplenomegaly on examination.
- Main sites of relapse are bone marrow, CNS, and testes.

Investigations
- Normochromic normocytic anaemia with low reticulocyte count.
- High white cell count due to lymphoblasts; neutropenia may be present.
- Thrombocytopenia.
- Bone marrow is hypercellular and dominated by lymphoblasts (usually >50%).
- Cytogenetic abnormalities may be present, e.g. hyperdiploidy or the Philadelphia chromosome (Ph).
- Urate high.
- LDH high.
- Calcium, potassium, and phosphate may also be raised.
- Mediastinal mass on chest X-ray in T cell-ALL.
- Cerebrospinal fluid examination may show lymphoblasts, increased pressure, and increased protein.

FAB classification of ALL

- L1: small cells, homogenous, small or absent nucleoli, scanty cytoplasm
- L2: large cells, heterogenous, occasional large nucleoli, more cytoplasm
- L3: large cells, homogenous, prominent nucleoli, abundant cytoplasm

Fig. 37.6 The French–American–British (FAB) classification of acute lymphoblastic leukaemia (ALL.). Note that ALL may also be classified according to phenotype (B cell, T cell, common, null). (ALL, acute lymphoblastic leukaemia.)

Features of bone marrow failure

Cells affected	Result	Manifestation
red cell precursors	anaemia	lethargy, dyspnoea, pallor
white cell precursors	neutropenia	recurrent infections, fever
platelet precursors	thrombocytopenia	bleeding, bruising, purpura

Fig. 37.7 Features of bone marrow failure.

Treatment

Treatment should be managed in a specialized unit and include:

- Supportive care with antibiotics and blood products.
- Allopurinol to prevent tumour lysis syndrome.
- Cytotoxic chemotherapy (induction, consolidation, maintenance).
- CNS prophylaxis: cranial irradiation, intrathecal methotrexate.
- Testes: no prophylaxis but often a site of relapse.
- Treat with radiotherapy if relapse occurs.
- Bone marrow transplantation (allogeneic or autonomous) can be curative; it is used in poor risk patients.

Prognosis

- Children: 60% 5-year survival.
- Adults: 30% 5-year survival.
- Poor prognostic indicators include increasing age, increasing white cell count, null-cell or T-cell phenotype, male sex, and abnormal karyotype.

Acute myeloid leukaemia and acute non-lymphocytic leukaemia

Epidemiology

Acute non-lymphocytic leukaemia (ANLL) and AML account for 20% of all leukaemias, and 85% of adult leukaemias.

Aetiology

- Genetic predisposition: concordance in twins, Down syndrome, Bloom's syndrome, Fanconi's anaemia, and ataxia telangiectasia.
- Ionizing radiation: survivors of Hiroshima, and military personnel involved in nuclear test explosions.
- Chemical exposure: leather and rubber workers (benzene) or cigarette smokers.
- Previous chemotherapy: alkylating agents.
- Other drugs: chloroquine, LSD.
- Predisposing diseases: myeloproliferative diseases, multiple myeloma, aplastic anaemia, myelodysplasia.

Pathology

- Accumulation of immature haemopoietic cells in the bone marrow, which can cause bone marrow failure.

- Blasts can infiltrate the gums, liver, spleen, skin, and less commonly the CNS.
- Classified as shown in Fig. 37.8.

Presentation

- More frequent with increasing age (median age at presentation is 50).
- Symptoms are due to marrow failure (Fig. 37.7, particularly skin infections) or infiltration by leukaemic cells.
- Bone pain, joint pain, and malaise may be prominent symptoms.
- Hepatomegaly and moderate splenomegaly are common.
- Lymphadenopathy is rare with except in subtype M5.
- Gingival hypertrophy and skin lesions are features of subtypes M4 and M5.
- When the circulating white cell count is very high, leucostasis may occur, resulting in a cerebrovascular event or acute pulmonary deterioration.

Investigations

- Normochromic normocytic anaemia with low reticulocyte count.
- High white cell count due to circulating blasts; neutropenia may be present.
- Blasts may contain Auer rods.
- Thrombocytopenia.
- Bone marrow is hypercellular and normal marrow is replaced by blast cells.
- Cytogenetic abnormalities may be present in around 50% patients.
- Urate high.
- LDH high.
- Hypokalaemia may occur.
- Calcium and phosphate may also be raised.

Treatment

Treatment should be managed in a specialized unit and include:

- Supportive care with antibiotics and blood products.
- Allopurinol to prevent tumour lysis syndrome and gout.
- Intensive cytotoxic chemotherapy (induction, consolidation).
- Bone marrow transplantation in some patients.

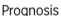

Prognosis

- 25% Long-term survivors (may be improved with transplantation).
- Poor prognostic factors include increasing age, very high white cell count, secondary leukaemia (e.g. previous myelodysplasia), cytogenetic abnormalities, and the presence of disseminated intravascular coagulation (DIC).

Chronic lymphocytic leukaemia

Epidemiology and aetiology

Chronic lymphocytic leukaemia (CLL) is the most common leukaemia in the Western Hemisphere (30% all leukaemias). Its aetiology is unknown.

Pathology

- Proliferation of small lymphocytes in bone marrow, blood, and lymphoid tissues.
- These are morphologically mature but functionally abnormal.
- 95–98% of CLL patients have B cell phenotype (remainder are T cells).

Incidence and presentation

- The most common type of leukaemia is in the Western World.
- Uncommon in the Far East.
- Increasing incidence with age (90% cases >50 years).
- More common in males.
- Some patients are asymptomatic; others may describe malaise, weight loss, night sweats, recurrent infections, bleeding, or symptoms of anaemia.
- Lymphadenopathy is usually found (60%).
- Hepatosplenomegaly may also be present.

Investigations

- Monoclonal lymphocytosis with 'smear' or 'smudge' cells seen on film.
- Anaemia may be due to marrow infiltration or autoimmune haemolysis (Coombs positive).
- Thrombocytopenia may be due to marrow infiltration or autoimmune destruction.
- Bone marrow shows accumulation of mature lymphocytes.
- Hypogammaglobulinaemia (monoclonal gammopathy may occur).

Treatment

- Observe only if asymptomatic mild disease.
- If there is symptomatic and progressive disease use oral alkylating agents (e.g. chlorambucil or cyclophosphamide).
- Intravenous fludarabine (antimetabolite) can be used in disease resistant to alkylating agents.
- Autoimmune phenomena are responsive to oral prednisolone.
- Radiotherapy may be beneficial in symptomatic, localized disease.
- Splenectomy is sometimes used in refractory hypersplenism.

French–American–British (FAB) classification of AML		
FAB subtype	**Name (predominant cell type)**	**Specific clinical features**
M1	undifferentiated myeloblastic	–
M2	myeloblastic	most common
M3	promyelocytic	DIC may cause fatal bleeding
M4	myelomonocytic	gingival, skin and meningeal infiltration
M5	monocytic	gingival, skin and meningeal infiltration lymphadenopathy and DIC may occur
M6	erythroleukaemia	particularly older patients
M7	megakaryocytic	–

Fig. 37.8 The French–American–British (FAB) classification of AML. (AML, acute myeloid leukaemia; DIC, disseminated intravascular coagulation.)

Prognosis
- Dependent on extent of disease (survival ranges from 1.5 years to over 12 years).
- In around 10% of CLL, Richter transformation to high-grade lymphoma occurs as a terminal event.

Chronic myeloid leukaemia
Incidence and aetiology
The incidence of CML is 1 per 100 000 (20% of all leukaemias). It can be due to ionizing radiation in some patients, but often the cause is unknown.

Pathology
Malignant proliferation of myeloid cells.

Presentation
- Presents in middle age, most commonly between 40 and 60 years, with a male preponderance.
- Symptoms include lethargy, weight loss, sweats, and left hypochondrial discomfort (enlarging spleen).
- Symptoms of anaemia or thrombocytopenia may be present.
- On examination there is splenomegaly, which may be massive.
- Hepatomegaly is present in 50% of cases but lymphadenopathy is uncommon.
- The natural history is characterized by a chronic phase lasting several years, followed by an acute, aggressive phase.
- Leucostasis may occur in the acute phase.

Investigations
- High white cell count with full range of immature and mature myeloid cells.
- Anaemia may be due to marrow infiltration or hypersplenism.
- Thrombocytosis is common.
- Bone marrow demonstrates accumulation of myeloid cells.
- 95% of patients have a chromosomal translocation called the Philadelphia chromosome (Ph), which is a reciprocal translocation between chromosomes 9 and 22 producing the chimeric bcr/abl gene.
- Neutrophil alkaline phosphatase is low.
- Urate is high.
- LDH is high.
- Serum vitamin B_{12} is high.

Treatment
- Allopurinol orally.
- Cytotoxic chemotherapy with hydroxyurea (drug of choice) or busulphan.
- α-Interferon achieves good haematological control and reduction in the presence of Ph.
- Allogeneic bone marrow transplantation may be curative and should be considered in young patients with an HLA-matched sibling.
- Leucopharesis will reduce the white count quickly in leucostasis.

Prognosis
- Chronic phase: median time 2–6 years.
- Acute phase: median survival <3 months.
- Transformation is to AML in two-thirds of patients and to ALL in the remainder.

MULTIPLE MYELOMA

Incidence and aetiology
The incidence of multiple myeloma is 5 per 100 000 (1% of all malignancies, 10–15% of all haematological malignancies). Its aetiology is unknown though ionizing radiation may be important in some patients.

Pathology
- Neoplastic proliferation of a single clone of plasma cells (a plasma cell is a terminally differentiated B cell)
- The malignant cells secrete a monoclonal immunoglobulin or light chain and normal immunoglobulin production is suppressed.
- Osteoclast activity is increased resulting in bone reabsorption.
- AL (systemic) amyloidosis affects 10% cases.

Presentation
- Disease mainly of the elderly with a peak incidence in the 7th decade.
- Bone pain due to osteolytic lesions and pathological fractures affect two-thirds of patients.
- Recurrent infections result from impaired antibody response and hypogammaglobulinaemia.
- Symptoms of anaemia may be present.
- Examination usually reveals pallor alone.
- Hepatosplenomegaly is occasionally present.

- Peripheral neuropathy occurs with amyloidosis.
- Spinal cord compression and radiculopathy can result from compression by tumour or vertebral collapse.
- Polymerization of the monoclonal antibody occasionally results in hyperviscosity.
- Abnormal bleeding is caused by platelet dysfunction.

Investigations
- Normochromic normocytic anaemia.
- Rouleaux (RBCs sticking together) and background immunoglobulin staining may be seen on the blood film.
- ESR: usually high.
- Serum protein electrophoresis demonstrates a monoclone often with immune paresis.
- Bence Jones protein may be found in the urine.
- Skeletal survey reveals generalized osteopenia, 'punched-out' lytic lesions, and pathological fractures.
- Over 10% of bone marrow cells are plasma cells.
- Calcium high (increased osteoclastic activity), alkaline phosphatase is normal.
- Urate high.
- Renal failure may result from a number of factors (Fig. 37.9).

Treatment
- Observation only in asymptomatic, uncomplicated disease.
- Supportive treatment with antibiotics, blood products, analgesics, and correction of hypercalcaemia where necessary.
- Melphalan and prednisolone usually controls symptoms and reduces tumour burden.
- Combination cytotoxic chemotherapy can be used in refractory disease.

- High-dose chemotherapy with autologous stem cell rescue can lead to durable remission.
- Radiotherapy may be useful where there is localized disease causing bony pain.
- The role of α-interferon is not yet defined.

Prognosis
- Median survival is 3 years.
- Poor prognostic factors include high β_2-microglobulin levels (most accurate), high urea, low haemoglobin, increasing age, and low albumin.

N.B. A monoclonal gammopathy may be present in the absence of myeloma in monoclonal gammopathy of uncertain significance (MGUS). These patients should be monitored under long-term review.

MALIGNANT LYMPHOMAS

Malignant lymphomas are neoplastic proliferations of lymphocytes which form solid tumours within lymphoid tissue. They are split into two broad categories on the basis of histological findings: Hodgkin's disease (Reed–Sternberg [RS] cells present) and non-Hodgkin's lymphoma (all others).

Hodgkin's disease
Incidence and aetiology
The incidence of Hodgkin's disease (HD) is 6 per 100 000 (one of the most common malignancies in young adults). Its aetiology is unknown but there is a definite link with Epstein–Barr virus (EBV).

Pathology
- Characteristic RS cells in a background of inflammatory infiltrate.

Causes of renal failure in multiple myeloma

- hypercalcaemia
- hyperuricaemia
- precipitated light chains
- amyloidosis
- NSAIDs prescribed for bone pain

Fig. 37.9 Causes of renal failure in multiple myeloma. (NSAID, non-steroidal anti-inflammatory drug.)

The three principle features of multiple myeloma are:
- Skeletal abnormalities.
- Production of a monoclonal protein.
- Accumulation of plasma cells in the bone marrow.

- RS cells are large bi- or multinucleated cells with prominent 'owl-eyed' nucleoli.
- HD is divided using the Rye classification into four histological subgroups (Fig. 37.10).

Presentation

- Bimodal age at presentation with peaks at 20–29 and above 50 years with a male preponderance in children.
- Principally affects white populations and is more common in higher socioeconomic groups.
- Symptoms are due to painless lymph node enlargement (particularly cervical, axillary, and mediastinal) and/or 'B symptoms' (Fig. 37.11).
- Lymphadenopathy is supradiaphragmatic in 90% of patients and mediastinal disease may cause dry cough and exertional dyspnoea.
- Some patients describe pruritis and alcohol-induced lymph node pain.
- Affected lymph nodes feel rubbery.
- Pallor and hepatosplenomegaly may also be found on examination.

Investigations

- The diagnosis is usually made on lymph node biopsy (reviewed by haematopathologist); staging of disease is then performed to determine the extent of disease and is central to planning appropriate treatment (Fig. 37.12).
- Normochromic normocytic anaemia, neutrophilia, eosinophilia, and thrombocytosis.
- Alkaline phosphatase raised (serum Ca^{2+} may be high).
- LDH raised in bulky disease (prognostic indicator).
- Urate high.
- ESR may be raised.
- Chest X-ray: mediastinal lymphadenopathy.
- Computed tomography (CT) scan of the thorax, abdomen and pelvis to stage the extent of the disease.
- Bipedal lymphogram may demonstrate pelvic lymphadenopathy not detectable on CT scan (rarely performed).
- Bone marrow examination in some patients usually shows reactive marrow only.
- Staging laparotomy with splenectomy, which used to be performed for early stage disease, is now almost never necessary.

Treatment

- Localized disease (stage IA–IIA): radiotherapy (usually mantle).
- Stage IIB–IIIA: treatment is controversial (?combined radiotherapy and chemotherapy).
- Extensive disease (stage IIIB–IVB): chemotherapy (MOPP—mustine, oncovin, procarbazine, and prednisolone which is the gold standard although other regimens are available).
- Relapse after radiotherapy: chemotherapy as above.
- Relapse after chemotherapy: alternative chemotherapy regimen, high-dose chemotherapy with autologous bone marrow or stem cell transplant in selected patients.

Prognosis

- Overall 5-year survival 75% but this is greatly affected by histological type and stage of disease at presentation.
- Poor prognostic indicators include B symptoms, high stage, lymphocyte depleted histology, increasing age, high ESR, and high LDH.

The Rye classification of Hodgkin's disease		
Subtype	**Percentage**	**Prognosis**
lymphocyte predominant	10	excellent
mixed cellularity	30	intermediate
lymphocyte depleted	<5	poor
nodular sclerosis	60	variable

Fig. 37.10 The Rye classification of Hodgkin's disease.

'B symptoms'

- weight loss >10% of initial weight over previous 6 months
- drenching night sweats
- fever >38°C

Fig. 37.11 'B symptoms'.

Non-Hodgkin's lymphomas

Incidence and aetiology

Non-Hodgkin's lymphomas (NHL) account for 4% of all cancers, and the incidence is increasing for reasons which are unclear. Incidence increases with age (uncommon before 40, median age is 50) and the condition is more common in males. The aetiology is probably multifactorial including the following:

- Genetic predisposition.
- Immunosuppression, e.g. HIV infection, transplant recipients.
- Viruses, e.g. EBV (particularly Burkitt's lymphoma).
- Ionizing radiation, e.g. survivors of the atomic bomb.

Pathology

- Neoplastic proliferation of B (usually) or T lymphocytes within the lymphoid system forming solid tumours which do not have RS cells.
- Heterogenous group of conditions with many different subtypes.
- A number of different classification schemes have been developed in an attempt to identify groups of patients with similar clinical, histological, and genetic features. The most recent scheme is called the REAL (Revised European American Lymphoma) classification.
- In practical terms, NHL can be broadly divided into two groups: low-grade NHL and high-grade NHL.

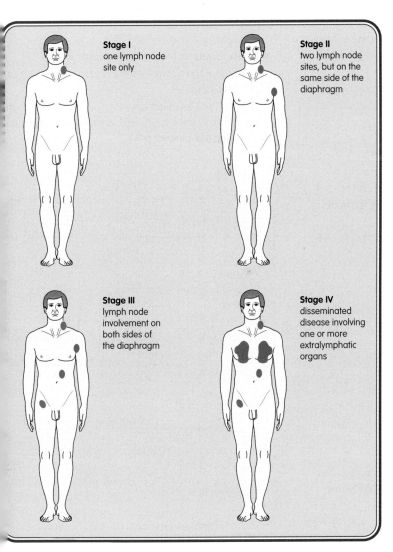

Stage I
one lymph node site only

Stage II
two lymph node sites, but on the same side of the diaphragm

Stage III
lymph node involvement on both sides of the diaphragm

Stage IV
disseminated disease involving one or more extralymphatic organs

Fig. 37.12 Ann Arbor staging of malignant lymphomas. Diagram shows stages I to IV. When you stage a patient you give a number (I–IV) and a letter (A or B). The letter A denotes the absence of B symptoms and B denotes the presence of B symptoms. Patients at stage IIA, for example, have stage II lymphoma without B symptoms.

Presentation
- Most common haematological malignancy.
- Usually presents with painless lymphadenopathy or 'B' symptoms.
- May also involve extranodal sites including skin, lung, bowel, CNS, and bone.
- Low-grade NHL has an indolent course but is not curable; high-grade NHL presents aggressively but may be cured in up to 40% of patients.
- Lymphadenopathy, hepatosplenomegaly, pallor, and involvement of Waldeyer's ring or extranodal sites should be looked for on examination.

Investigations
- The diagnosis is usually made on lymph node biopsy (and should be reviewed by a haematopathologist as diagnosis can be difficult); staging investigations should then be performed to determine the extent of disease using the Ann Arbor system (Fig. 37.12).
- Normochromic normocytic anaemia is often present.
- Circulating lymphoma cells are sometimes seen on the peripheral film.
- Bone marrow is not uncommonly infiltrated by lymphoma cells and may cause bone marrow failure.
- LDH high in bulk disease.
- Urate high.
- Chromosomal translocations are characteristic of certain subtypes.
- CT scan of the thorax, abdomen and pelvis: will determine the stage of the disease.

Treatment
Low-grade NHL
- Asymptomatic: observation only.
- Localized disease: radiotherapy.
- Symptomatic or progressive disease: oral chemotherapy (chlorambucil or cyclophosphamide).
- Combination chemotherapy can be given in refractory disease.

High-grade NHL
- Localized lesion: radiotherapy.
- Most patients require cytotoxic chemotherapy (CHOP is the gold standard).
- The role of high-dose chemotherapy with autologous bone marrow or stem cell transplantation is currently under evaluation.

Prognosis
- Low-grade NHL: median survival is around 8–10 years.
- High-grade NHL: 40% 5-year survival.
- Poor prognostic factors include increasing age, high LDH, extensive disease, T cell phenotype, certain extranodal sites, poor performance status, and low-grade NHL that has transformed into high-grade NHL.

BLEEDING DISORDERS

An increased tendency to bleeding can result from abnormalities of platelets, the coagulation pathway, or of blood vessels. The differential diagnosis, clinical findings, and investigation of these disorders are discussed in detail in Chapter 23. Specific conditions and their management are considered here.

Haemophilia A
Incidence and aetiology
Haemophilia A affects 1 in 8000 males. It is an inherited condition (X-linked recessive).

Pathology
Decreased plasma factor VIII activity.

Presentation
- Severity of bleeding correlates with level of factor VIII activity (lower levels correspond to more severe symptoms).
- Bleeding may be spontaneous or secondary to trauma.
- Recurrent haemarthroses and intramuscular haematomas cause long-term disability due to arthopathy and contractures.
- Haematuria and intracranial bleeding may also occur.
- Bleeding from small cuts is usually minor (due to normal platelet function) but easy bruising occurs and bleeding following surgery may be fatal.
- After trauma, bleeding may be delayed as initial haemostasis is maintained by platelets.
- GI bleeding is uncommon.

Investigations
- APTT: prolonged.
- PTT: normal.

- TT: normal.
- Bleeding time: normal.
- Factor VIII assay: low.

Treatment

- Usually managed in specialized haemophilia centres.
- When there is bleeding or the patient requires surgery, factor VIII levels can be increased in two ways—mild haemophilia with desmopressin (DDAVP); moderate or severe haemophilia with factor VIII concentrates.
- Other aspects of management include analgesia (avoiding aspirin), joint replacement, synovectomy for arthropathy, regular dental care, and psychosocial support.

Prognosis

Life expectancy should be normal with current therapies.

Complications

Complications of receiving factor VIII concentrates include exposure to HIV, hepatitis B and C, and the development of inhibitors to infused factor VIII.

Haemophilia B (Christmas disease)
Incidence and aetiology

Incidence is 1 per 30 000. It is an inherited condition (X-linked recessive, and therefore affects males).

Pathology

Decreased plasma factor IX activity.

Presentation

Identical to haemophilia A.

Investigations

- APTT: prolonged.
- PTT: normal.
- TT: normal.
- Bleeding time: normal.
- Factor IX assay: low.

Treatment

Treatment is with factor IX concentrates (DDAVP has no effect on factor IX levels). Otherwise treatment is the same as for haemophilia A.

Prognosis

With current therapies life expectancy should be normal.

Von Willebrand's disease
Incidence and aetiology

Von Willebrand's disease (VWD) occurs in 1% of the general population. It is an inherited (autosomal dominant) condition.

Pathology

- Deficiency of von Willebrand's factor (VWF).
- VWF is a plasma protein that acts as a cofactor in platelet adherence to the subendothelium and platelet aggregation; it is also a carrier protein for factor VIII.

Presentation

- Both sexes equally affected.
- Severity of disease is variable.
- Most patients present with mucosal bleeding (epistaxis, bleeding gums, GI bleeding).
- Menorrhagia and bleeding following surgery, dental extractions, trauma, and delivery are common.
- Haemarthroses and intramuscular haematomas are rare.

Investigations

- APTT: prolonged (may be normal).
- PTT: normal.
- TT: normal.
- Bleeding time: prolonged.
- VWF assays: low.
- Ristocetin platelet aggregation: abnormal.

Treatment

Treatment is with desmopressin (DDAVP) or concentrates (usually cryoprecipitate) in haemorrhage or perioperatively.

Prognosis

Usually normal life expectancy.

DISSEMINATED INTRAVASCULAR COAGULATION

Aetiology

DIC may be caused by:

- Malignancy: mucus-secreting adenocarcinomas,

prostate, pancreatic carcinoma, acute promyelocytic leukaemia.
- Infection: Gram-negative septicaemia, meningococcal septicaemia, *Clostridia*, toxic shock syndrome.
- Obstetric: amniotic fluid embolism, placental abruption, eclampsia, septic abortion.
- Tissue damage: rhabdomyolysis, fat embolism, severe trauma, burns.
- Immunological: incompatible blood transfusion, drug reaction, anaphylaxis.
- Liver disease: acute fatty liver of pregnancy, fulminant liver failure.
- Others: snake bites, acute pancreatitis, aortic aneurysm.

Pathology
- Intravascular coagulation is precipitated by release of tissue factor or procoagulant substances into the circulation from injured cells, malignant cells, or damaged endothelium.
- Microthrombi form throughout the microcirculation causing ischaemia and infarction.
- Platelets, fibrin, and clotting factors are consumed by the thrombotic process and the fibrinolytic system becomes activated; these two processes result in a tendency to bleed, and haemorrhage may be significant.

Presentation
- DIC may be mild and chronic (e.g. adenocarcinoma), or severe and life threatening.
- Thrombosis can cause ischaemia or infarction in the lungs, kidneys, liver, heart, brain, or skin.
- Bleeding is often into the skin or recent venepuncture sites.
- GI and pulmonary haemorrhage may also occur.

Investigations
- Platelet count: low.
- PTT: prolonged.
- APTT: prolonged.
- TT: prolonged.
- Fibrinogen: low (may be normal as acute phase reactant).
- D-dimers (fibrin degradation products): high.
- Blood film: fragmented RBCs due to microangiopathic haemolysis.

Treatment
- Treatment of the underlying disease usually resolves the DIC.
- Supportive care, e.g. fluids, antibiotics, debridement of gangrene.
- Replacement of platelets and clotting factors (using fresh frozen plasma or cryoprecipitate) may be used if there is haemorrhage or risk of haemorrhage, e.g. in surgery.
- Pharmacological inhibitors of coagulation or fibrinolysis e.g. heparin or tranexamic acid, may be beneficial in certain circumstances but their use is controversial.

Prognosis
Mortality is 80% in severe DIC and is usually due to the underlying disease.

THROMBOTIC DISORDERS

Aetiology
Risk factors for venous thrombosis are outlined in Fig. 37.13.

Pathology
- Venous thrombosis can be caused by abnormal vein walls, venous stasis, or hypercoagulable blood.
- Thrombosis may be precipitated by a specific provoking event such as surgery or a physiological state such as pregnancy.
- The lower limbs are the most common site of thrombosis.
- Small clots may break off and cause pulmonary embolus or, very rarely, cerebral infarction by paradoxical embolus in patients with a patent foramen ovale.

Presentation
- Deep vein thrombosis (DVT) causes local pain and swelling.
- The diagnosis can be difficult to make on clinical grounds.
- Pulmonary embolus (PE) causes sudden onset of pleuritic chest pain, dyspnoea, and haemoptysis.
- Inherited hypercoagulable states present with recurrent venous thromboses often at an early age, spontaneous abortions, and warfarin-induced skin necrosis.

- Antiphospholipid syndrome and hyperhomocysteinaemia may cause arterial as well as venous thromboses.

Investigations

- Every effort should be made to confirm the diagnosis of suspected venous thrombosis by radiological tests as it has important implications for long-term management; these tests include venous doppler, venogram, ventilation/perfusion scan and pulmonary angiogram.
- Careful clinical examination should be performed looking for an underlying cause such as malignancy and investigated as appropriate.
- If the patient is young, ask if there have been recurrent episodes, recurrent spontaneous abortions, or a family history of thromboembolism, and consider hereditary thrombophilia. Assays are available to detect these abnormalities.
- A baseline platelet count and clotting screen should always be done.

Treatment if thrombosis is proven

- Full anticoagulation with heparin for 5 days (low molecular weight heparin can be used for lower limb DVT, unfractionated heparin for PE and other thromboses).
- Oral warfarin should be given simultaneously and monitored using the INR (International Normalised Ratio) which should be maintained between 2 and 3.
- Heparin should be continued until the INR is therapeutic.

Treatment period

The length of time a patient should be anticoagulated is controversial and currently under review, but as a general rule:

- Lower limb DVT: warfarin for 3 months.
- PE: warfarin for 6 months.
- Two or more unprovoked and documented thromboses: lifelong warfarin.

Risk factors for venous thrombosis		
Aetiology	**Risk factor**	**Example**
inherited	antithrombin deficiency protein C deficiency protein S deficiency activated protein C resistance homocysteinuria dysfibrinogenaemia	
acquired	physiological	pregnancy and childbirth obesity elderly
	provoking events	surgery trauma
	pathological	immobility malignancy venous trauma/obstruction oestrogen therapy nephrotic syndrome antiphospholipid syndrome hyperviscosity syndromes

Fig. 37.13 Risk factors for venous thrombosis.

INTRODUCTION

Infections affecting specific systems have been discussed in the appropriate chapters. This chapter considers in detail two important multisystem infections, human immunodeficiency virus (HIV) and malaria.

HIV AND AIDS

Epidemiology

28 000 people in the UK are infected with HIV, of which 13 400 have the acquired immunodeficiency syndrome (AIDS). Approximately 1 400 000 cases have been reported worldwide but the true prevalence is likely to be much higher than this. Eighty per cent of cases are found in the developing countries, particularly Africa. The World Health Organization estimates that 30–40 million people will be infected by HIV by the year 2000.

Aetiology

HIV-1 (i.e. the first type discovered, also once called HTLV-III, for human T cell lymphotropic virus III, and LAV, for lymphadenopathy-associated virus) is found throughout the world.

HIV-2 (similar to a monkey virus, simian immunodeficiency virus, hence SIV) is uncommon except in West Africa.

The original source of the virus is unknown but it may have been Central Africa. HIV can be transmitted by sexual, parenteral, or vertical routes (Fig. 38.1).

Pathology

HIV is a lentivirus, which is a subgroup of the human retroviruses. Its genetic information is stored in a single strand of ribonucleic acid (RNA). Three specific genes produce proteins essential for HIV survival (Fig. 38.2). The virus can infect any cells expressing CD4+, notably T helper cells, lymphocytes central to the immune response. Macrophages and monocytes also express CD4+ and can serve as a reservoir for HIV. CD4+ acts as

Routes of HIV transmission	
Route	**Examples**
sexual	vaginal intercourse, anal intercourse
parenteral	intravenous drug abuse, blood transfusion, needlestick injury
vertical (i.e. from mother to fetus)	during gestation or delivery, via breast milk

Fig. 38.1 Routes of HIV transmission.

HIV genes and the proteins they encode	
Gene	**Protein**
pol	reverse transcriptase (makes DNA copies of the viral RNA)
gag	core protein p24
env	external (envelope) glycoprotein (for attachment of HIV to target cells)

Fig. 38.2 HIV genes and the proteins they encode.

a receptor for glycoprotein on the virus envelope allowing the virus to enters the cell.

The enzyme reverse transcriptase makes DNA copies of the virus RNA, which become integrated into the host cell's genome resulting in constant production of more viruses. The normal function of the infected cells is disrupted and the host cells are eventually destroyed.

Because the principal cells affected are those of the immune system, HIV infection is characterized by diseases resulting from immunodeficiency, e.g. infections and malignancies.

Presentation

There are four recognized phases of HIV infection (Fig. 38.3).

Seroconversion

Seroconversion usually occurs after 6–8 weeks incubation and severity varies significantly. Symptoms include mild 'glandular fever-type' illness, arthralgia, fever, headaches, rash, generalized lymphadenopathy, and neurological abnormalities. The illness is self limiting and usually resolves within 8 weeks.

Asymptomatic phase

The patient may remain well and asymptomatic for up to 15 years.

Generalized lymphadenopathy

Rubbery, mobile lymphadenopathy develops in multiple sites for at least 3 months prior to the onset of symptomatic disease. Biopsy shows non-specific reactive histiocytosis.

Symptomatic infection

This stage is characterized by constitutional symptoms (weight loss, diarrhoea, and fever), recurrent infections, malignancies, and neurological abnormalities (Fig. 38.4). Specific criteria for the diagnosis of AIDS exist based on the development of certain indicator diseases with or without laboratory confirmation of HIV infection. Malignancies seen with increased frequency in HIV infection are often associated with specific viral infections (Fig. 38.5).

Investigations

All investigations for HIV infection should be performed under the strictest of confidentiality. The diagnosis has immense social, financial, health, and psychological implications; counselling prior to testing is very important.

The activity of HIV infection can be assessed by the measurement of viral antigens (p24), the immune response to the infection (anti-HIV antibodies), or the effects of the infection (CD4+ counts). Fig. 38.6 summarizes the findings at the different stages.

In practice, the diagnosis is usually made using HIV antibody tests. Several different methods of detection are now commercially available. If a result is positive, the test should be repeated using a different method. If that is also positive, a further serum sample should be taken and the tests repeated before the diagnosis is confirmed. In this way, false positive results are reduced to a minimum.

Note that HIV antibodies may be undetectable for up to 3 months after infection and that this is a window for false negative results.

Once the diagnosis is made, progress can be assessed by monitoring CD4+ counts. Fig. 38.7 lists other illnesses that may reduce the CD4+ count and it is important to look at the general trend rather than individual counts.

Other tests for detection of HIV include viral culture and polymerase chain reaction detection. These may have specific clinical indications, such as in children and after occupational exposure, but are not routinely performed.

Anaemia, leucopenia, and thrombocytopenia may be found; β_2-microglobulin levels may also be raised.

Treatment

Treatment falls into three broad categories: treatment of opportunistic infections, treatment of malignancies, and treatment of the HIV infection itself. There are many clinical trials currently in progress looking at these different aspects. It is likely that, as the results of these

Phases of HIV infection	
Phase	**Features**
I	seroconversion
II	asymptomatic phase
III	persistent generalized lymphadenopathy
IV	symptomatic infection including AIDS

Fig. 38.3 Phases of HIV infection.

studies become available and with the emergence of drug-resistant organisms, the management of HIV patients will change. Management should be based in specialist centres.

Treatment of opportunistic infections

Treatment of opportunistic infections is summarized in Fig. 38.8.

Treatment of malignancies

- Kaposi's sarcoma: local treatment includes camouflage, vinblastine, or interferon injections into the tumour, and radiotherapy. For widespread disease α-interferon, or vincristine plus bleomycin may be given.
- Cerebral lymphoma: whole brain irradiation and corticosteroids.

Features of symptomatic HIV infection		
Organ/ body system	**Feature**	**Examples**
mouth	infection	*Candida*, abscesses, gingivitis, periodontitis
	premalignant	hairy leukoplakia
	malignancy	**Kaposi's sarcoma** of hard palate
	others	aphthous ulceration
lungs	infection	*Pneumocystis carinii* pneumonia, pneumococcal pneumonia, *Haemophilus influenzae, Staphylococcus aureus, Pseudomonas aeruginosa, Mycobacterium tuberculosis, Mycobacterium avium-intracellulare* complex, fungal pneumonia (*Aspergillus*)
	malignancy	**Kaposi's sarcoma**, lymphoma
neurological	infection	**toxoplasmosis** (intracranial abscess, encephalitis), **cryptococcal meningitis, cytomegalovirus** (encephalitis, ascending polyradiculopathy, transverse myelitis), herpes simplex (encephalitis), herpes zoster (transverse myelitis), bacterial abscesses, tuberculomas
	malignancy	**cerebral lymphoma**
	HIV-related	**encephalopathy**, meningitis, myelopathy, peripheral neuropathy (sensory), proximal myopathy, inflammatory demyelinating polyneuropathy (e.g. Guillain–Barré syndrome)
gastrointestinal	infection	oesophagitis (*Candida*, **herpes simplex, cytomegalovirus**), liver disease (mycobacteria, hepatitis B, cytomegalovirus, microsporidia), biliary disease (cytomegalovirus, *Cryptosporidium*, microsporidia), enterocolitis (*Campylobacter, Salmonella, Shigella, Cryptosporidium, Giardia*, **cytomegalovirus**, microsporidia)
	malignancy	**Kaposi's sarcoma**, lymphoma
	HIV-related	enteropathy, gastropathy, malabsorption
skin	infection	viral (**herpes simplex**, herpes zoster, molluscum contagiosum), bacteria (*Staphylococcus*), fungi (*Candida*, tinea cruris, and tinea pedis)
	malignancy	**Kaposi's sarcoma**, basal cell carcinoma, squamous carcinoma
	others	seborrhoeic dermatitis, psoriasis
eyes	infection	retinitis (**cytomegalovirus**, herpes virus, toxoplasmosis)
joints	mono/polyarthropathy	cause unclear

Fig. 38.4 Features of symptomatic HIV infection. Conditions seen in AIDS (indicator diseases) are in **bold**.

- Non-Hodgkin's lymphoma: local radiotherapy or CHOP chemotherapy for widespread disease. (CHOP—cyclophosphamide, doxorubicin, vincristine, and prednisone.)

Treatment directed at the HIV virus itself

Treatment directed at the HIV virus itself is usually started when the CD4$^+$ count is 200–500 $\times$ 10^6/L. Two different classes of drugs are currently available (Fig. 38.9). Combination treatment with azidothymidine (AZT) with either dideoxyinosine (DDI) or zalcitabine (DDC) has been shown to be more effective than monotherapy.

The role of other drugs is the focus of ongoing clinical trials.

Prevention

As there is no 'cure' for HIV infection, preventative measures must remain a high priority. Such measures include education, the provision of clean needles for intravenous drug abusers, the use of condoms, the screening of blood products and organs donated for transplantation, and avoidance of breastfeeding in HIV-positive mothers.

Prognosis

Survival of up to 3 years, from the onset of symptomatic disease, can be achieved with the use of combination anti-HIV treatment and prophylaxis against infection.

MALARIA

Epidemiology

Worldwide, malaria affects over 100 million people each year. It causes around 1 million deaths each year (particularly of children) and is endemic in the tropics and subtropics. It is seen in temperate zones when imported by people who have visited or come from endemic areas.

Aetiology

The disease is caused by protozoal infection with one of the species of the genus *Plasmodium* (*P. vivax*, *P. ovale*, *P. malariae*, or *P. falciparum*).

Pathology

Malaria is spread from an infected person to a non-infected person by the female *Anopheles* mosquito. At schizogony the red blood cell bursts, releasing malaria parasites, malaria antigen, malaria pigment,

Malignancies seen with increased frequency and associated viruses	
Tumour	**Associated virus**
Kaposi's sarcoma	human herpesvirus 8
cerebral lymphoma	Epstein–Barr virus
non-Hodgkin's lymphoma	Epstein–Barr virus
Hodgkin's disease	not determined
cervical carcinoma	human papillomavirus
anal carcinoma	human papillomavirus

Fig. 38.5 Malignancies seen with increased frequency and associated viruses.

Investigation at different stages of HIV infection				
Phase	Viral replication	p24	HIV antibodies	CD4$^+$ count
seroconversion	high	detectable until HIV antibodies appear	detectable 3 weeks to 3 months after exposure	transient fall due to high viral load, but returns to normal when HIV antibodies appear
asymptomatic phase	low	undetectable as antibody in excess to antigen	detectable	normal
symptomatic phase	high	detectable	detectable	falls; when <200 $\times$ 10^6/L risk of infection is very high

Fig. 38.6 Investigation at different stages of HIV infection.

Differential diagnosis of a low $CD4^+$ count
• HIV infection • acute viral infections • TB • SLE • sarcoidosis • steroids

Fig. 38.7 Differential diagnosis of a low $CD4^+$ count (HIV, human immunodeficiency virus; SLE, systematic lupus erythematosis; TB, tuberculosis.)

haemoglobin, and other constituents of the red blood cells, into the blood stream causing the typical clinical picture.

This occurs every 72 hours in *P. malariae* (quartan malaria), every 48–72 hours in *P. vivax* and *P. ovale* (tertian malaria) and every 48 hours in *P. falciparum* (subtertian malaria). *P. vivax, P. ovale*, and *P. malariae* invade up to 2% of the circulating red blood cells. *P. falciparum* may affect over 10% of cells, producing a more severe clinical picture.

Fig. 38.10 demonstrates the life cycle of malaria.

Treatment and prophylaxis of opportunistic infections

Infection	Treatment	Treatment alternatives	Indication for prophylaxis	Prophylactic drug regimes
Pneumocystis carinii	high-dose intravenous cotrimoxazole steroids may be beneficial	intravenous pentamidine, or clindamycin + primaquine, or dapsone + trimethoprim	secondary prevention or $CD4^+ <200 \times 10^6/L$	oral cotrimoxazole, or nebulized pentamidine, or dapsone + pyrimethamine
toxoplasmosis	sulphadiazine + pyrimethamine + folate	clindamycin replacing sulphadiazine	secondary prevention or $CD4^+ <200 \times 10^6/L$ positive serology	pyrimethamine + sulphadiazine, or clindamycin, or cotrimoxazole, or dapsone
cytomegalovirus	ganciclovir or foscarnet	—	secondary prevention	ganciclovir or foscarnet
herpes simplex	aciclovir	valaciclovir or foscarnet	secondary prevention	aciclovir
herpes zoster	aciclovir	valaciclovir or foscarnet or famciclovir	—	—
cryptococcal meningitis	fluconazole or amphotericin B and/ or flucytosine	—	secondary prevention	fluconazole
Mycobacterium avium-intracellulare	rifampicin + ethambutol + clarithromycin	rifabutin replacing rifampicin	secondary prevention	rifabutin
Candida	fluconazole	ketoconazole or itraconazole	secondary prevention	fluconazole

Fig. 38.8 Treatment and prophylaxis of opportunistic infections.

Anti-HIV drugs

Class	Action	Examples
reverse transcriptase inhibitors	DNA copy of viral genome not made and therefore not integrated into the host cell genome	azidothymidine (AZT) dideoxyinosine (DDI) zalcitabine (DDC)
protease inhibitors	prevents cleavage of a structural protein producing defective viruses	saquinavir ritonavir indinavir

Fig. 38.9 Anti-HIV drugs.

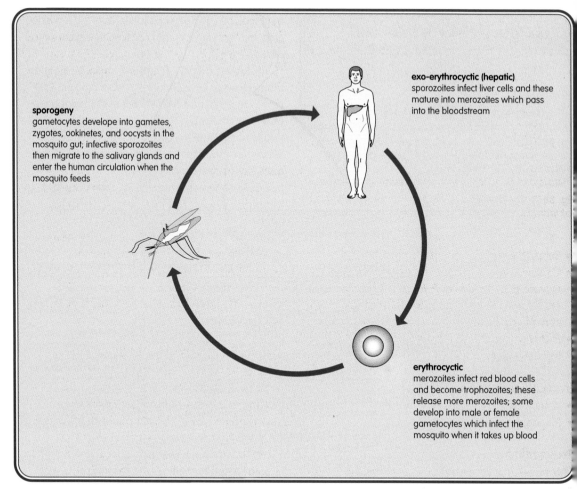

sporogeny
gametocytes develop into gametes, zygotes, ookinetes, and oocysts in the mosquito gut; infective sporozoites then migrate to the salivary glands and enter the human circulation when the mosquito feeds

exo-erythrocyctic (hepatic)
sporozoites infect liver cells and these mature into merozoites which pass into the bloodstream

erythrocyctic
merozoites infect red blood cells and become trophozoites; these release more merozoites; some develop into male or female gametocytes which infect the mosquito when it takes up blood

Fig. 38.10 The malaria transmission cycle.

Presentation

Malaria is characterized by periodic fevers, sweating, and rigors, which coincide with schizogony. Nausea, vomiting, abdominal pain, headache, cough, and arthralgia may also be present. Splenomegaly is commonly found but mild icterus and hepatomegaly may also be present.

  P. falciparum can produce severe illness ('malignant' malaria), characterized by a high level of parasitaemia, which causes the occlusion of small blood vessels by adherence to their endothelium. Fig. 38.11 summarizes the complications of *P. falciparum* malaria.

Investigations

- Thin and thick blood films stained with Giemsa: thick films allow parasites to be identified, thin films are useful in species identification.

- Anaemia, leucocytosis, and thrombocytopenia may occur.
- Coagulopathy: may be a feature of *P. falciparum* infection.
- Liver function tests: including bilirubin often become abnormal.
- Hyponatraemia: *P. falciparum.*

Treatment

The treatment of malaria is under constant review as resistant strains develop. Up-to-date information regarding prophylaxis and treatment of malaria can be obtained from local infectious disease centres.

The acute episode
Management of the acute episode includes:

Complications of infection by *Plasmodium falciparum*

- cerebral malaria (hyperpyrexia, coma, death)
- hypoglycaemia
- non-cardiogenic pulmonary oedema
- seizures
- severe intravascular haemolysis with haemoglobinuria ('blackwater fever')
- acute tubular necrosis
- hepatic necrosis
- jaundice

Fig. 38.11 Complications of infection with *Plasmodium falciparum*.

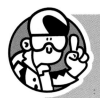

Even though a patient may take malaria prophylaxis, he or she may still develop malaria.

- Supportive care as appropriate.
- Chloroquine for *P. vivax*, *P. ovale*, and *P. malaria*.
- Quinine and fansidar for *P. falciparum* as most cases are chloroquine resistant; mefloquine or halofantrine can also be used.
- Exchange transfusion may be useful when there is a high level of parasitaemia.

Eradication of liver parasites
- Is necessary in *P. ovale* and *P. vivax*.
- Primaquine is used.

Prevention
With the emergence of resistant organisms, the avoidance of mosquito bites and mosquito control take on greater importance.

Chemoprophylaxis
For chemoprophylaxis, refer to up-to-date information, e.g. the British National Formulary (BNF) or the London School of Hygiene and Tropical Medicine's helpline. It should be started 1 week prior to travel and continued for at least 4 weeks after return.

Where there is a low risk of chloroquine-resistant malaria, either chloroquine or proguanil should be used, but where there is a high risk, both chloroquine and proguanil should be used.

Other drugs are available but should be prescribed on expert advice.

Avoidance of mosquito bites
- Mosquito nets.
- Mosquito repellents.
- Wear appropriate clothing, particularly long-sleeved/trousered and light-coloured clothes around dawn and dusk, which is when the female *Anopheles* mosquito is most active.
- Spray bedroom with insecticide last thing in the evening.

Prognosis
Prognosis is excellent with *P. vivax*, *P. ovale*, and *P. malariae* infection but *P. falciparum* is still a life-threatening condition.

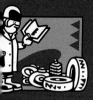

39. Drug Overdose

EPIDEMIOLOGY

Drug overdose results in 10% of all acute hospital admissions and 4.7% of all hospital admissions in 12–20 year olds.

AETIOLOGY

Overdose may be due to the following:
- Accidental: particularly in children.
- Deliberate: self-administration in suicide or parasuicide, homicide, or child abuse, e.g. Munchausen's by proxy.
- Iatrogenic: uncommon, e.g. interacting drugs.

PRESENTATION

History

Drug overdose in many patients may result in a mild illness requiring little intervention. However, some patients take many tablets or cocktails of drugs causing a life-threatening state requiring intensive care and may be fatal. Around 80% patients are conscious and able to provide a history. In all patients, particularly the unconscious, make every effort to talk to family, friends, and the ambulance staff. Always consider overdose in any unconscious patient. Where possible, try to establish the following facts.

Features indicating a high suicide risk
• elderly • male • previous suicide attempts • unemployed • socially isolated (single, living alone) • chronic debilitating illness (psychiatric or physical) • drug or alcohol abuse

Fig. 39.1 Features indicating a high suicide risk.

What drugs were taken and when?

It is very common for more than one drug to be taken, and alcohol is often also used. Try to establish which tablets were taken, how many and how long ago in order to establish the likely ongoing risk. However, it is good policy to treat the patient and not the history as this may be unreliable.

Try to assess the suicidal risk

Have they taken an overdose before? What events led to the overdose? Did the patient intend suicide at the time or was it a reaction to acute stress such as an argument? Was the act premeditated, e.g. were tablets collected over a period of time, was a suicide note left, were the tablets taken when the patient expected to be alone for a while? What did they do after taking the tablets—did they ring for their partner or ambulance immediately? Does the patient feel suicidal now? Would they do it again?

Fig. 39.1 summarizes features indicating a high suicidal risk.

Examination

The examination should be in three stages: assess how ill the patient is, look for evidence to suggest the likely drug(s) involved, and look for complications of overdose.

How ill is the patient?

The first priority is ABC—ensure the patient has an adequate Airway, Breathing (respiration) and Circulation. Assessment of coma scale, pulse, blood pressure, temperature, and BM (glucose estimation) should then be assessed.

Is there any evidence to suggest underlying cause?

Relatives or ambulance staff may have brought bottles from the scene. Look for evidence on the patient such as diabetic cards or hospital appointment cards, e.g. it may be an insulin overdose. Also look for:
- Pinpoint pupils: opiates, organophosphates.
- Dilated pupils: tricyclic antidepressants, amphetamines, cocaine.
- Nystagmus: phenytoin, alcohol.

- Papilloedema: carbon monoxide.
- Burns around the mouth: corrosives.
- Hyperventilation: aspirin.
- Hypothermia: chlorpromazine.
- Needle marks: opiates, benzodiazepines, stimulants.

Have any complications occurred?

Fig. 39.2 summarizes complications of drug overdose.
N.B. Use a low-reading thermometer to detect
hypothermia.

INVESTIGATIONS

- Paracetamol and salicylate levels should be
  measured in all patients.
- Urea and electrolytes, blood glucose, serum
  osmolarity.
- Baseline clotting and liver function tests in
  paracetamol overdose.
- Drug levels can be measured in the blood, gastric
  contents, and urine, but this is not necessary in the
  majority of patients.
- Electrocardiogram: if clinically indicated, e.g.
  arrhythmia.
- Chest X-ray: if evidence of aspiration.

MANAGEMENT

The management of drug overdose can be divided into
three parts: general measures for all patients, specific
measures according to the drug taken, and psychiatric
assessment and social input when the patient recovers
physically.

Complications of drug overdose

- coma
- respiratory depression
- hypotension or hypertension
- arrhythmias
- seizures
- head injury
- hypothermia or hyperthermia
- aspiration pneumonia
- rhabdomyolysis
- gastric stress ulceration

Fig. 39.2 Complications of drug overdose.

General approach
Supportive care

- If unconscious, clear airway and give oxygen via a
  face-mask.
- If no gag reflex, call anaesthetist as the patient may
  need endotracheal intubation.
- Some patients may require assisted ventilation.
- Gain intravenous access, keep patient with
  head downwards, and give intravenous fluids
  for hypotension unless there is cardiogenic
  shock (central venous pressure monitoring may
  be necessary).
- Nurse semiprone and measure observations
  regularly—some patients who walk into A&E may
  deteriorate rapidly.
- Attach cardiac monitor if arrhythmia is suspected or
  the patient is known to have taken tricyclic
  antidepressants.
- In arrhythmia, correct hypoxia, acidosis or electrolyte
  balance; antiarrhythmic agents should be used with
  caution as they can exacerbate the arrhythmia.
- Convulsions should be treated with intravenous
  benzodiazepines.

Prevent gastrointestinal absorption

Gastrointestinal absorption may be prevented by
either emptying the stomach or preventing bowel
adsorption.

Emptying stomach

- Indications: consider gastric emptying within 4 hours
  for most drugs; within 6 hours after opiates and
  anticholinergics; within 12 hours after tricyclic
  antidepressants, salicylates, and aminophylline.
- Contraindications: ingestion of caustic, corrosive, or
  petroleum derivatives.

There are two methods of gastric emptying: induced
emesis (vomiting) or gastric lavage:

- Induced emesis—syrup of ipecacuanha; particularly
  useful in children; should not be given if the patient i
  drowsy or likely to become drowsy because of the
  risks of aspiration; is of limited value in preventing
  absorption.
- Gastric lavage—used where induced emesis is
  refused, contraindicated, or unsuccessful (usually in
  the unconscious patient whose airway is protected
  by a cuffed endotracheal tube).

Preventing absorption in the bowel

- Activated charcoal binds poisons in the stomach preventing absorption.
- More effective the sooner it is given.
- Doses may be given every 4 hours to increase the elimination of certain drugs (aspirin, carbamazepine, phenobarbitone, quinine).
- Contraindicated in drowsy patients (risk of aspiration).
- Ineffective for iron, lithium, potassium, alcohol, and cyanide.

Specific measures in the management of drug overdose		
Drug	**Toxic side effects**	**Specific management**
opiates	respiratory depression, drowsiness or coma, pinpoint pupils, hypotension, bradycardia, hypothermia, pulmonary oedema	naloxone 0.8–2 mg intravenously (may need to be repeated every 2–3 minutes to a maximum of 10 mg due to its short half-life); can be administered by continuous intravenous infusion
benzodiazepines	drowsiness, dysarthria, nystagmus, ataxia, coma, respiratory depression; fairly safe if taken alone but potentiate the effects of other sedative drugs which are often taken at the same time	flumazenil 200 µg over 15 seconds, then 100 µg every 60 seconds until response (maximum dose 1 mg); should be used cautiously
paracetamol	nausea and vomiting in the first 24 hours; acute hepatocellular necrosis may develop after 3 days with as few as 20 tablets causing jaundice, encephalopathy, hypoglycaemia and abdominal pain; renal tubular necrosis may also occur	monitor prothrombin time, glucose, U&Es; check paracetamol levels from 4 hours onwards (treatment may begin before result is available if significant overdose suspected); use nomogram to determine whether antidote should be given if less than 24 hours since tablets were taken give acetylcysteine (Parvolex) by intravenous infusion oral methionine may be given instead if overdose less than 12 hours before
aspirin	nausea, vomiting, tinnitus, deafness, sweating, hyperventilation, tachycardia, delirium, seizures, coma, impaired clotting, hypokalaemia, hypoglycaemia, metabolic acidosis (respiratory alkalosis initially)	correct dehydration, hypokalaemia and hypoglycaemia if plasma salicylate levels >500 mg/L (3.6 mmol/L), the patient should have forced alkaline diuresis under close supervision in severe poisoning (>700 mg/L or 5.1 mmol/L), haemodialysis may be life-saving
iron	usually accidental affecting children causes haemorrhagic enteritis (corrosion) with nausea, vomiting, abdominal pain, haematemesis, bloody diarrhoea, acute hepatocellular necrosis, metabolic acidosis, peritonitis, hypotension, coma	desferrioxame by intravenous or intramuscular injection
digoxin	nausea, vomiting, diarrhoea, hyperkalaemia, bradyarrhythmias, tachyarrhythmias, altered colour vision, delirium	correct electrolyte disturbance temporary ventricular pacing in atrioventricular block digoxin-specific antibody fragments (Digibind) in severe overdose
β-blockers	bradycardia, hypotension, cardiac failure, convulsions, coma, asystole	atropine intravenously for bradycardia glucagon intravenously in severe overdose
heparin	haemorrhage	intravenous protamine sulphate
warfarin	haemorrhage	intravenous vitamin K, intravenous infusion of concentrates of factors II, VII, IX, and X, or fresh frozen plasma

g. 39.3 Specific measures in the management of drug overdose with certain of the more common drugs. (U&Es, urea nd electrolytes.)

Increase elimination of drug

Elimination of drugs can be increased using forced alkaline diuresis or dialysis

Forced alkaline diuresis

- Increases renal drug excretion.
- Used in severe salicylate, phenobarbitone, and amphetamine overdose.
- Can cause fatal fluid overload, electrolyte disturbance, or acid–base disturbance, and should be monitored very carefully.

Dialysis

Dialysis should be used in severe overdose when other methods are contraindicated or unsuccessful. The techniques include peritoneal or haemodialysis and haemoperfusion.

Specific antidotes

Advice for overdose of any drug or ingestion of any poisons can be obtained 24 hours a day from a number of poisons information centres. Each A&E department and hospital switchboard will have a list of national numbers.

Fig. 39.3 summarizes the specific management of overdose of some of the more common drugs.

Psychiatric and social assessment

Once the acute event and medical management is completed, an assessment of the patient's psychiatric state (ongoing suicidal risk) and social circumstances should be made, however trivial the overdose may have appeared. Where appropriate, psychiatrists and social care workers should be involved.

All suicide threats should be taken seriously.

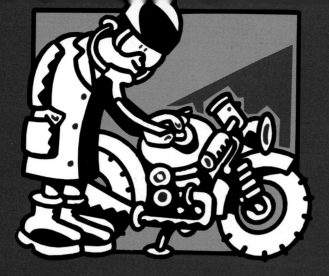

SELF-ASSESSMENT

Multiple-choice Questions

Indicate whether each answer is true or false.

1. The pulse:

a) In pulsus paradoxus the rate slows during inspiration.
b) Pulsus alternans indicates a poorly functioning left ventricle.
c) A tachycardia of 150 beats per minute in a resting patient usually implies an underlying cardiac arrhythmia.
d) A collapsing pulse may be noticed in thyrotoxicosis.
e) Corrigan's sign supports a diagnosis of aortic stenosis.

2. Heart murmurs:

a) A low rumbling diastolic murmur with presystolic accentuation may be heard in mitral stenosis accompanied by atrial fibrillation.
b) Causes of a pansystolic murmur include mitral regurgitation and ventricular septal defect.
c) A systolic murmur heard over the whole praecordium associated with a thrill usually indicates aortic stenosis.
d) Left heart murmurs are best heard during expiration.
e) An early blowing diastolic murmur at the left sternal edge indicates aortic incompetence.

. Pulsus paradoxus:

a) The volume of the pulse increases in inspiration.
b) Can be confirmed by detecting >10 mmHg difference in systolic pressure during the breathing cycle.
) Is a sign of severe asthma.
d) Is called paradoxus because it is the opposite of what normally happens to the pulse.
e) Can occur in cardiac tamponade.

. The jugulovenous pressure:

a) Is raised if it is 2 cm from the sternal angle with the patient seated at 45°.
) Tall 'a' waves may be seen in pulmonary hypertension.
 Irregular cannon waves indicate complete heart block.
 Regular cannon waves may indicate a nodal rhythm.
 Giant 'v' waves and a pulsatile liver indicate tricuspid stenosis.

. The physical signs of an uncomplicated large pneumothorax include:

 The trachea deviated to the opposite side.
 A clicking sound synchronous with the heart beat.
 Symmetrical expansion of the chest.
 Increased breath sounds over the pneumothorax.
 Increased percussion note over the pneumothorax.

6. The following would help distinguish between a kidney and a spleen in the left upper quadrant:

(a) Dull to percussion over the mass.
(b) A well-localized notched lower margin.
(c) Moves with respiration.
(d) A ballottable mass.
(e) A family history of renal failure.

7. Nystagmus:

(a) Vertical nystagmus usually indicates a lesion of the medulla oblongata.
(b) Horizontal nystagmus is usually ipsilateral to an irritative lesion of the labyrinth.
(c) Ataxic nystagmus indicates a lesion of the medial longitudinal bundle.
(d) May be absent in a lesion of the cerebellar vermis (the central part).
(e) Pendular nystagmus may indicate partial blindness.

8. The following would suggest an upper rather than a lower motor neuron lesion:

(a) Fasciculation.
(b) Increased tone.
(c) An absent plantar reflex.
(d) Clonus.
(e) Relatively little wasting.

9. Hand signs:

(a) Clubbing may be caused by uncomplicated chronic bronchitis.
(b) Koilonychia usually indicates liver disease.
(c) Osler's nodes and Heberden's nodes both occur in osteoarthritis.
(d) Splinter haemorrhages are due to embolic rather than immunological phenomena.
(e) Psoriatic arthritis affects most joints in the hand but usually spares the distal interphalangeal (DIP) joints.

10. The face:

(a) A malar flush may indicate mitral valve disease or hypothyroidism.
(b) A butterfly rash in the face is seen in dermatomyositis.
(c) Bell's palsy can cause ptosis due to paralysis of orbicularis oculi.
(d) Herpes labialis may be associated with pneumococcal pneumonia.
(e) An expressionless face and drooling could indicate Parkinson's disease.

11. The electrocardiogram:

(a) The PR interval is measured from the peak of the P wave to the start of the QRS complex.
(b) Right axis deviation is indicated by a QRS axis of -35°.
(c) Q waves in S-II, S-III and aVf indicate a transmural inferior myocardial infarction.
(d) Left bundle branch block is suggested by broadening of the QRS complex to 0.10 seconds (two and a half little squares), and positive RSR' waves in V_4–V_6.
(e) P mitrale is suggested by a P wave taller than 2.5 mm.

12. The chest X-ray:

(a) Loss of the right heart border indicates consolidation in the right lower lobe.
(b) Cardiomegaly is suggested by a cardiothoracic ratio of >0.5 in a posteroanterior (PA) film.
(c) Notching of the ribs posteriorly may be seen in coarctation of the aorta.
(d) Upper venous congestion, Kerley B lines and bat wing's shadowing are typical features of left ventricular failure.
(e) Perihilar eggshell calcification is a feature of sarcoidosis.

13. Serum electolytes and creatinine:

(a) A potassium level of 3.0 mmol/L and a bicarbonate level of 38 mmol/L may indicate Cushing's or Conn's syndromes.
(b) A creatinine level of 125 µmol/L would be normal in elderly people.
(c) A urea level of 20 mmol/L and a creatinine level of 95 µmol/L may indicate an acute gastrointestinal bleed.
(d) A sodium level of 125 mmol/L is within the normal range.
(e) A high chloride level may indicate primary hyperparathyroidism.

14. Hypercalcaemia:

(a) Can be caused by thiazide diuretics.
(b) Can be caused by frusemide.
(c) Is usual in secondary hyperparathyroidism.
(d) Could indicate the presence of breast carcinoma or myeloma.
(e) Can be caused by sodium etidronate.

15. In the full blood count:

(a) A haemoglobin of 10.0 g/dL would be considered normal in a premenopausal woman.
(b) Polycythaemia rubra vera is usually indicated by elevation not only of the haemoglobin but also of the white cell count and platelets.
(c) A low platelet count could indicate a flare-up of systemic lupus erythematosus (SLE).
(d) High platelets can be seen in gastrointestinal bleeding.
(e) A raised mean corpuscular volume is usual in significant alcohol excess.

16. Anaemia:

(a) A high urinary urobilinogen, spherocytes on the blood film, and low haemopexins are all features of a haemorrhagic anaemia.
(b) Hypochromic, microcytic anaemia indicates iron deficiency.
(c) Macrocytic anaemia could be caused by *Diphyllobothrium latum*.
(d) A Schilling test can differentiate pernicious anaemia from malabsorption.
(e) Low serum iron and TIBC (total iron binding capacity) indicate anaemia of chronic disease.

17. Myocardial infarction:

(a) The usual criteria for diagnosis include three out of the following four: ECG changes, myocardial distribution of pain, cardiac enzymes, duration of pain.
(b) A pleuritic nature of the chest pain could indicate pericarditis as an alternative diagnosis.
(c) Non-specific T wave changes within 24 hours are an indication for thrombolytic therapy.
(d) Reinfarction can be prevented to some degree by both β–blockade and verapamil.
(e) A prolonged PR interval and left bundle branch block (LBBB) are together an indication for temporary pacing in the setting of an acute myocardial infarction.

18. Asthma:

(a) Is a clinical diagnosis based on episodic wheezing, cough and shortness of breath.
(b) The asthma triad syndrome includes aspirin sensitivity, nasal polyps, and a family history.
(c) In the emergency situation the clinical features of acute asthma are better signs of severity than blood gases.
(d) A 12% improvement in forced expiratory volume (FEV$_1$) indicates a good response to β$_2$-agonists.
(e) A good pointer to poor control is diurnal variation of >20% in the peak expiratory flow rate (PEFR).

19. Heart failure:

(a) The clinical features of left heart failure include: tachycardia, basal crepitations, pulsus alternans and a raised JVP.
(b) Congestion of the pulmonary veins alone does not result in orthopnoea.
(c) Chronic congestive heart failure leads to secondary hyperaldosteronism.
(d) Causes of heart failure include ischaemic heart disease, hypertension, and thiamine deficiency.
(e) Clinical features of right heart failure include a raised JVP, ankle oedema, and hepatomegaly.

20. Acute renal failure:

(a) Anaemia and small kidneys on ultrasound support a diagnosis of acute on chronic renal failure.
(b) A creatinine level of more than 450 μmol/L is an indication for dialysis.
(c) The ECG may show tall T waves and absent P waves.
(d) Accelerated hypertension, eclampsia, and SLE are all causes of intrinsic renal parenchymal disease.
(e) A persistent urine flow of <20 ml/h after correction of hypovolaemia may indicate the onset of tubular necrosis.

21. Hepatitis:

(a) Causes of hepatitis include alcohol abuse, hepatitis C, and delta agent in combination with hepatitis B surface antigen (HbsAg).
(b) The presence of HbsAg is the first manifestation of hepatitis B virus infection and precedes clinical evidence of hepatitis.
(c) In viral hepatitis there are usually prodromal, icteric, and convalescent phases.
(d) In hepatocellular damage the aspartate transaminase and ALT (alanine transaminase) are not as elevated as the alkaline phosphatase and γ-glutamyltransferase.
(e) The prothrombin time is a sensitive marker of liver dysfunction.

22. Pleural effusion:

(a) A protein level of >40 g/L indicates a transudate.
(b) Tapping of >1 L at a time may result in pulmonary oedema.
(c) The signs of a pleural effusion include stony dullness, absent breath sounds, and increased whispering pectoriloquy at the margin of the effusion.
(d) Malignant effusions are exudates but are rarely blood stained.
(e) Causes of a pleural effusion include Meig's syndrome.

3. Stroke:

(a) Cerebral haemorrhage accounts for more than 40% of acute strokes.
(b) In supratentorial strokes with homonymous hemianopsia, patients cannot see on the hemiplegic side.
(c) Vertigo, vomiting, dysphagia, and Horner's syndrome indicate occlusion of the vertebrobasilar circulation.
(d) Pinpoint pupils and bilateral upgoing plantars could signal a brainstem stroke.
(e) Carotid endarterectomy should be considered for patients with more than 70% stenosis because this is more effective than medical treatment.

24. Pulmonary embolus:

(a) One of the earliest signs is a persistent tachycardia.
(b) Is associated with carcinoma of the pancreas.
(c) Results in unmatched defects in the ventilation–perfusion isotope scan.
(d) The diagnosis must be confirmed before starting full anticoagulation.
(e) Full anticoagulation should be used for 3 weeks to lyse the clot before warfarin is introduced.

25. Respiratory failure:

(a) Type I failure results in a partial pressure of oxygen (pO_2) <8 kPa and a partial pressure of carbon dioxide (pCO_2) of >6.5 kPa.
(b) In respiratory failure associated with chronic bronchitis, the level of carbon dioxide (CO_2) determines the respiratory rate.
(c) Respiratory failure as defined in (a) would be an indication for ventilation in pure asthma.
(d) Doxapram is a respiratory stimulant used in respiratory failure associated with chronic obstructive pulmonary disease.
(e) The main aim in type II failure is to keep the pO_2 >7.0 kPa without worsening of the acidosis or pCO_2.

26. Graves' disease:

(a) Is associated with thyroid microsomal antibodies.
(b) Describes a triad of goitre, exophthalmos, and pretibial myxoedema.
(c) Should be considered when a patient presents with atrial fibrillation.
(d) Results in an elevated thyroxine and thyroid-stimulating hormone.
(e) Carbimazole is an effective antithyroid drug.

27. Cushing's syndrome:

(a) May give rise to hypertension, diabetes, and truncal obesity.
(b) Is usually diagnosed by estimation of the urinary free cortisol followed by an overnight dexamethasone suppression test.
(c) Could be associated with pigmentation.
(d) The most common cause is probably iatrogenic.
(e) Nelson's syndrome is a complication of bilateral adrenalectomy for pituitary-dependent Cushing's disease.

28. Diabetes mellitus:

(a) Is diagnosed if the fasting blood sugar is 6.5 mmol/L.
(b) May occur in acromegaly.
(c) Impotence, nocturnal diarrhoea, and postural hypotension are features of autonomic neuropathy.
(d) Can usually be treated effectively in young patients with sulphonylureas, e.g. glibenclamide.
(e) Diabetic ketoacidosis should be treated with intravenous fluids, high-dose insulin, potassium, and bicarbonate infusions.

29. Leukaemia:

(a) The common presenting triad is infection, bleeding, and fatigue.
(b) Acute myeloid leukaemia (AML) may result spontaneously or follow on from CML, polycythaemia rubra vera or myelosclerosis.
(c) The usual development of chronic lymphocytic leukaemia is a transformation to acute lymphoblastic leukaemia.
(d) A platelet count of 40×10^9/L would not normally give rise to spontaneous bleeding.
(e) Bone marrow transplantation is a recognized treatment for AML.

30. Lymphoma:

(a) The Rye classification of Hodgkin's lymphoma includes lymphocyte depleted, mixed cellularity, nodular sclerosing, and lymphocyte predominant.
(b) Painless enlargement of a group of nodes, fever, and pruritus are all features of Hodgkin's disease.
(c) The 5-year survival of Hodgkin's disease is about 80%.
(d) Reed Sternberg cells are typical of non-Hodgkin's lymphoma.
(e) Laparotomy with splenectomy continues to be a standard method of staging lymphomas.

31. Hypertension:

(a) An average diastolic blood pressure of >90 mmHg over prolonged observation is an indication for drug treatment in uncomplicated hypertension.
(b) Thiazide diuretics are the least effective antihypertensive drugs.
(c) Thiazide diuretics work on the loop of Henle in the kidney.
(d) Resistant hypertension is defined as a failure to control the blood pressure adequately with a good three-drug regimen.
(e) Thiazide diuretics are contraindicated in gout and diabetes.

32. Angiotensin-converting enzyme inhibitors:

(a) Work by inhibiting the conversion of renin to angiotensin II.
(b) Relieve symptoms but do not prolong life in heart failure.
(c) Are safe in pregnancy.
(d) May cause hyperkalaemia.
(e) Reduce proteinuria in diabetic nephropathy.

33. Migraine:

(a) Can be treated with subcutaneous sumatriptan, a 5-HT$_1$ agonist.
(b) May be helped by β–blockade.
(c) Ergotamine is useful prophylaxis for migraine.
(d) Methysergide is effective but leads to retroperitoneal fibrosis.
(e) May cause hemiplegia.

34. Parkinson's disease:

(a) Tremor can be treated by antimuscarinic drugs.
(b) Can be treated with major tranquillizers.
(c) Levo-dopa should be combined with a peripheral decarboxylase inhibitor to prevent adverse effects.
(d) Lysuride is an antiparkinsonian drug with effects similar to bromocriptine.
(e) Can be treated effectively by prochlorperazine.

35. In the treatment of asthma:

(a) Intal and Inderal are both effective treatments.
(b) The new, long-acting β$_2$-agonists are largely replacing shorter-acting agents as standard treatment.
(c) Inhaled corticosteroids alone are probably as effective as inhaled β$_2$-agonists alone for maintenance treatment.
(d) Aminophylline is a phosphodiesterase inhibitor.
(e) Measurement of serum theophylline is of little value in clinical practice.

36. Antibiotics:

(a) Flucloxacillin and fusidic acid are both very effective against *Staphylococcus aureus*.
(b) Legionnaire's disease can be treated with erythromycin.
(c) Penicillins work by inhibiting bacterial cell wall synthesis.
(d) The rashes caused by cotrimoxazole are usually due to the trimethoprim component and not the sulphonamide.
(e) Patients with valvular heart disease do not need antibiotic prophylaxis for dental polishing.

37. Oral corticosteroids:

(a) Are an effective treatment for SLE.
(b) In the long term may cause cataracts.
(c) Should be avoided in sarcoidosis because they induce pulmonary oedema.
(d) May be stopped abruptly after 2 weeks of 40 mg prednisolone daily in patients who are not exposed to repeated courses.
(e) May reveal that 15% of patients labelled as having chronic bronchitis, in fact have reversible airways disease.

38. Tricyclic antidepressants:

(a) In overdose may cause a divergent strabismus.
(b) Are effective for chronic pain syndromes.
(c) Can cause dry mouth and blurred vision.
(d) Are inferior to benzodiazepines for treating panic disorder.
(e) Have their metabolism decreased by cimetidine.

39. Paracetamol overdose:

(a) Ipecacuana followed by oral methionine is effective for most patients who are just over the treatment line.
(b) Can cause renal failure.
(c) Intravenous N-acetylcysteine frequently causes anaphylaxis.
(d) The serum paracetamol level is of most value between 1 and 4 hours after ingestion.
(e) In co-proxamol (distalgesic) overdose, sudden death is likely to be due to hypoglycaemia caused by paracetamol.

40. Aspirin therapy:

(a) Decreases the incidence of stroke in patients suffering from transient ischaemic attacks.
(b) Is very effective in unstable angina.
(c) Reduces 25% of cardiovascular events in individuals at high cardiovascular risk.
(d) Must not be combined with dipyridamole.
(e) May cause an iron-deficiency anaemia.

41. Treatment of myocardial infarction:

(a) Aspirin and streptokinase are more effective than either alone after myocardial infarction.
(b) Thrombolysis improves short-term complications but not mortality after myocardial infarction.
(c) Tissue plasminogen activator and anistreplase are more effective than streptokinase but not used because they are far more expensive.
(d) ACE inhibitors improve outcome after myocardial infarction for patients with ventricular dysfunction.
(e) HMGCo-A reductase inhibitor therapy is contraindicated for patients after myocardial infarction.

42. For angina, the following are of proven value:

(a) Weight loss.
(b) Treatment with thyroxine in hypothyroidism.
(c) Verapamil treatment.
(d) Constant plasma levels of long-acting nitrates for maintenance treatment.
(e) α-blocker treatment.

43. For self-poisoning:

(a) Gastric lavage is recommended for most drugs up to 12 hours after ingestion.
(b) Naloxone is the specific antidote for benzodiazepine overdose.
(c) Patients with tricyclic antidepressant overdose need cardiac monitoring for up to 48 hours.
(d) All patients should be assessed by a qualified psychiatrist.
(e) Pinpoint pupils could indicate opiate overdose.

44. Ethanol:

(a) Causes loss of finer grades of judgement and attention even at low doses.
(b) Causes increased secretion of antidiuretic hormone.
(c) Is subject to saturation or zero order kinetics.
(d) In excess over prolonged periods may cause a cardiomyopathy.
(e) The legal blood alcohol limit for driving in the UK is 100 mg/100 mL blood.

45. Digoxin:

(a) Is the treatment of choice for ventricular extrasystoles.
(b) May cause xanthopsia.
(c) Is excreted by the kidneys.
(d) Adverse effects are reduced by hypokalaemia.
(e) Must not be coadministered with an ACE inhibitor.

46. Complications of bronchial neoplasm include:

(a) Pancreatitis.
(b) Hyponatraemia.
(c) Hypercalcaemia.
(d) A hoarse voice.
(e) Episcleritis.

47. Dementia may result from:

(a) Parkinson's disease.
(b) Huntington's chorea.
(c) Hypothyroidism.
(d) Acquired immune deficiency syndrome (AIDS).
(e) A cerebral tumour.

48. The following statements regarding human immunodeficiency virus (HIV)/AIDS are correct:

(a) The incidence of AIDS in the UK is now decreasing.
(b) The risk of seroconversion from a needlestick injury from an HIV-positive patient exceeds 10%.
(c) The median time from HIV infection to AIDS is usually less than 5 years.
(d) Zidovudine is of proven value for symptomatic HIV-positive patients.
(e) The median life expectancy following AIDS diagnosis exceeds 12 months.

49. Oxygen:

(a) Should be administered with a high inspired concentration (>50%) in the treatment of type II respiratory failure.
(b) Should not be used at high concentration in patients with pulmonary embolism because respiration may be severely impaired when the hypoxic drive is reduced.
(c) Continuous long-term (domiciliary) oxygen improves survival in patients with respiratory failure caused by chronic bronchitis and emphysema.
(d) Is needed when respiratory failure is diagnosed by finding a pO_2 of less than 11 kPa in an arterial blood sample.
(e) Comprises 21% of atmospheric air.

50. Multiple sclerosis:

(a) May be treated in some cases with β-interferon.
(b) Is a recognized cause of ataxic nystagmus.
(c) Causes demyelinating lesions in different sites and at different times, usually with some capacity for regeneration and restoration of function.
(d) Presents most commonly in patients over 50 years old.
(e) Is a recognized sequela of bacterial meningitis.

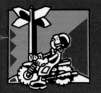
1. List the findings on lumbar puncture that distinguish bacterial from viral meningitis.

2. What electrocardiographic changes are seen in acute myocardial infarction and what is the time sequence of these changes?

3. Describe the common infections that can give rise to diarrhoea.

4. What angiographic results during coronary angiography would be indications for surgical as opposed to medical treatment in coronary heart disease?

5. Describe the differential diagnosis and initial investigations for a patient presenting with polyuria and polydipsia.

6. Discuss briefly the treatment of Parkinson's disease.

7. List the diseases or treatments that may result in a patient being immunocompromised.

8. What factors predispose to the development of venous thromboembolism?

9. Describe the clinical features and investigations that support a diagnosis of chronic active hepatitis.

10. Discuss briefly the management of a patient with suspected giant cell (temporal) arteritis.

11. How does the knowledge of the cell type in lung cancer affect the management and prognosis?

12. Describe the clinical features and investigations that help to distinguish ulcerative colitis from Crohn's disease.

13. What investigations are appropriate for a 63-year old patient presenting with recurrent syncopal episodes?

14. How is the nephrotic syndrome defined and what are the common causes of this syndrome?

15. Outline the use of the Schilling test for vitamin B12 deficiency.

16. How may diabetes mellitus affect the eye?

17. Discuss briefly the investigations that help to distinguish haemolytic, hepatic, or obstructive jaundice.

18. What is the differential diagnosis of a young patient presenting with cervical lymphadenopathy?

19. List four drugs that may cause or worsen renal disease and describe briefly how this occurs.

20. Describe briefly the clinical features and investigations for Addison's disease.

Case-based Questions

1. A 50-year old man presents to you with a chronic productive cough, weight loss, and a previous history of tuberculosis as a child. How would you confirm your suspicion that this man has reactivation of tuberculosis? Discuss the further management of the patient after the diagnosis is established.

2. A young woman aged 25 years old attends your clinic because she was found at a health club screening to have a cholesterol of 6.9 mmol/L. Does she need lipid-lowering treatment with a statin? In the same clinic you see a man aged 58 years old who is recovering from a myocardial infarction whose cholesterol is 5.6 mmol/L. Should he be on a statin? In your answers to these questions you should clarify in your own mind the role of lipid-lowering treatment for primary and secondary prevention of coronary heart disease.

3. A 64-year old woman presents to your clinic with anaemia. Which features in the history, clinical examination, and investigations will help you to determine the cause of the anaemia?

4. A patient aged 48 years old is referred to you by his general practitioner with acute renal failure. How will you manage this patient?

5. A previously healthy young man of 23 years presents with diabetic ketoacidosis. Describe the management of the acute episode and the subsequent treatment of his diabetes.

6. A 72-year old woman complains to you of acute low back pain. Initial investigations reveal hypercalcaemia and a high erythrocyte sedimentation rate. What is your differential diagnosis? What investigations should be performed to establish the diagnosis?

7. A man aged 61 years old is referred to you by his general practitioner for assessment of dyspepsia. What features in the history would suggest peptic ulcer disease as the cause for his symptoms? He is found to have a duodenal ulcer on endoscopy and has a positive test for *Helicobacter pylori*. How should his peptic ulcer be managed?

8. A patient is admitted unconscious to your Accident and Emergency department. Discuss your management of this patient.

9. A 34-year old woman is referred to you with painful joints and early morning stiffness. What features in the history, examination, and investigations would support a diagnosis of rheumatoid arthritis? What is the drug treatment of rheumatoid arthritis?

10. A 70-year old man is admitted severely short of breath. You confirm on clinical examination that he has left ventricular failure. Discuss your management of his acute pulmonary oedema and the therapies available for chronic heart failure.

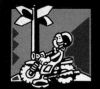

MCQ Answers

1. (a)F, (b)T, (c)T, (d)T, (e)F
2. (a)F, (b)T, (c)T, (d)T, (e)T
3. (a)F, (b)T, (c)T, (d)F, (e)T
4. (a)F, (b)T, (c)T, (d)T, (e)F
5. (a)F, (b)T, (c)F, (d)F, (e)T
6. (a)F, (b)F, (c)F, (d)T, (e)T
7. (a)F, (b)F, (c)T, (d)T, (e)T
8. (a)F, (b)T, (c)F, (d)T, (e)T
9. (a)F, (b)F, (c)F, (d)F, (e)F
10. (a)T, (b)F, (c)F, (d)T, (e)T
11. (a)F, (b)F, (c)T, (d)F, (e)F
12. (a)T, (b)T, (c)T, (d)T, (e)T
13. (a)T, (b)F, (c)T, (d)F, (e)T
14. (a)T, (b)F, (c)F, (d)T, (e)F
15. (a)F, (b)T, (c)T, (d)T, (e)T
16. (a)F, (b)T, (c)T, (d)T, (e)T
17. (a)F, (b)T, (c)F, (d)T, (e)T
18. (a)T, (b)T, (c)F, (d)F, (e)T
19. (a)F, (b)F, (c)T, (d)T, (e)T
20. (a)T, (b)F, (c)T, (d)T, (e)T
21. (a)T, (b)T, (c)T, (d)F, (e)T
22. (a)F, (b)T, (c)T, (d)F, (e)T
23. (a)F, (b)T, (c)T, (d)T, (e)T
24. (a)T, (b)T, (c)T, (d)F, (e)F
25. (a)F, (b)F, (c)T, (d)T, (e)T

26. (a)T, (b)T, (c)T, (d)F, (e)T
27. (a)T, (b)T, (c)T, (d)T, (e)T
28. (a)F, (b)T, (c)T, (d)F, (e)F
29. (a)T, (b)T, (c)F, (d)T, (e)T
30. (a)T, (b)T, (c)T, (d)F, (e)F
31. (a)F, (b)F, (c)F, (d)T, (e)T
32. (a)F, (b)F, (c)F, (d)T, (e)T
33. (a)T, (b)T, (c)F, (d)T, (e)T
34. (a)T, (b)F, (c)T, (d)T, (e)F
35. (a)F, (b)F, (c)T, (d)T, (e)F
36. (a)T, (b)T, (c)T, (d)F, (e)F
37. (a)T, (b)T, (c)F, (d)T, (e)T
38. (a)T, (b)T, (c)T, (d)F, (e)T
39. (a)F, (b)T, (c)F, (d)F, (e)F
40. (a)T, (b)T, (c)T, (d)F, (e)T
41. (a)T, (b)F, (c)F, (d)T, (e)F
42. (a)T, (b)F, (c)T, (d)F, (e)F
43. (a)F, (b)F, (c)T, (d)F, (e)T
44. (a)T, (b)F, (c)T, (d)T, (e)F
45. (a)F, (b)T, (c)T, (d)F, (e)F
46. (a)F, (b)T, (c)T, (d)T, (e)F
47. (a)T, (b)T, (c)T, (d)T, (e)T
48. (a)F, (b)F, (c)F, (d)T, (e)T
49. (a)F, (b)F, (c)T, (d)F, (e)T
50. (a)T, (b)T, (c)T, (d)F, (e)F

1. The inflammatory response in bacterial meningitis is usually more pronounced than in viral meningitis. This leads to a higher cerebrospinal fluid (CSF) pressure, a higher protein content, and a more dense inflammatory cell infiltrate, which results in a more turbid CSF. These changes are suggestive but not diagnostic for bacterial meningitis. Stronger evidence for a bacterial cause is provided by polymorphonuclear cells on microscopy, rather than mononuclear cells, and a CSF glucose level of less than two-thirds of the blood glucose level. Confirmatory evidence of bacterial meningitis is given by the presence of organisms on a Gram-stain (or a Ziehl–Neelsen stain for tuberculosis) and culture of the organism. (See Chapter 34, Fig. 34.7)

2. The changes seen after a transmural myocardial infarction are as follows:
   - Tall arrowhead T waves occurring very early after infarction—the so-called hyperacute T waves.
   - Convex elevation of the ST segments within hours of infarction.
   - The development of pathological Q waves within about 6–24 hours.
   - T wave inversion occurring between 12 and 48 hours.

   These changes are observed in leads II, III and aVf in inferior myocardial infarction, V_1–V_6 and usually I plus aVl in anterior myocardial infarction, and V_1–V_3 in antero-septal infarcts. The time sequence for recovery from these changes is recovery of the T wave inversion within days, followed by the ST segment. If the ST segment remains elevated at 6 months, this suggests the presence of a ventricular aneurysm as a complication of a large infarction. Persistence of the pathological Q waves is usual and may signal to a physician a previous infarction even years after the event.

3. Infectious diarrhoea can be caused by many organisms by different pathological processes, which include toxin production, enteroadherence of organisms, mucosal invasion, or as part of a systemic infection. *Staphylococcus aureus*, *Bacillus cereus* and *Clostridium perfringens* all have a preformed toxin and give rise to food poisoning starting with vomiting and then leading to diarrhoea. Organisms that give rise to diarrhoea by enterotoxin production are enterotoxigenic *Escherichia coli* and *Vibrio cholerae*, whereas *Clostridium difficile* and *E. coli O157:H7* produce a cytotoxin. Enteroadherence is observed with *Cryptosporidium* and *Giardia*. Mucosal invasion is a feature of infection with viruses, e.g. rotavirus and *Campylobacter sp.*, *Salmonella*, *Shigella* and *Entamoeba histolytica*. Systemic infections that can cause diarrhoea include viral hepatitis, Legionnaire's disease, measles and toxic shock syndrome.

4. Patients who are at very high risk of coronary events have an improved survival with coronary artery bypass surgery as opposed to medical treatment. These patients can be identified with coronary angiography by the presence of three-vessel disease, left main stem disease, or proximal left anterior descending artery disease. Patients with one- and two-vessel disease can be treated by both methods or by coronary angioplasty. Surgery may be better for relief of angina for these patients but has a higher short-term mortality related to the surgery.

5. See Chapter 12.

6. The treatment of Parkinson's disease depends to some extent on which of the three clinical syndromes (idiopathic, drug-induced, or postencephalitic), and on which symptoms (bradykinesia, rigidity, and tremor) predominate. Idiopathic Parkinson's, bradykinesia, and rigidity respond best to a combination of levadopa with a dopa decarboxylase inhibitor, whereas drug-induced or postencephalitic Parkinson's and tremor respond best to an antimuscarinic drug, e.g. orphenadrine. As Parkinson's disease is progessive, many patients will eventually require combinations of drugs. The other classes available include dopamine agonists (e.g. bromocriptine, lysuride, pergolide, and apomorphine), amantidine which enhances the release of dopamine, and the monoamine oxidase-B inhibitor selegiline. It was suggested that selegiline may delay the progression of the disease but early hopes were unfounded. Indeed, the most recent studies showed a slightly increased mortality with long term use but this requires confirmation. Long-term complications of levadopa therapy are common and include end-of-dose deterioration, freezing episodes, painful dystonias, on–off phenomena, and peak-of-dose dyskinesia, akinesia, and delerium.

7. Diseases such as leukaemia and lymphoma often result in immunosuppression through specific lesions such as problems with phagocytosis, humoral immunity, and cellular immunity, resulting from deficiency of granulocytes, antibodies, and T cells. Infections, e.g. human immunodeficiency virus (HIV), also result in immunosuppression and acquired immune deficiency syndrome (AIDS) has brought to prominence organisms such as *Pneumocystis carinii*, *Cryptosporidium sp.* and *Mycobacterium avium*, which do not normally cause disease in immunocompetent people. Doctors now commonly immunosuppress patients to treat neoplastic (with cytotoxic drugs) and inflammatory diseases (e.g. with corticosteroids, azathioprine, methotrexate) and to prevent the rejection of transplants (e.g. with cyclosporin).

8. Many conditions are risk factors for venous thrombo-embolism. They can be divided into inherited and acquired conditions. Inherited disorders include defective inhibition of coagulation factors (factor V Leiden [activated protein C resistance], antithrombin III deficiency, protein C deficiency and protein S deficiency), impaired clot lysis (dysfibrinogenaemia), and homocystinuria. Acquired diseases include previous thromboembolic disease, malignancy, myeloproliferative disorders, oestrogen treatment, nephrotic syndrome, and congestive heart failure. Some physiological states also result in an increased risk of venous thromboembolism, e.g. pregnancy, immobilization, old age, and postoperative states. Cigarette smoking is a risk factor for arterial but not for venous thromboembolism.

9. Autoimmune chronic active hepatitis is a chronic disorder featuring hepatocellular necrosis and inflammation, usually with fibrosis. It tends to progress to cirrhosis and liver failure, but has a wide spectrum of severity. The clinical features include an onset of disease that may be insidious or abrupt and be confused initially with acute viral hepatitis. One group of patients with autoimmune hepatitis have distinct features and are young to middle-aged women with markedly raised immunoglobulins and high titres of antinuclear antibodies. Other autoimmune features are common in this group and include malaise, anorexia, amenorrhoea, arthralgias, and jaundice. Occasionally, arthritis, rashes (including cutaneous vasculitis and erythema nodosum), colitis, pleurisy, pericarditis, anaemia, and keratoconjunctivitis sicca may also occur. Many patients have normal levels of serum bilirubin, alkaline phosphatase, and globulin with only a slight increase of the apsartate transaminase and ALT levels. In severe cases, the bilirubin is moderately elevated (50–150 μmol/L). A low albumin level occurs in patients with very active or advanced disease, but serum alkaline phosphatase levels may be moderately elevated or near normal.

10. Giant cell (or temporal) arteritis is a medical emergency because of the risk of blindness. The diagnosis should be made quickly, but because the treatment is high doses of corticosteroids, it should be made as accurately as possible. Headache is the predominant symptom and may be associated with a tender, thickened artery. Scalp pain and claudication of the jaw and tongue may occur. In untreated patients, ischaemic optic neuritis may lead to serious visual symptoms including sudden blindness. Other manifestations include malaise, fatigue, anorexia, weight loss, sweats, and arthralgias. The diagnosis of temporal arteritis can often be made clinically by the demonstration of the classical picture of fever, anaemia, and high erythrocyte sedimentation rate with or without symptoms of polymyalgia rheumatica in an elderly patient. The diagnosis should be confirmed by biopsy of the temporal artery obtained as quickly as possible, especially in the context of eye signs and symptoms. Therapy with high-dose prednisolone should not be delayed while awaiting a biopsy. A dramatic clinical response to steroid therapy can confirm the diagnosis.

11. See Chapter 31, Figs 31.8 and 31.9.

12. The clinical features more common in ulcerative colitis include rectal bleeding, toxic megacolon, and malignancy with long-standing disease. In Crohn's disease, palpable abdominal masses, strictures, small bowel involvement, and fistulas are more likely. The barium enema in ulcerative colitis shows: loss of the normal haustral pattern, the bowel is smooth like a 'hose pipe', ulcers and pseudopolyps may be seen, and oedema of the colonic wall produces widening of the presacral space. In Crohn's disease it may show skip lesions, a coarse cobblestone appearance of the mucosa, and fibrosis producing narrowing of the intestine—'string sign'—with proximal dilatation. Biospy of the affected mucosa via sigmoidoscopy or colonoscopy is usually the best way of distinguishing between the two. Transmural segmental involvement, with granulomas, fibrosis, fistulas, and mesenteric fat and lymph node involvement, supports Crohn's disease. In ulcerative colitis there is continuous mucosal inflammation with neutrophilic infiltration and epithelial damage resulting in multiple ulcerations. Infiltration of the crypts by neutrophils leads to crypt microabscesses, loss of goblet cells, and submucosal oedema.

13. See Chapter 18, Fig. 18.3.

14. The nephrotic syndrome is a clinical condition characterized by a number of renal and extrarenal features with the most prominent being proteinuria of >3.0 g/24 hours, plus hypoalbuminaemia and oedema. Hyperlipidaemia, lipiduria, and hypercoagulability also coexist. The key component is proteinuria, which results from an altered permeability of the glomerular filtration barrier for protein. The common causes of the nephrotic syndrome are shown in Chapter 13, Fig. 13.1.

15. The Schilling test is useful in the differential diagnosis of malabsorption and is frequently carried out in three stages with vitamin B_{12} being given:
    - Without intrinsic factor.
    - With intrinsic factor.
    - After a course of treatment with antibiotics or anti-inflammatory drugs.

    Vitamin B_{12} is absorbed primarily in the distal ileum. Therefore, an abnormal response to a Schilling test without intrinsic factor indicates pernicious anaemia, but with intrinsic factor indicates pathology of the distal small bowel. When the terminal ileum is involved such as in Crohn's disease and lymphomas, the first -and second- stage Schilling tests are often abnormal because ileal receptor sites appear to be damaged in these disorders. The impaired absorption of vitamin B_{12} is not corrected by the addition of intrinsic factor or the use of antibiotics.

16. Diabetes mellitus may affect the eye in many ways. When examining the eye in a diabetic patient one should examine the visual acuity, which may be impaired. The iris may show rubeosis, a cataract may be present, and the retinal changes include background retinopathy (dot and blot haemorrhages, hard exudates, cotton wool spots), proliferative retinopathy (new vessel formation, scars, vitreal haemorrhages, retinal detachments), macular oedema, and the laser coagulation burns of previous therapy.

17. See Chapter 10.

18. Painful lymphadenopathy suggests local pyogenic infection or local or systemic viral infection. Painless enlargement of glands in the neck may be a manifestation of lymphoma, sarcoidosis, or HIV infection. Chronic infections presenting with cervical lymphadenopathy include tuberculosis, actinomycosis, and toxoplasma.

19. The list of drugs that can cause or worsen renal impairment is very long and beyond the scope of this short answer. As a general principle, before prescribing drugs to patients with renal disease, it is wise to check whether you are likely to do more harm than good. In the UK this can be done by looking up the drug in the British National Formulary appendix on prescribing for renal disease. Four examples of drugs that may impair renal function are:
- Angiotensin-converting enzyme inhibitors in the presence of bilateral renal artery stenosis, resulting in renal failure.
- Analgesics during long-term use, causing analgesic nephropathy characterized by papillary necrosis and tubulointerstitial inflammation.
- Gold for the treatment of rheumatoid arthritis, causing nephrotic syndrome.
- Chemotherapy for leukaemias and lymphomas, causing hyperuricaemic acute tubular necrosis. Renal failure occurs because of intratubular deposition of uric acid crystals.

20. Addison's disease results from progressive destruction of the adrenal glands, which must involve more than 90% of the glands before adrenal insufficiency appears. The clinical features are an insidious onset of fatiguability, weakness, anorexia, nausea and vomiting, weight loss, cutaneous and mucosal pigmentation, hypotension, and, occasionally, hypoglycaemia. Early in the disease there may be no abnormalities detectable in routine laboratory tests. However, as the adrenal reserve is decreased despite a normal basal steroid output, a subnormal increase occurs after stress. Adrenal stimulation with synthetic adrenocorticotrophic hormone (Synacthen test) uncovers abnormalities at this stage of the disease, eliciting a subnormal increase of cortisol levels or no increase at all. With more advanced disease, serum sodium, chloride, and bicarbonate levels are reduced and the serum potassium level is elevated. The hyponatraemia is due both to loss of sodium into the urine due to aldosterone deficiency and to movement into the intracellular compartment, which accentuates hypotension. About 50% of patients will also have circulating adrenal antibodies.

Index

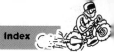

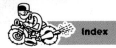